RELATIONAL CARING AND PRESENCE THEORY IN HEALTH CARE AND SOCIAL WORK

A Care-Ethical Perspective

Andries Baart
Guus Timmerman

First published in Great Britain in 2025 by

Policy Press, an imprint of
Bristol University Press
University of Bristol
1-9 Old Park Hill
Bristol
BS2 8BB
UK
t: +44 (0)117 374 6645
e: bup-info@bristol.ac.uk

Details of international sales and distribution partners are available at policy.bristoluniversitypress.co.uk

British Library Cataloguing in Publication Data
A catalogue record for this book is available from the British Library

ISBN 978-1-4473-7572-2 hardcover
ISBN 978-1-4473-7573-9 ePub
ISBN 978-1-4473-7574-6 ePdf

Cover design: Robin Hawes
Front cover image: Erik-Jan Ouwerkerk
Bristol University Press and Policy Press use environmentally responsible print partners.
Printed and bound in Great Britain by CPI Group (UK) Ltd, Croydon, CR0 4YY

FSC
www.fsc.org
MIX
Paper | Supporting responsible forestry
FSC® C013604

To our friend and colleague Frans Vosman (1952–2020), moral theologian and care ethicist, whose life, work and death gave us much food for thought.

Contents

List of figures, tables and case fragments

Figures

Tables

Case fragments

About the authors

A.J. (Andries) Baart PhD is Extraordinary Professor in the field of ageing and generational dynamics at the North-West University in South Africa, former visiting professor at the Department of Psychiatry of the University Medical Center Utrecht (2018–23), and Professor Emeritus of the University of Humanistic Studies (2012–15), Tilburg University (2007–12), and Catholic Theological University Utrecht (1991–2006) in the Netherlands. In 2004 he founded with others the Presence Foundation. In 2025, he will publish *Iemand voor iemand: Handboek presentie*, Bussum: Coutinho. See: www.andriesbaart.nl, www.presentie.nl, www.ethicsofcare.org.

A.B. (Guus) Timmerman PhD has worked as a care ethicist and qualitative researcher at the Presence Foundation since 1 November 2014. Together with Professor Andries Baart, he publishes on relational caring and presence in healthcare and social work and on the methodology of qualitative research. He has researched the care and practical wisdom of general practitioners at the sick- and death-beds of their patients; the life-world of people in the Dutch city of Rotterdam who use the bed-bath-bread provision for irregular migrants and rejected asylum seekers; and what it is like to be a person with advanced dementia. His current research is on narrative accountability in care for older persons: giving insight to relevant interlocutors through stories. See: www.presentie.nl, www.ethicsofcare.org.

Acknowledgements

We wish to thank, first of all, all those professionals, clients, patients, pupils and residents who allowed us and our colleagues to enter their practices and lives, and to study their living and living together, their undergoing, acting and refraining, their perceiving, weighing, deliberating and evaluating, their more or less succeeding in giving good care, learning and accounting.

We are particularly grateful to the two outreach chaplains in the Dutch city of Utrecht, in whose practices in particular the presence theory in its original formulation was grounded.

We thank fellow travellers and critical friends, especially Jaco Hoffman (North-West University, South Africa), Mieke Grypdonck (Professor Emerita Ghent University, Belgium), Harry Kunneman (Professor Emeritus University of Humanistic Studies, The Netherlands), Annelies van Heijst (Professor Emerita Tilburg University, The Netherlands) and the late Frans Vosman (Professor Emeritus University of Humanistic Studies, The Netherlands) to whom we dedicate this book.

We thank former and current colleagues of the Presence Foundation, from its start in 2004, for sharing their questions, insights, doubts and answers, and challenging us to be clearer. We are particularly grateful to the Presence Foundation's first managing director, Marjanneke Ouwerkerk, for her unwavering support and critical questions during the process of writing this book; and her brother, Erik-Jan Ouwerkerk, for taking the photo on the cover of the book.

Furthermore, we want to thank Maurice Hamington (Portland State University, United States), Vanessa Nurock (Côte d'Azur University, France) and Maggie FitzGerald (University of Saskatchewan, Canada) for giving feedback on a previous version of the book.

We also want to thank the six anonymous reviewers for Policy Press, in two rounds, for their comments, encouragement, criticisms, questions and suggestions. The book has substantially profited from these.

We thank Brian Heffernan for his invaluable language editing.

Finally, we want to thank our editors at Policy Press, Jen McGall and Isobel Bainton.

Preface

This book addresses a deep and globally felt dissatisfaction, among citizens in general but also among professionals. Namely, that in healthcare, the social domain, in education, in the domain of housing, but also in psychiatry, youth care and, for example, public administration, things have too often gone off course. As a result, there is a growing gap between the regime of competent professionals and managers, on the one hand and the lifeworld of patients, clients, pupils and residents with their needs, concerns and longings, on the other. And also a gap between the institutional logic of organisations and their administration and quality systems, on the one hand, and the everyday practice and practical wisdom of front-line professionals, on the other. In these interrelated gaps, disconnected competences, bureaucracy, aloofness, mismatches and distrust are proliferating. In short: 'Many are busy with you, but few are looking after you.' The relentless improvements since the 1980s hardly repair these deficits because they are producing more of the same: the same pragmatism and distancing, the same type of thinking, perceiving and knowing, the same rationality and market-driven organisation that are at the root of the difficulties. People, both as citizens and as professionals, hardly feel seen. Their distrust toward fellow citizens, their dissatisfaction with their work and their receptivity to populism are growing.

This book summarises over 30 years of research into the practices of practitioners who are recognised by care receivers and colleagues as good practitioners, to present a realistic and empirically grounded alternative. At its heart is radical relational caring, connecting with and attuning one's practice to the other person before applying expert knowledge. What relational caring entails and how it works has been practically and theoretically explored in different domains and is described in detail. But the book goes further and shows its payoff. It analyses what kind of professionalism is required for this way of working, and how practitioners can be trained and formed to work in increasingly radical, relational ways. It presents the practice of relational caring in a broad range of domains – the presence approach – but also the underlying theory, ethics and philosophy – the multidisciplinary presence theory. It pays attention to its foundations – in care ethics – and the methodology, qualitative research and politically oriented critiques on which it relies. To this end, it coins its own concepts, which challenge professionals, managers and researchers to stay on track.

Although much of the research was done in the Netherlands, this book is international in scope and actively engages in numerous international discussions. It targets scholars and researchers, but certainly also professionals and change specialists in healthcare and social work, from practitioners to trainers, and from quality officers to managers. In the Netherlands, Belgium,

Germany and, for example, South Africa, this kind of presence is practised by social workers, healthcare workers (caregivers, nurses, psychiatrists, doctors), youth care workers, by professionals in the care of people with intellectual disabilities, and at places where people with a serious addiction who avoid any form of care, homeless people or early school leavers need to be reached. The book elaborates the thesis that no form of care, help or support can do without this relational core, with the risk that mismatches arise and seekers of help are abandoned. It is precisely this experience of not being included that fuels discontent worldwide. And not being allowed to practise relational caring is conducive to satisfaction fatigue and burnout of front-line professionals.

The book aims at providing a broad and critical introduction to relational caring in healthcare, social work, education and so forth to interested scholars, professionals, administrators, trainers, quality officers, policy makers and researchers. The book is about professional caring and the required knowledge, attitude, morality, quality frameworks, learning models and so forth. We do not go into the subject of unpaid and family carers, however topical and relevant it certainly is worldwide, especially after the COVID-19 pandemic, criticism of neoliberal efficiency thinking in healthcare and social work, labour market shortages and, for instance, in the light of current thinking on 'communities' and civil society. Something for another book.

To give the reader a sense of what we mean by relational caring and practising presence, the book begins with a case description from residential social work and points out a few features which are remarkable, considering the contemporary emphasis on methodical interventionism. The description also introduces some of the terms that will later be explained more fully. In Part I, the concept, practice and theory of presence and relational caring as we understand it are presented, related to other approaches and discussed. We argue that if we are to study complex, dynamic and emergent practices of healthcare and social work, it is necessary to bring about an empirical turn in care-ethical research and a practice turn in theoretical thinking. This results in the theoretical perspective of presence, a complex, rather unusual but fruitful and revealing way of looking at care practices and issues that emerge in these practices and are relevant to its participants.

In Part II, six major topics in relational caring are discussed by looking at it from the presence-theoretical perspective: the political context, perception, relationality and 'finality' (that is, the ultimate aim of the practice), practical wisdom, quality and the continuing formation of relationally caring professionals. A note on relational caring and technology is added after the three quintessential aspects of good care are discussed: freely perceiving and imagining, properly attuning one's practice to the person in need of care and practising practical wisdom. Instead of offering a conclusion, in the final chapter we discuss the meta-theoretical and political background theories of the presence-theoretical perspective.

Andries Baart and Guus Timmerman
Nieuwegein/Amersfoort, The Netherlands
17 May 2024

Prologue: 'Somewhere between a scream and silence'

This book is about relational caring, conceptualised as practising presence, the core or heart of all good professional care, help and support in healthcare and social work. To give the reader a sense of what we mean by relational caring and practising presence, we will begin the book with a case description from residential social work and point out a few features.[1] The description also introduces some of the terms that will later be explained more fully in the book.

Case description

Hein-Jan Hagen is a coach and personal supervisor at the Schoonhegge residential hotel in the Dutch city of Rotterdam. Schoonhegge is a form of sheltered housing and assisted living for clients with a (very) intensive or specific need for supervision. It is a facility of Perpektief, a social care organisation. An employee of Perspektief, Hagen offers help and shelter to people who are stuck in life and who are accommodated in Schoonhegge in modest apartments. Here he reflects on Sharon and his care for her (paragraphs are numbered to assist in later discussion).

> Sharon is 27, has a mild intellectual disability and is streetwise. Neglected, beaten and raised in youth institutions, she ended up in a criminal environment. She has three children with different men; she wanted to take care of them but couldn't. Her children are in various foster homes. [1]
>
> She came to us at Schoonegge like hunted game. She hadn't lived anywhere for longer than a few months. At first, she could barely get out of bed. The peace here caused her fears and traumas to surface. Sharon refused any treatment; she perceives this as a judgement, a rejection. You have to make her feel that she is allowed to speak, swear and fail. She doesn't have to show her best side, there is room for 'this is me and this is it for the moment'. Two sides of Sharon have become visible: on the one hand, she is a quiet, timid child who literally lies down until the storm has passed; on the other hand, she is a survivor who throws herself into battle screaming, without a thought for the consequences. There is a yawning gap between these two sides. [2]
>
> When we first met, Sharon immediately showed me pictures of her children. They live with foster families; in her eyes, they have been taken away from her. She attacked the guardian who told her she will

never have her children back: 'I will hit back at anyone who touches my children.' Other forms of problem solving are alien to her. [3]

It was only during a car ride through Rotterdam that I got to know her a little better. The stories emerged from the cityscape. So, we took car rides more often, and the route brought out her life story: where she had lived, what she had done and where. There was always a certain pride in her voice. She was a bit of a rascal, tough and vulnerable at the same time. [4]

Unexpectedly her boyfriend was released from detention and moved in with her. That was not what we wanted. But sending him away would have meant sending her back into a criminal milieu. So then there were two of them in her single-room apartment – not an ideal situation. But the bottom line was: they were two people who care about each other. They lived there with a budgie, a small tortoise and a dog – and this despite the rule banning pets … I had to stretch the boundaries once more. Because what do you do if you don't agree? Refuse, hit out, scream? I had no option but to set an example: be patient, accepting and interested. I didn't try to plan or know everything in advance, I just kept talking, inquiring and explaining, both towards Sharon and towards colleagues from inside and outside my organisation who had a stake in the case. [5]

Meanwhile, Sharon and I would continue to talk together about the kids. That was what she wanted, she wanted to get on with restoring contact with her children. Sharon had already arranged a visit herself, and this went well. She showed me the pictures and I reacted enthusiastically and thought perhaps things were taking a turn for the better. But I celebrated too soon. The guardian called and told me the visit had had adverse effects on the children: they were wetting the bed, were anxious and were having nightmares. The guardian was going to tell Sharon that she wasn't allowed to see the children for the time being. A high-risk decision: if she were to explode, there was a chance that she might have to be expelled and might be detained. [6]

Of course, Sharon got angry when I told her about the upcoming ban. She blamed everyone, especially the guardian and the foster parents: 'When I see them, I will go for them.' I emphasised to her the fact that it had been right of her, not wrong, to visit her children. That she was not to blame for her children's reaction. That it was not her fault, but that we, as professionals, had rushed the whole thing. Then we started to prepare for her meeting with the guardian. We agreed that if the guardian had something negative to say, Sharon would leave together with my colleague, and I would stay. And she managed to do it, she was able to restrain herself – how smart of her! I had further consultations with the guardian. I said that if we wanted to give Sharon a chance, we would have to move cautiously, we would first have to see the foster parents and then proceed step by step towards success. The guardian agreed. Once outside, Sharon and I celebrated with cake. [7]

The next problem was the pace: if we wanted to achieve something, all parties (Sharon, the guardian, the foster parents and the children) would have to keep pace with each other. That is fine-tuning with tweezers. I had to make sure I didn't get ahead of Sharon, but that I would follow her. I had to wait for her to take the initiative, but I would have to be prepared for it. There was plenty of time for that. I discovered that her pace was slower than I thought. When she started talking about getting in touch with her children again, I pointed out there was so little I could do for her. She absolutely did not want anyone to have consultations about her children without her being there. And rightly so: she is and remains their mother. I kept saying that to her. This created some space to explain that caring for children is not the same thing as being their mother. Sharon is and remains their mother. She also determines what I can and cannot do for her. That was stressful for me. I needed more leeway from her to be able to continue. And a small miracle happened: she allowed me to try something. She had come to this point from being the Sharon who never trusted anything or anyone … Another moment for cake! [8]

We could continue, but how? The children live in different foster families, and my first conversations there were tense: I was seen as another care worker who was trying to enforce contact between parent and child. I strongly stressed the importance of care: the foster parents and the guardian are the ones who are taking care of the children, so they decide when it is time for the next step. We follow Sharon, she must lead the way. The fact that she has a slow pace does not mean she isn't involved. Her motherhood develops in small steps; this is the only way she can be successful as a mother. [9]

Sixteen months have passed. Sharon has already seen two of her three children, and we are still waiting for the green light to see the youngest. The next challenge is continuing on this course. Sharon is not doing so well: her traumas are deep, her relationship is over. However big the problems are, we just have to make the next appointment with the children. Because that is going well. What remains is a single mother, who lives somewhere between a scream and silence. [10]

Some features

We believe that this case description from residential social work shows relational caring as standing at the heart of what professionals do. Let us point out some features.[2]

Relationship first

Everything that is of value to Sharon is more or less ruined, unavailable or unacceptable. She does not fit into the normal regime at all, and measured by ordinary standards she is barely teachable. And yet the professional does not leave Sharon to her fate. He engages in an endless process of inquiry into what is good for Sharon, with only one guideline: entering into and maintaining a relationship with her. It is not about what the professional thinks is important. It is not about success or making steady progress. It is about preventing or at least limiting damage, and about not abandoning Sharon, ever. It is also about wasting time professionally, on practical wisdom, on love, on composure: by going at her pace, going down the path she takes, staying with her stories. Above all, it means never accusing, never disapproving, never taking over, never escalating. The professional learns what is at stake for Sharon by taking this approach: her honour, her motherhood. What the professional does here is let her be who she fatefully is, create the space for this and, above all, create suitable opportunities for this. The professional's only means to do this is relational caring work.

Sharon, a mother

Sharon's life has taken many turns, many of which have severely damaged her, and she has arrived at an institution that does not promise to solve her problems, but that offers help and shelter. The difference between solving problems and offering help and shelter may seem minor, but it is not. The latter is not about the professional's own professional goals, honour or ambitions, but about professionals taking it upon themselves to offer help to another person in the life she is trying to live. This means immediately giving Sharon the position she desires to occupy: she is a mother. Yes, a mother with a low IQ, with troubles, traumas, fears, a stigma and a big mouth [paragraph 2], but still a mother. This means admitting not an individual, detached client, but a woman-in-relationships, with loyalties and with an identity to be respected. She has an aversion to 'treatments' [2] and the professional refrains from opposing this, from attempting to persuade her, from pushing his own aims and punishing the client's refusal to accept these. On the contrary, the client is carefully helped to emerge: she is given the opportunity to find rest, there is no pushing or pulling, she is allowed to show herself as she is at that moment, she does not have to be 'consistent' – contradictions are permitted – and she can be sure of the interested attention of the professionals. And in this context, she shows what is at stake for her: being a mother to her children [3]. She shows the bandwidth of her repertoire ('other forms of problem solving are alien to her') [3] and what her fears are (never seeing the children again).

Remarkably, Sharon is allowed to show herself 'freely': there is no mention of tests, intake forms or diagnostic instruments. The professional has a basic notion of her 'disorders' [1] and that apparently suffices. No 'explanation' from experts at a distance is required. The main thing is to let her speak and to give her the opportunity to show herself, with her desires and struggles, especially through her stories. This happens outside the framework of institutional arrangements, be they forms or interviews: it happens as she and the professional sit in the car and drive through the city, as she points out important places and recounts what she experienced there and what this means for her [4]. This is what we call 'diluted seriousness': discussing highly serious matters lightly, mixed with fun. Sharon can also show what makes her proud: she knows how to survive! This permits two images of Sharon to develop: the analytic image (diagnosis, the disorders and their causes) and the narrative image (her identity, her lifeworld and the meanings it contains).

The professional as Sharon's spare self

The story quoted earlier is told by a professional, Hein-Jan Hagen, and it shows how he defines professionalism: it is not about falling back on diagnoses and intervention plans, but about being an expert in relationships, building a relationship with Sharon, maintaining and growing that relationship into a source of knowledge that informs his actions, using the relationship to determine the pace, tone and topic of the conversation, making it the stage on which Sharon can gradually show herself [3–4]. This helps him to understand who she is and what she needs. His task is far from simple: Sharon is a complicated woman for whom help and support might easily increase the pain and mistrust even further.

Hein-Jan is a professional and understands how to let Sharon take the lead [4, 8], how to interact with her, what methodical knowledge and expertise he should or should not take out of his backpack and deploy. And when he deploys his knowledge and expertise, he knows how and when to do this. Any aid must be tailor-made. He uses his knowledge on the basis of his relationship with Sharon, and the relationship develops thanks to his skilled approach. There is no hint that he presents this complex case as an essentially simple problem that can be solved by following some straightforward step-by-step plan. On the contrary [5]. One of the less obvious aspects is that Sharon is undeniably vulnerable, someone who has been hurt often in the past. And the help she has received may well have contributed to making her even more vulnerable. She is vulnerable, has been hurt and has been *made* vulnerable. And yet the picture is even more complex: she herself is now hurting others: her children, the guardian of her children, the foster parents [7]. There is not one, single image of Sharon that Hein-Jan can rely on.

Of course, according to the ideal of social work that currently prevails, Sharon should actually be able to do everything herself. But Hein-Jan's estimation is that this is not true, and he takes a different approach in this case. If you have a leg injury, the doctor will prescribe an orthopaedic brace; if you are deaf, a hearing aid. If your teeth are rotten, you will be given a crown and if your ankle is sprained, you will have to use crutches. These devices represent what Hein-Jan is to Sharon: a brace, a hearing aid, a dental crown and a crutch. External instruments that almost become natural extensions of Sharon herself, to help her do what she cannot do herself, see what she does not see herself, say what she cannot say herself, hear what she cannot hear herself [6]. Such aids are preferably temporary, but many people live with a hearing aid or glasses for the rest of their lives. This is not the point. The point is that it is an intimate thing to become a 'part' of the other to preserve what would otherwise be lost: honour and motherhood [7]. It is a great struggle for the professional to enter into and remain in such a relationship, despite many moments of rejection, to become her alter ego, her spare self. An analysis of the phronetic nature of professionalism can be found in Chapter 11.

Sharon in the lead

The help and support offered may seem clumsy: it appears to follow no methodical, straightforward path, but instead resembles a meandering course, a kind of muddling through, always trying to respond as best as possible to what presents itself (boyfriend from prison [5], guardian who refuses further visits [6], and so on) and what is or is not possible [8]. The story is full of expressions that prove that the professional is trying to connect with and become attuned to Sharon ('That is fine-tuning with tweezers') [8]. Ultimately, the aid offered did not result in any resounding success [10]. But nor did it inflict any further damage or hurt on Sharon, and she did not fall out of care [10]. Despite her expressed intentions, she did not harm anyone, and she gained confidence in the help and support [9]. She is seeing her children again and her motherhood is developing [9]. Perhaps not all has been achieved as planned, but things are on the rails. It seems that the professional has a clear idea of what his work is ultimately about [8]. Sharon must benefit from the help. Following the path she lays out herself, the professional must discover what is of value to her [8]. It is her life, and she therefore takes the lead [9]. She also has to experience the benefit herself. We see that Hein-Jan constantly thinks and acts from that perspective, and not from self-devised goals that he regards as worth pursuing (achieving independence, safety, work, daily routine, and so on).

We may assume that this is also the reason why Hein-Jan says that he is happy to account for his actions to his colleagues at work, but that Sharon is the first person to whom he is accountable. It should work *for her*. Given this ultimate goal, the professional activities of inquiring, deliberating, thinking, becoming inventive and testing possibilities are defined. This is how relational caring develops. Seeing a possibility, discussing whether this might be something for Sharon and then allowing Sharon to be in the lead again. If we consider the details of the case, we can indeed conclude that Sharon leads the way, and sets the pace and the direction. The professional goes down the path she sets out, while at the same time knowing very well where he wants to go with her. He points out openings, compromises and possibilities ('The next challenge is continuing on this course') [10]. He pursues what might be good for Sharon, but he is by no means her unwilling servant. He tries his best to do at least something sensible in the minefield that this case is, by using his expertise, his knowledge, his methodical skills, his intuition and sense of direction. He is not blindly obedient to Sharon, but neither does he simply follow all kinds of rules and protocols that the sector and the organisation impose. He finds the space that is required, and makes such space if necessary. This asks a lot of the organisation, its management and its quality system, but there is next to nothing about this in this case description. It appears to be of secondary importance. There is more about the quality of good care and how to determine it in Chapter 12.

Her concerns, not just society's problems with her

It is striking that Hein-Jan's account focuses on Sharon's problems (her multiple vulnerabilities and her having the appearance of 'hunted game') [2], or better: her needs (forming a family) [5], or even better: her concerns (including: how do I get access to my children, given all these professionals who are blocking my way?). Importantly, problems, needs and concerns are not simply different words for the same thing – 'problems' is a detached word that reflects an uninvolved way of thinking, while 'concerns' are personal and relate to Sharon's suffering and struggles. Problems are usually identified more or less objectively at the beginning of a trajectory, and they are subsequently there only to be dealt with, either successfully or not. Concerns, on the other hand, come and go according to the complications, opportunities and setbacks encountered during the process. They continuously challenge the professional to keep looking at the care receiver and her relatives and to come up with adjusted responses. In this case, it is not objective problems that are to the fore, but Sharon's concerns, and through those concerns Hein-Jan also touches on her problems. Apart from the difficulties that are at hand, it is noticeable that the recounting also mentions that good things are celebrated: the car rides are pleasant (and informative) and are therefore repeated [4]. Hein-Jan is happy when Sharon keeps her cool during the meeting with the guardian and they celebrate the drawing up of a good plan with cake [7], and later again: 'Another moment for cake!' [8]. This professional celebrates, is proud and counts his blessings.

Still other goods emerge and are realised in this way. The professional's relationship with Sharon has an instrumental quality: things get done, thanks to that relationship. But we also see that that relationship involves recognition for Sharon: I see you, you count for me, I am following you, you can trust me, that's not your fault and I am not holding you accountable for it, I am proud of you and celebrate what we achieve, your desire to be a mother is important to me, I will always adjust my plans if that is better for you, you are allowed to be the way you are, and so on. In that sense, Sharon not only experiences good things after or as a result of the relationship, but also within the relationship itself, no matter what its outcomes are. It does her good that she has this relationship and that she receives the recognition that she receives within it; perhaps this in itself is a more healing experience than any external outcome could be. It is a fundamental thing that appeals to horrific trauma and deep desire. In the case described at the start of this Prologue, value is not attached only to the outcomes achieved, but also very much to the realisation of these 'social goods', the goods that the care receiver immediately experiences and that heal her. In this sense, the help and care in this account are not only useful but also beneficial, because they humanise and constitute a form of solicitude. Even if few concrete goals are achieved, this relational good is acquired. Moreover, this method also has a political meaning, because the underlying (here: silent) message is: she may be a difficult woman who causes trouble, does irresponsible things (like having children) and refuses to listen, but she still counts – at least for the professional, and therefore also for society. For more on concerns and responses, see Chapter 10.

Objections

It is possible to raise objections against relational caring as we conceptualise it on the basis of cases like the one presented here as the core or heart of all good professional care, help and support. The main objection is surely: relational caring – practising presence – is for virtuoso practitioners, professionals who have all the time in the world and have the full support of their organisation. In other words: this is not practically viable for most professionals, who have full caseloads, goals to be achieved, deadlines and so on. And although it may be an attractive perspective for outreaching social workers, it is not advisable for brain surgeons. We will return to these objections in greater detail later (see Chapter 4). Suffice it here to make the following remarks. In our empirical research, we have seen relationally caring professionals in all domains of healthcare and social work, including in hospitals. Our training of professionals in healthcare and social work has taught us that relational caring can be learned and developed further, although it is not for everyone. Indeed, it has to be facilitated and managed relationally, but we have observed that there are professionals who practise relational caring also in institutional contexts that are not themselves particularly receptive to relational caring. But above all, we think that care, help and support should be about the good of the resident, the client, the patient, the pupil and their relatives. Continuous inquiry into the life, lifeworld and concerns of the other or others is required to find out what that good is. Of course, the good to which the professional can contribute has to be in accordance with the ultimate object of the professional's practice. But this inquiry is the be-all and end-all of relational caring.

1

Introduction

We have been studying practices of caring in the domains of healthcare and social work for more than 30 years. We have seen and keep seeing many practices, situations and processes that present us with puzzles. These can be understood and solved, either easily or with some effort, using existing theoretical or practical perspectives, but these leave us unsatisfied. We feel that many of these perspectives remain on the outside, are not sufficiently empirically grounded, ideologically open and morally sensitive. For these reasons, they fail to get to the heart of what we think we are seeing in healthcare and social work. What exactly do we see, hear, perceive when we study actual practices, situations, processes or organisations? What do residents, patients, clients, pupils and their relatives value as good care, help and support? What practices do practitioners engage in who are acknowledged to be good practitioners by residents, patients, clients and pupils and their relatives, as well as by their colleagues and managers? What makes social workers good social workers, nurses good nurses, youth workers good youth workers, doctors good doctors? And managers good managers and teachers good teachers? Also, what makes care, help and support good enough, and what is deficient or lacking when we see care, help and support that are not so good? Asking these questions is not to criticise existing care practices, let alone caregivers, but to search for how to adequately and appropriately perceive, describe and, when necessary, evaluate these practices. This book is about practices of care, help and support in the domains of healthcare and social work – and other domains too, such as education and the 'care for the world'. We approach these practices as instances of the practice of care, in the sense in which care ethics uses the word 'care': the effort to sustain life when it is weak, fragile, dependent or not yet fully developed, especially when it is in danger, threatened, in pain or broken.

In search of good care

We have just mentioned puzzles, but this is not to say that we have no clues, answers or solutions. Much of this book is about the insights we have gained. We categorise them collectively as 'relational caring', especially the 'practising of presence', a specific conceptualisation of relational care, namely, a strongly relational one (for more on relational caring and strong relationality, see Chapter 10). The first author, Andries Baart, developed his 'theory of presence' in a longitudinal qualitative study of a particular practice: outreach pastoral care in deprived urban neighbourhoods (Baart, 2001; Baart and Vosman, 2011; Timmerman and Baart, 2016b; Schaftenaar et al, 2018). 'Presence' is how he came to thematise the heart of all good professional care, help and support in the areas of health, welfare and a habitable world. It must essentially be understood as a qualified, efficacious way of being for others by being with others. The consequent practising of presence results in a 'presence approach' that has been methodically extensively elaborated, but remains fundamentally open. 'Presence theory' elaborates on how to understand this approach and why it is so efficacious; it is an empirically grounded, care-ethical theory about presence as the heart of all good work with and for people. It is not without significance, incidentally, that the particular practice from which this theory of presence was developed is a very weakly institutionalised practice. In this book we present the current state of the theory of presence, which continues to develop in interaction with theory, practice and research and to integrate more and more issues and domains, including newly emerging ones.

When we use the word 'puzzle', what we are saying is that the search for good care in healthcare and social work is a continuing inquiry into what makes specific care practices good in a wide variety of domains, each in their own time-specific circumstances, and regardless of formal standards; practices that are highly contextual, situated, complex, dynamic and emergent, and whose quality has to be validated locally. It is a continuous inquiry for care receivers and their relatives, as well as for caregivers and their organisations and for researchers. This inquiry again and again places all who partake in relational caring before surprises, incongruities, hypotheses and new insights, and that in turn raises questions and presents intriguing puzzles: if this is good, how must we understand this?

These questions do not occupy us, as researchers and scholars, in a disengaged, detached way, as if there is nothing at stake for us. On the contrary, these are urgent questions, at least in our analysis of the precarious situation in which both clients and professionals in healthcare and social work – and also, for example, in education – find themselves in today's late modern societies in the Global North. Our analysis engages with the relevant international literature from diverse disciplines such as ethics, philosophy, sociology and political science, and it is based primarily on our inquiries into healthcare and social work in the Netherlands (Baart, 2001; 2018c), but also, as if in contrast to the former, in South Africa (Baart, 2018a; Baart and Hoffman, 2021). We consider the situation of healthcare and social work in the Netherlands an exemplary case of healthcare and social work in the Global North, due to the historically conditioned, international orientation of our country and its receptivity to management and market thinking, in its institutions and society (de Vries, 2007; Dwarswaard, Hilhorst and Trappenburg, 2011).

Instead of presenting a complete analysis of the situation of healthcare and social work in the Netherlands, which would be beyond the scope of this chapter, we will make six disturbing observations.

1. There is frequent, more or less compulsory and ideological use of terms such as autonomy, self-reliance, self-control, resilience, co-creation, participation, self-strength and self-development with regard to patients, clients, pupils, residents, citizens and neighbourhoods, combined with exaggerated but obligatory ideas about positivity and the manufacturability of society. This actually keeps vulnerable people dependent on themselves and their equally vulnerable relational networks, ensuring that they rely as little as possible on professionals and organisations paid by public money and the government.
2. There is a focus, partially impelled by austerity measures, on short-term problem solving, which induces professionals and organisations to choose the most promising patients, clients or residents, and to refer other, less promising patients to other professionals and organisations, ultimately abandoning the least promising, most difficult, most complex of them, including their relatives.
3. There is a strong aversion among organisations and authorities to risk, tragedy and partiality, leading them to distrust professionals and, in an attempt to manage this distrust, causing domestication of professionals and protocolisation of their practice. This in turn leads to – often unrecognised – mismatches in care for people who need care, dissatisfaction among patients, clients, pupils and residents, and moral distress, compassion fatigue and exhaustion among professional caregivers in healthcare and social work.
4. There is a strong, often algorithm- or protocol-driven emphasis on efficiency and safety, which suppresses substantive, moral understandings of what good care, help and support are.
5. The dominant understanding of the quality of care is quantitative, requiring the measurement and monitoring of performance indicators that create their own abstract world and a lot of work, but that remain external to the concrete relationships in which care is given and received, and thus obfuscate the actually experienced benefits and harm for clients, patients, pupils, residents and their relatives in their lives and lifeworld.
6. The dominant approach to professionals in healthcare and social work is to see them as agents of effective procedures, which they are entitled to implement because they have a sufficient degree of accumulated knowledge, learned skills and acquired competencies.

In contrast with these observations, this book reports on our engaged quest to understand instances of good care, good-enough care and not-so-good care in healthcare, social work and other domains, and to contribute to facilitating and promoting practices of good care, especially by training and educating professional caregivers. In other words, this book does not claim to provide the conclusive answer to these questions, but instead offers a state-of-the-art account of an ongoing inquiry and its intriguing results so far. We are engaged in this inquiry together with the many participants in caring practices – professionals as well as clients and their relatives – in healthcare, social work, education and other domains in which professionals work with and for people. It is an inquiry in which we have learned a lot, struggled with countless puzzles, solved many of them and are continuously encountering new ones.

Puzzles of good care

What kinds of intriguing situations, cases and practices in healthcare and social work have challenged and continue to challenge our concepts and understanding of good care? We will now present seven not entirely arbitrary examples. It is not insignificant, incidentally, that two of these are about hospitals, a very strongly institutionalised site of caring.

CASE FRAGMENT 1.1

Deferred care is expensive care

Michelle van Tongerloo, a general practitioner who also sees and treats people living on the streets, recounts the following: 'My patient is sitting in front of me. Clammy, sweaty. Sick. He didn't come of his own accord. My assistant saw that he suddenly ordered morphine via the prescription line. "What happened here," she wondered. I open his file and see an old letter from a hospital. It only says that he has broken a number of ribs in a scooter accident. "I'm in so much pain," he says on the phone, "I can hardly breathe." He sounds confused and I invite him to come and see me. He has a fever, a rapid pulse and an open wound. For weeks he has been indicating at the hospital that things are not going well. He is always told that the wounds have to heal by themselves. He doesn't feel they are taking him seriously. I call the surgeon, express my concerns and ask if he would like to see the patient today. He refuses and dismisses me saying, "Call my assistant for an outpatient appointment." As if I am trying to sell a vacuum cleaner. But the next patient is already knocking on my door at this point. And I, too, send the man home. Against my better judgement – his pulse isn't that fast either, this is how I justify it to myself. I call him at the end of the day. It's not going well, he says, the wound has opened and is bleeding. I call the surgeon again. "How heavily is it bleeding?" he asks. No idea. "Is there enough for a cup or a puddle, or is it streaming?" No idea! I'm getting angry. "Perhaps you should see for yourself what's going on; I wanted to send this patient to you this morning!" I reply, to which he says, a little irritated, that he will call him. The patient goes to see the surgeon the next day. He is told he'll have to continue to rinse the wound, and is sent home without further examination. The following day, his condition goes from bad to worse. When he becomes very grey and short of breath, his wife calls the emergency room. He is refused again: they're too busy. She drives him to another hospital, where he is seen. First they have to wait in the waiting room. Then they see a nurse, then a doctor. Then he is examined, and there is more waiting. Three hours later, it turns out things are very bad. His lung is filled with pus and he needs surgery. But not there. He is a patient of the first hospital – that's where he will have to go. He is urgently transferred by ambulance, and upon arrival, all the examinations are repeated. In the early hours of the morning, finally, he is put to bed, exhausted, in a hospital ward. The infection has affected his ribs to such an extent that they don't heal properly. His lungs are damaged. If it had been diagnosed earlier, a simple course of antibiotics might have cured it – in fact, he has to see three different specialists every week.' How could this happen?[1]

The puzzle here is how it is possible, in our highly advanced system of healthcare and social work, that even experienced professionals are unable to arrange good care for certain categories of patients, clients or residents. This puzzle calls for a political conception of care, help and support, also in response to the second observation made in the numbered list earlier in this chapter.

CASE FRAGMENT 1.2

Being attentive in a general hospital

In a general hospital, a PhD student observes physicians' consultations with patients. She notices a physician being very attentive to one patient and, a few moments later, very inattentive to another patient. The same doctor, the same hospital, the same day. Why the difference? What is attentiveness? What is the influence of the institutional context on attentiveness? How does it contribute to good care?[2]

The puzzle is which concepts we need so as to understand how a professional can be attentive to one patient, client or resident, and inattentive to another. This puzzle prompts the question of the relational and social inclusion of all human beings, also in response to the third observation.

CASE FRAGMENT 1.3

Crossing but disconnected storylines in youth care

A national newspaper carries a fly-on-the-wall article featuring youth protection agent Sylvana and her working week. Her story provides penetrating insight into her work as a 'youth protection agent, lawyer, mediator and scapegoat all at once', as she calls herself. It is a familiar story in Dutch youth care: a social worker who has to deal with many complicated cases in the space of three working days. Sylvana has been working as a youth protection agent for almost 20 years. She takes care of 12 families, is the legal guardian of several children placed with foster parents and supervises a number of other children. She works hard and clocks up long days, and agonises over difficult issues. She wasn't asking for it, but her story evokes admiration for her commitment and for how she keeps it up. The article mentions a case Sylvana took over from a colleague, a home visit she makes standing in for a colleague who was unable to come, and a case that Sylvana has not been involved in for very long and that has been going on for a decade. At this point, the narrative intersects with a second dominant storyline in youth care, exemplified by the story of Monique, the mother of a 15-year-old daughter with serious psychological problems. Over the years, they and their family have had to deal with many different caregivers, and this has led to mismatches, delays and deteriorating conditions; finally, the daughter was placed in a secure youth care facility. This is a frequently heard complaint in the stories of many clients, ex-clients, parents, foster parents and family home parents. We see these two storylines often in youth care. Narratives that intersect but are unfortunately barely connected. How could these two storylines be linked?[3]

The puzzle here is why professionals who work hard are experienced not only as unhelpful but even as harmful. This raises the question of what their profession ultimately is about (its ultimate end), how professionals answer that question and how they can bring their actual practice into accordance to their answer to that question. This can also furnish a response to the fourth observation.

CASE FRAGMENT 1.4

'Fortunately, they're not professionals!'

In a longitudinal, extensive study of the practice of two urban neighbourhood outreach chaplains, the residents are interviewed about how they value these professionals. It turns out that they appreciate the chaplains highly, and compare them favourably to the other professionals in their neighbourhood. They tell the interviewer, 'Fortunately, they're not professionals!' What is it that they appreciate and why do they dissociate the benefit they experience from what 'professionals' do?[4]

The puzzle is how it is possible that professionals whose task it is to help people are experienced as not helpful. Or, more specifically, why certain categories of patients, clients or residents experience no benefit at all from any individual intervention or specific policy. This puzzle asks for a substantive, normative conception of care, help and support, also in response to the first observation in the numbered list earlier in this chapter.

CASE FRAGMENT 1.5

Practical wisdom at the end of life

In a case study, general practitioners (GPs) were interviewed about a particular case of their care for their dying patients. The researchers wanted to understand how the GPs perceive, assess, consider, act and evaluate, and they reconstructed it as an instance of practical wisdom. They concluded that the GPs practise a medical profession and, within this profession, know and apply the rules and regulations. But they do this in such a way that the patient and their relatives are acknowledged as relational beings. As a consequence, these GPs show considerable freedom in how they deal with rules and regulations. How do they do this?[5]

The puzzle is how excellently trained GPs, who are strictly monitored and held to account by various bodies, can deviate so far from the rules, and yet be appreciated by family and the inspectors. This puzzle calls for professionals who are able to act in case of uncertainty and conflicting duties, also in response to the first and the fourth observations.

CASE FRAGMENT 1.6

Complexity reduction through constant renewal

In a general hospital, the executive leadership 'has to deal with government and insurance company policies which not only change rapidly, but can also be internally inconsistent or even contradictory with one another. Both the board and higher management spend vast amounts of time coping with these external policies. Although certain managers remain confident with regard to complexity reduction via systems, as some seem to entertain the phantasm that the insoluble can by grasped and managed, many however are critically aware of the feasible, the insoluble and the simply tragic. For instance, certain managers (...) tried to give physicians and nurses a shared responsibility as 'co-operators' on a ward, rather than pursuing a hierarchical model of work, hierarchy that might lead to tensions and wouldn't tap into the (different forms of) available knowledge. At the same time these managers were also busy contributing to the increase of complexity, for example by introducing three 'renewals' at the same time: (1) integrating two teams of nurses, of two completely different medical wards, into one single multi applicable team, (2) trying to introduce and manage the merger of two different hospitals while also (3) trying to intensify the Lean approach of working processes among employees. Thus as complexity reduction in the hospital reached a certain level of stability, this was paradoxically achieved through a state of constant renewal: all partakers accepted that they and all processes are ultimately, constantly on the move. One of the top managers of the hospital literally depicted this state: "as long as we keep the matter liquefied we are doing a good job".'[6]

The puzzle is which concepts we need to understand how pursuing the reduction of complexity leads to never ending processes of complex, far-reaching and interfering innovations. The puzzle is why the reduction of complexity is being pursued. This puzzle calls for a qualitative, narrative understanding and evaluation of quality of care, also in response to the fifth observation.

CASE FRAGMENT 1.7

The coordinates of the physician

As part of a major transition and research project in a general hospital, a researcher is observing the work of a physician. The physician is going to see a woman who has cancer and her husband in a regular follow-up consultation. The doctor asks the patient whether she is taking her medicine regularly and is sticking to her diet. The patient reassures the doctor that she is following the instructions for her medication and diet. The doctor is satisfied and invites her to go to a sectioned-off part of the room for a physical examination. When they have gone, the patient's husband leans over to the researcher and whispers to him: 'It's not true! She is not doing that at all!' What made the doctor ask those questions and be satisfied by his patient's first response, preventing himself from obtaining true information about the patient's condition?[7]

The puzzle is how the doctor expects to become properly informed if he does not let the patient speak. This puzzle prompts the question how professionals can be trained and formed to be capable of relational caring, also in response to the sixth observation.

Each one of these case fragments presents a puzzle. A successful solution to these puzzles would be a meaningful explanation, that is, an account that makes sense or a 'figure' that provides insight. These puzzles are not like jigsaw puzzles that can be solved only in one way by finding the right place for each piece. We regard them as conundrums that can be solved in many ways by forming different configurations or shapes that each have a more or less understandable meaning – like a tangram puzzle with its seven geometrical pieces. The question then is: which of these shapes is the most adequate, rich, multilayered, satisfactory and helpful, at least for the moment, to participants in caring practices? In other words, which image or shape gives the best account of what the fragment is about? We think these puzzles are not easily solvable. We are also eager not to unduly simplify, abstract, individualise or decontextualise these issues, because that would be to skirt around the core issue at stake.

Once all these puzzles tentatively have been solved, the question is what connection there is between the different solutions. Assuming, as we do, that all these puzzles are about the same phenomenon – care, in a care-ethical sense – then they can be regarded as pieces of one and the same big puzzle, even if some are so by way of contrast, as a photographic negative. If these were pieces of a large jigsaw puzzle, it could be asked: what is the image that becomes visible when they are all put together? We think it is more adequate to see these puzzles as pieces of an overarching puzzle that can be solved in many ways, by forming different shapes. Again, it can be asked which image or shape gives the best account of what good care, help and support is. In terms of the philosophy of science: which empirically grounded theory offers the best explanatory model of what good care, help and support is and accomplishes?

Looking at these seven puzzles, and based on our inquiries into caring practices and the resonance validation of our findings by practitioners, any such account will have to involve a conception of care that is first of all *relational*, that is, that does justice to the relationality, dependence and interdependence of the resident, patient, pupil or client and their relatives, the care professional, often a team member, and the care organisation. It should also be *empirical*, do justice to what participants in care practices actually do, say, use, refrain from doing and undergo. And it must be *theoretically informed*, acknowledge that nothing is as practical as good theory. The conception of care that we are looking for must be *complex*, that is, must not carelessly simplify the complexity of care, as a practice that is intersected by other practices and that takes place within its organisational, institutional and societal context. It should also be *critical*: critical of its own presuppositions and of simplifications, distortions and the depoliticisation and commodification of care. And it must be *morally scrutinised*, stripped of inappropriate, external, ideologically motivated morality. Finally, the conception of care we are developing must be *political*, must acknowledge that good care, good-enough care and not-so-good care happen in 'the political', the 'flow of coming together, chafing, understanding and conflict' (Vosman, 2023: 40). It must contribute to the living together of people in society and its structures. Only if it is relational, empirical, theoretically informed, complex, critical, morally scrutinised and political can a conception of care do justice to the actual caring of professionals and citizens in complex organisations in late modernity. In this book we will be showing how far we have come with developing such a conception of care.

Relational caring

We call the conception of care we have developed and which is relevant to both healthcare and social work, 'relational caring'. We did not coin this term. Others, although not many, are using it too (Miller, 2014; Ray and Turkel, 2014; Dupuis et al, 2016). We deliberately chose the gerund 'caring' instead of the noun 'care' to designate the dynamic and emergent character of care as a practice. Our conception of relational caring is predicated on the practising of 'presence', which must essentially be understood as a qualified, efficacious way of being there for others by being with them. In the practising of presence, the relationship between the professional or professionals and the persons whom they work with and for is very important (van Heijst, 2011). But relational caring should not be understood as meaning: first establish a caring relationship and then start to care. Relational caring is a way of perceiving, interpreting, programming, evaluating and so forth, and must be understood as the steering principle of establishing and maintaining relationships that embed, support and limit caring with and for others – and, where necessary and possible, terminating it, but doing so in a relational way.

As we want our conception of care to be relational, empirical, theoretically informed, complex, critical, morally scrutinised and political, we position ourselves in particular academic fields that are inhabited by dialogue partners, fellow travellers and critical friends. A relational and empirical conception of care is interested in both the general and the particular. That requires qualitative empirical research and the development of theories and theoretical concepts, on the one hand, and ethical reflection, on the other, without carelessly introducing external theories or moral principles into the practice. An empirical and complex conception of care requires theories and theoretical concepts that enable us to perceive well and understand what we are perceiving in our inquiry into care practices in healthcare and social work. Practice theory and complex thinking are helpful in this respect. We frame our critical-political conception of care in a care-ethical way. We take care ethics, a body of theory with critical impact that started with the work of Carol Gilligan in the 1980s, as a political-ethical discipline, in discussion with political phenomenology and critical sociology.

In late modernity, which is the current stage of modernity, institutions such as healthcare and social work are under increasing pressure from rule-based systems derived from utilitarian, goal-directed, production-oriented and bureaucratic management models (van Heijst, 2011). This systemic pressure burdens the work with and for people that is being performed within these institutions, increasingly modelling it as the production of commodities. That is why it is not insignificant that the practice that was the site of discovery of our care-ethical presence theory is a very lightly institutionalised practice.

The issue that occupies us in this book can be formulated as follows: what characterises activities that turn out to be essential in healthcare and social work and that have shown themselves to be good and helpful in late modern society, in the first place for the care receiver and their relatives? If relational caring is inevitably at the heart of good professional care, help and support, how do professionals deal with situations in which entering into and maintaining relationships is subject to high systemic pressures that predicate on and are additional to the ambiguities of late modernity? And how can good care, help and support be maintained and promoted in late modern, complex and dynamic contexts? In our view, the beginnings of an answer to these questions can be found by studying what advanced, deliberating and practically wise professionals who are acknowledged as such by care receivers, colleagues and managers do when they deliver good, good-enough and not-so-good care, help and support, and what organisational and systemic forces they have to face and deal with.

This book presents the newest insights from empirical research, theory development and ethical reflection about relational caring from a presence-theoretical perspective. Throughout the book, we will use the expression 'presence-theoretical perspective' in order to remind ourselves and our readers that we are trying to inquire into and theorise about the world in all its complexity, with its dynamic and emerging aspects. Although the presence theory has proven to be adequate, we want to keep our perspective open to aspects, processes and events that do not easily fit into this theory but are nevertheless real, that is, relevant to, but not at the disposal of, carers, institutions, clients, patients, residents, pupils and their relatives, and/or society. We invite the reader to join us on our quest, our inquiry into good care, good-enough care and not-so-good care. We do not know where it will bring us, as the world, including ourselves, is always changing and will always continue to change.

Structure of the book and how to read it

In this book, we present the state of the art of our inquiry from a presence-theoretical perspective into practices of healthcare and social work in the Netherlands. In Part I, we present and discuss the concept, practice and theory of presence and relate these to other approaches. We argue that if we are to study complex, dynamic and emergent practices of care and social work, it is necessary to effect an empirical turn in care-ethical research and a practice turn in theoretical thinking. This results in the theoretical perspective of presence, a complex, rather unusual but fruitful and revealing way of looking at care practices and issues that emerge in these practices and are relevant to its participants.

Part II contains six chapters about major topics in relational caring that each discuss a particular issue by looking at it from this presence-theoretical perspective. The case fragments in this chapter have already introduced the issues. Each of the chapters in Part II starts with a new case fragment that illustrates what the chapter is about. The reader will note that these case descriptions often also illustrate what is discussed in other chapters. After all, everything is at issue in everything else. That is why complex issues require complex, non-reductive thinking. To manage this everything-is-at-issue-in-everything-else and the reader's expectations, each chapter has its own motto.

We recommend that the reader first read Part I in its entirety and that they then choose the chapter or chapters in Part II that interest them. Reading Part I is helpful – and reading Chapters 3 and 4 is even necessary – to understand and appreciate the meaning, relevance and scope of the empirical findings, the insights and the 'stepping stones' that we are offering professionals, managers and scholars in the domains of healthcare and social work.

Throughout the book we will use words and expressions in a way that might not be familiar to native English speakers. And we sometimes use familiar words and expressions in non-familiar ways. This is not just a translation issue. We do the same in our native language, Dutch. It starts with the word 'presence', which we use, in combination with other words or not, in a very specific, qualified and yet very broad meaning. It can be compared to the word 'care' in 'care ethics'. Other examples are expressions such as 'connecting with and attuning your practice to' and 'diluted seriousness'. We do this to express – and to remind ourselves and our readers – that we are inquiring into and thinking about caring practices in theoretical terms that are grounded in empirical material. The effect is that both professionals and scholars are invited to look beyond their jargon and search together for the meaning and usefulness of such empirically grounded theoretical terms in their concrete practice, situation or context.

PART I

Presence, practice and theory

2

Presence: the concept

This chapter and the next two deal with 'presence', the word we use to thematise the heart of all good professional care, help and support in the areas of health, welfare and a habitable world. The current chapter is about presence as a concept used in different domains in healthcare and social work. The next two chapters address presence as a particular practice and as a theory.

Why presence?

The concept of presence has appeared in scholarly literature on missionary pastoral care, nursing, psychotherapy and other domains since the 1960s. It is often referred to as the centre, heart or core of the practice in question, and especially as a quality standard for good care. It has increasingly become the subject of qualitative research since the 1990s. While it may not be easy to explain why this happened, we think the main cause lies in the development of modernity. In the current stage of modernity – late modernity – institutions such as healthcare and social work are coming under increasing pressure from rule-based systems derived from utilitarian, goal-directed, production-oriented and bureaucratic management models (van Heijst, 2011). This systemic pressure burdens the work with and for people that is being done within these institutions, increasingly modelling it as the production of commodities. Many professionals as well as scholars feel that this is problematic in light of what care, help and support are and should be.

The question to which presence is an answer may be formulated as follows: what characterises activities that are regarded as essential in the social, therapeutic, nursing and medical professions and that have shown themselves to be beneficial to care receivers and their relatives in today's late modern society? If working relationally stands at the heart of good social, therapeutic, nursing and medical professional practice, how then should we deal with situations where entering into and maintaining relationships are subject to high systemic pressures? And how can good care, help and support – care, help and support that are experienced as good and beneficial to care receivers – be maintained and promoted in complex and dynamic late modern contexts? An answer to these questions can be obtained only by empirically studying what professionals actually do when they deliver good care, help and support, and what organisational and systemic forces they face.

In this chapter we will explore presence, first as a word and then as a concept as it occurs in scholarly literature on missionary pastoral care, nursing, psychotherapy and other domains. The purpose of this exercise is to set the background for an understanding and appreciation of the way in which we will use the word presence in this book, that is, as the common denominator of a particular kind of practice that is at the core of good professional care. Used in this particular way, the term presence can be succinctly defined as 'being there for others by being there with others', or as 'being there with others, leading to being there for others'.

Meaning, origin and relation to other concepts

The English noun 'presence' comes from the Anglo-Norman and Old French nouns *presence, presens, presance* (French *présence*), which in turn stem from the Latin noun *praesentia*. It means 'the existence of someone or something in a particular place and/or at a particular time'.[1] The Latin noun *praesentia* is derived from the adjective *praesēns*, which means 'being here, being there', and more particularly 'being here, being there instantly, immediately' and 'effectively, strongly, powerfully'. *Praesēns* is the translation of the Greek word *parōn*, the present participle of *páreimi*, which means 'to be with someone', and more particularly 'to stand at someone's side, to help someone', and is the opposite of *ápeimi*, which means 'to be absent', and more particularly 'to stay away'. This brings us close to the moral injunction of care: 'not to turn away from someone in need' (Gilligan, 1987: 20) and to the main purpose of caring: 'the care-receivers' experience of being supported and not left on their own' (van Heijst, 2011: 3).

The late Latin verb *praesentāre* is similarly derived from *praesēns*, and means 'to make present, to show, to offer'. This is the root of the English verb 'to present', and the noun 'a present', meaning 'a gift, an offering'. Metaphysically, presence originates in a gift: the (helping) existence and impact of someone who is near to me comes to me from without.

From very early on, the term presence has also been applied to the spiritual level. The divine presence meant the appearance, communication and efficacy of God. The idea of the real presence of Christ in the Eucharist first appears in the work of Ignatius of Antioch, in the second century of the Common Era. In the English language, this use of the term can be found for the first time in the 12th century, initially with reference to God and subsequently also to humans. It also occurred in the 13th century with reference to inanimate objects (*Oxford English Dictionary*).

In the 19th and 20th centuries, existentialism turned presence from a thing of the gods into 'a matter of the time-bound, earth-bound creature. And presence enlarged its original meanings of being now, being here, and being a gift, to an immediacy, nearness, and bestowal that are subjectively construed' (Doona et al, 1997).

In the late modern history of the Christian churches, the term 'presence' has appeared before and after the Second World War in the quest for an authentic, effective manner of existence of Christians in a secularised, post-Christian, multiform society. It was advanced to oppose the idea that churches had to be 'planted'. But the term was also used in other areas. In nursing, for example, it appeared in the 1960s as a philosophical concept founded in the existentialism of Gabriel Marcel and Martin Heidegger and the religious philosophy of Martin Buber. There has been a tendency in nursing since the mid-1980s to understand presence as an intervention strategy, and, in opposition to this, nursing presence was defined in the 1990s as 'an intersubjective encounter between a nurse and a patient in which the nurse encounters the patient as a unique human being in a unique situation and chooses to "spend" herself on his behalf' (Doona et al, 1997) (see the next section). In the qualitative research of a particular practice that underpins Andries Baart's presence theory (which will be explained further in Chapter 4), 'presence' was the word used to describe 'the efforts of the chaplains to be meaningful to the local residents by being there with them and thus also being there for them' (Baart, 2001: 728).

Presence is part of a synonym group that also includes existence and being there. The term is used in this book in a sense that can be defined succinctly as 'being there for others by being there with them' or 'being there with others, leading to being there for them'. Closely related terms are care, attunement, connection, attentiveness and attention, understood as aspects, attitudes or practices of presence. Presence as a gift provokes wonderment. Gabriel Marcel associated presence with the term availability (*disponibilité*): to be present to the other by making one's own resources available and by being open and transparent to the other. In church history, presence is connected with urban mission, and in theology with testimony. Ill-considered associations of presence with certain psychological concepts such as mindfulness and empathy are not unproblematic.

The lexical antonym of presence is absence. But in the sense in which presence is used in this book, the opposite can also be hyper interventionism, that is, a practice in which interventions are self-referential – arising from the framework, disciplinary concerns and organisational tasks of the professionals themselves – and thereby in fact subtle, complex and ultra-modern instances of absence. Absence here in the sense of not responding to the care receiver's needs, concerns and longings.

Presence in scholarly literature

In their discussion of the research of nurses' judgements which they carried out independently from each other, Mary Ellen Doona, Lois Haggerty and Susan Chase observed a number of common themes, especially a phenomenon inextricably linked with nurses' judgements which they have reluctantly called 'presence' (Doona et al, 1997). Their initial reluctance disappeared after the tragic death of a woman due to a medical error during experimental treatment for breast cancer. They recognised that it would have made a difference in this case if the nurse had been present rather than absent. They also realised that nurses' presence is coming under pressure because of the pragmatic cost/benefit focus of many employers in healthcare. Scholars more generally have identified presence as a core element of practice in late modern society, not only in nursing, but also in psychotherapy, online communication and management. We will see that the way this core element is understood has been determined mainly by qualitative research. We will begin with the context from which the idea of presence as we understand it emerged.[2]

Missionary pastoral care

As said before, the term 'presence' has appeared before and after the Second World War in the quest for an authentic, effective manner of existence of Christians in society. Developments in Germany in the first half of the 20th century were important, as theologians such as Dietrich Bonhoeffer and Karl Barth criticised the entanglement of church and state, while at the same time in France the process of *laïcisation* provoked a renewal of theology among theologians such as Marie-Dominique Chenu (Stoppels, 1996) as well as a defensive reaction. Presence appeared as a threefold response: (a) to the experience of a non-authentic manner of existence of the church in the world, (b) to the experience of the absence of the church from the world of workers and factories and from deprived urban neighbourhoods, and (c) to the encounter with other religions. In *Présence au monde moderne* (1948), Jacques Ellul advocated a Christian presence that is about 'being' rather than 'doing'. In 1964, the World Student Christian Federation (WSCF) introduced presence as a concept to express the centre of the Christian faith as well as WSCF's response to this faith. The statement they issued explained that '"Presence" for us means "engagement", involvement in the concrete structures of our society. It indicates a priority. First, we have to be there before we can see our task clearly. In one sense of the word, presence precedes witness. In another sense, the very presence is witness' (cited in Stoppels, 1996: 46).

The Little Brothers of Jesus were founded in 1933, inspired by Charles de Foucauld (1858–1916), whose spirituality was nourished by the presence of Jesus in the lowly, the poor, the miserable and the little ones. They decided to enter the world of workers and factories. Similarly, the Little Sisters of Jesus and lay people such as the social worker Madeleine Delbrêl searched for ways to live with the poor. In 1941, the Dominican Father Jacques Loew started to work in a shipyard in Marseille. This was the beginning of the movement of the so-called 'worker-priests' (*prêtres-ouvriers*). Their presence in the areas where workers lived was expanded to presence in factories and unions. Similar developments involving non-stipendiary ministers or priests in secular employment took place in the Church of England and the Episcopal Church in the United States. In 1954, the Roman Catholic movement of worker-priests was banned by the Holy See, the government of the Roman Catholic Church, but the Second Vatican Council reopened this possibility for priests. In Germany, priests began to work in factories for the first time in the late 1960s. In 1983, the German worker-priests opened up membership to non-ordained theologians, women religious and lay pastoral workers who lived from their own manual work (Straßner, 2005).

In the Netherlands, the term 'church presence' (*kerkelijke presentie*) was the slogan for the missionary work carried out by church ministers in deprived urban neighbourhoods. In 1990, Kor Schippers and others published a study based on their research of outreach chaplaincy (*buurtpastoraat*) in the deprived urban neighbourhood of 'Old West' (*Oude Westen*), an old city district of Rotterdam (Schippers and others, 1990). The objective of this church outreach service, based on altruism and reciprocity, was inspired by the principles of what was called 'urban mission': practical solidarity with actual poor people, in everyday life, in constant contact with the people who are actually at stake, going 'where God has already preceded us', as its protagonists would say.

It is crucial to this kind of neighbourhood pastoral care that the chaplains do not adopt the church's perspective on the people, but the people's perspective on the church. This 'Copernican revolution', as Herman IJzerman called it, can be made effective in practice through immersion or exposure. Supervised immersion in and exposure to everyday life in a deprived urban neighbourhood marked by an accumulation of social problems is 'a method of learning to perceive one's [own] socialisation, to reflect upon it and to become aware of it, in relation to the context of the big city, the neighbourhood and people in situations of deprivation' (IJzerman, 2002). In addition, IJzerman developed a scheme of what he calls A and B worlds, which is often used in training to help chaplains analyse their experiences in the neighbourhood and to reflect on the confrontation between their own world and the world of the local residents (van der Spek, 2010).

From 1991 to 2001, Andries Baart extensively studied what deprived urban neighbourhood chaplains actually do (Baart, 2001). He ultimately came to associate the work of neighbourhood chaplains with the word 'presence', thus connecting presence specifically with phased exposure, contrasting it with interventionism, placing it in the framework of care ethics and fleshing it out methodically. In a way, he recovered presence from its missionary context, and transformed criticisms of the church's insufficient presence or even absence into criticisms of inadequate social services (van der Spek, 2010). We will return to Baart's study and his theory of presence in the following chapters.

Nursing

In 1962, Sister Madeleine Clémence Vaillot introduced the phrase 'to be a presence to the patient' – that is, not an object – in nursing science, on the basis of Gabriel Marcel's existentialism. Drawing on the insights of Martin Buber, other authors further developed the term presence and turned it into a central, coherent concept in nursing science. However, multiple and mixed meanings were added in the mid-1980s. On the basis of phenomenological research, Jan Pettigrew (1990) distinguished five characteristics:

1. being available and at the disposal of the other;
2. listening to the other;
3. realising the privilege of participating in the experience;
4. giving oneself; and
5. being there with the other in such a way that the other person experiences it as meaningful.

According to Doona, Haggerty and Chase, the integrity of the concept was confused further by the 'penetration of utilitarianism'. In 1992, D. Gardner sees presence as an intervention. Doona et al, however, emphasise that nursing presence as they see it cannot be made into a technique (Doona et al, 1997).

Since the 1990s, the concept of nursing presence has attracted new attention due to increasing patient dissatisfaction, the falling number of nurses, as well as moral distress, compassion fatigue and exhaustion among nurses, particularly in 'holistic nursing' (Boeck, 2014). Doona et al have defined care presence as 'an intersubjective encounter between a nurse and a patient in which the nurse encounters the patient as a unique human being in a unique situation and chooses to spend herself on the patient's behalf, while at the same time the patient invites the nurse into his experience' (1997: 12). They have recognised that the patient's situation sometimes invites the nurse to take care of the patient. The key antecedents are the nurse's commitment to immersing herself in the patient's situation and the patient's willingness to allow the nurse to enter into their lived experience. As a consequence of nursing presence, both participants are confirmed as unique persons, the nurse as a professional and the patient as a person in need of care. According to Doona et al, nursing presence is essential to good care. It is the 'context' and 'reason' for the nurse's informed judgement. Knowing about the importance of nursing presence can be an antidote to the depersonalisation of healthcare, which seems to be on the increase as health systems are being restructured (Doona et al, 1997: 12).

In a hermeneutical analysis of their data on the nurses' judgements in three different contexts, Doona et al found six characteristics of nursing presence: (1) nursing presence is a unique moment in time, in which the uniqueness of the patient and the uniqueness of the nurse are undeniable; (2) the nurse connects with the experience of the patient as a whole person, not just as a sick person; (3) while collecting data from various sources, and connecting these facts with her own nursing experience, the nurse senses what is the case and what would be good to do or not do in this situation; (4) it goes beyond the theory and the scientific data; (5) it involves knowing in situations of uncertainty what will work and when to act – a knowledge the nurse owes to her immersion in the patient's situation; and (6) it involves being with the patient, that is, 'being exquisitely sensitive to the patient's subjective experience of mental illness' (Doona et al, 1999: 64).

Despite Doona's plea not to conflate being and doing, Pamela Renee Boeck has argued that nursing presence is not only an essential state of holistic nursing but also a core competency in today's nursing. She has defined nursing presence as 'being with another individual, deeply listening, not conditional on what to do or say next, while remaining in the intimacy of the moment' (Boeck, 2014: 5). Boeck argues that even if the nurse uses electronic technologies and is not therefore face to face with the patient, nursing presence remains an important therapeutic component.

According to Deborah Finfgeld-Connett, nursing presence requires a supportive environment, made up of 'individuals in management that value employees and diminish work-related stress', enabling nurses 'to work cooperatively' and have 'adequate time to enact presence and caring' (Finfgeld-Connett, 2008: 115).

Like pastoral presence, nursing presence has been substantively fleshed out through qualitative research. Doona et al identified their six characteristics of nursing presence through a hermeneutical analysis of 30 dense narratives of nurses' judgements, derived from three studies conducted and published independently from each other. They used ten transcripts from each database. The nurses' clinical contexts were significantly different, but each group was involved in supporting patients during significant transitions: one patient was being weaned off mechanical ventilation, another was transitioning from a psychotic to a nonpsychotic state, and yet another was going through labour to delivery. Doona et al shared the descriptions with a selection of nurses from the primary studies to confirm or refute the conclusions, and they found that these nurses agreed with their interpretation (1999).[3]

As we attempt to hone our own understanding of presence, we observe that scholars have conceptualised nursing presence as a core feature of nursing and have dissected it into different aspects. We also see that presence has been predominantly associated with the quality of a one-to-one relationship during the encounter between a nurse and a patient. We gather that the concept of presence is at risk of being regarded as a method or competence.

Psychotherapy

In 1963, the leading French psychoanalyst Sacha Nacht published his book *La présence du psychanalyste*. According to Nacht, it is crucial to the success of psychoanalytic therapy that the psychoanalyst is always available, is unconditionally friendly and unrestrictedly patient and is, above all, able to give (Veszy-Wagner, 1964). Fritz Perls, who founded Gestalt therapy together with his wife, Laura, was influenced by Martin Buber's concept of the I–Thou relationship. Presence is central to this relationship, unlike in the I–It relationship. Although both relationships are important in a therapeutic relationship, healing requires the mutual presence which is characteristic of the I–Thou relationship (Perls, 1969). In his later writings, Carl Rogers, one of the founders of humanistic psychology and client-centred, later person-centred, therapy, called the manner in which he was with his clients 'my presence' (Rogers, 1980: 129). Congruence, an unconditionally positive regard and empathic understanding are the three characteristics of this way of being, which unfolds when the therapist is present mindfully. According to Rogers, therapeutic presence is the foundation of these three basic conditions of a successful therapeutic relationship.

Geller and Greenberg have developed a working model for therapeutic presence based on a qualitative analysis of therapists' reports (2002; 2012). They asked seven experienced therapists who were authors on or advocates of the concept of presence about their experience of presence. They presented the therapists with the following definition of presence, taken from the literature: 'the quality of a therapist to be fully with the client in the moment, empty of thoughts of future or past, and unattached from ideas that she or he may have on what the client's issues are and even of the desire for the client to change' (2012: 41). The respondents were asked to reflect on their own experiences with presence after their therapy sessions for the duration of a few weeks. In a more in-depth interview, they were asked about the physical, emotional and cognitive aspects of their own experience of presence. The transcripts of the taped interviews were analysed and interpreted using a method that combined cutting and connotation categorising. After careful consideration and consultation, three higher-order categories were devised under which all the descriptive categories could be subsumed. These three broad categories formed the basis for a model of therapeutic presence.

Three domains emerged in the analysis: a first domain involves the process of preparing the ground for presence. It refers to both the preparation before the session and a more generalised preparation throughout the therapist's whole life. The second describes the process of presence. The processes or activities in which the therapist is engaged when he or she is therapeutically present are the practices of 'receptivity', 'inwardly attending' and 'extending and contact'. The third domain refers to the actual experience of presence during the session: 'grounding', 'immersion', 'expansion' and 'being with and for the client'. Based on this model, Geller and Greenberg used a quantitative study to develop a measuring instrument, the 'Therapeutic Presence Inventory', which can be used by therapists with respect to their presence, as well as by clients with respect to their perception of their therapist's presence. Based on these empirical studies, Geller and Greenberg developed a 'presence-based theory of the therapeutic relationship'. According to this theory, the experience of the therapist's presence makes it possible for the client to become present themselves, with their sorrows and suffering, so that a mutual relational presence can emerge. In this mutual, therapeutic presence, the therapist can attune themselves to the client and respond appropriately. This attuned sensitivity is a basic condition for the development of a positive therapeutic relationship and alliance, and forms the basis for the therapist's interventions, thus contributing to the positive outcome of the session.

Therapeutic presence also has paradoxical aspects. It involves 'a careful balance of contact between the therapist's own experience and the client's experience, while maintaining the capacity to be responsive from that place of internal and external connection' (Geller and Greenberg, 2012: 55). The therapist must simultaneously be fully present and reflect on what is happening, let go of their preconceptions and try to understand the client, abandon preconceived directions and allow a new direction to emerge naturally, and so forth. Geller and Greenberg have emphasised that therapeutic presence is not a substitute for technique, and that it is beneficial not only for clients but also for therapists themselves. The exercise of presence contributes to 'greater well-being, decreased burnout, greater self-care, improved interpersonal relationships, decreased anxiety, and heightened vitality' of the therapist (2012: 9). Although Geller and Greenberg have acknowledged that mindfulness is a powerful technique to cultivate therapeutic presence, they have distinguished therapeutic presence from mindfulness and therapeutic mindfulness techniques, because presence is a way of being with the client, and not a technique, nor is it rooted in Buddhism. Moreover, therapeutic presence does not necessarily produce mindfulness in the client (2012: 13).

As we seek to formulate our own understanding of presence, we note that scholars have understood therapeutic presence, like nursing presence, as a core feature of therapy and have dissected it into different aspects. Another point that we take from their work is that the therapist should not totally neglect their own needs and concerns, but should attend to themselves if they wish to be effective. In addition, therapeutic presence is also connected to the success of the therapy. Although the quality of the one-to-one relationship between the therapist and the client during the session is an important aspect, therapeutic presence also involves preparation before the session, the process of presence and the therapist's whole way of life. Geller and Greenberg have explicitly warned against understanding presence as a technique in general and as a mindfulness technique in particular.

Other domains

There are a few other domains in which presence has appeared as an important concept. We will mention only two: online communication and management.

Telepresence: technologically mediated presence

The term presence has also been used to describe subjective hallucinations, for example in cases where a schizophrenic person hears voices, or someone dreams about meeting someone else. Moreover, presence has been used as a shortened version of 'telepresence', which refers to subjective hallucinations, in which the individual in their perception does not correctly acknowledge the mediating role of technology in their experience. Presence occurs when the individual experience is mediated not only by the human senses and processes of perception but also by human-made technology, while the person perceives the experience as if it is mediated only by the human senses and processes of perception. Presence in this sense can vary in degree, and comes in various types: spatial, sensual, social and combined presence, for example, but also what is called the 'social actor within the medium' and the 'medium as social actor' (International Society for Presence Research, 2000). The term 'telepresence' was introduced in 1980 by the Massachusetts Institute of Technology (MIT) scientist Marvin Minsky, who was amazed at the nuclear industry's inability to handle the consequences of the partial meltdown of one of the two reactors of the Three Mile Island nuclear power plant in Pennsylvania, US. He used it to express the idea that it is possible by using remote control tools to give one's effective presence somewhere else 'the power of a giant or the delicacy of a surgeon' (Minsky, 1980).

The theory of 'social presence' was originally developed to explain the consequences of the use of telecommunication media for interpersonal communication. In 1976, Short, Williams and Christie defined social presence as the degree of salience (that is, the quality or state of meaningful existence) between two communicators who use a communication medium. They conceived of social presence primarily as a quality of communication media, which determined the way in which people interact and communicate with each other. Subsequent researchers, for example Gunawardena in 1995, recycled the theory of social presence to explain how computer-mediated communication in online learning can be personal and social. They drew attention less to the media and more to the people. Nowadays, scholars of social presence and online learning use a whole range of definitions of social presence. At one end of the spectrum, scholars tend to conceive of social presence as the degree to which a person is experienced as 'real' and 'really there'. At the other end, scholars focus on whether there is an interpersonal, emotional connection between communicators. Researchers of social presence have developed tools to measure social presence, for example through questionnaires, but also using multiple and mixed methods (Lowenthal, 2010).

As we attempt to formulate our own understanding of presence, we conclude that telepresence or social presence constitutes a challenge. The question is whether the technologically mediated presence of teachers, nurses, doctors or therapists, for example, can be understood as 'being-for-by-being-with'. We think that this is indeed possible, but will leave this question open for now.[4]

Presencing: leading from the emerging future

For the German MIT researcher and consultant Otto Scharmer, 'presencing' (from 'presence' and 'sensing') is a social technology. He has devised a theory called Theory U, in which he proposes a management method that respects the requirements of sustainability and global responsibility in management and provides the necessary management tools. His central idea is that the way in which a situation develops depends on how it is approached: specifically, whether it is approached from one's own attentiveness and mindfulness. Presencing or 'leading from the future' means acknowledging and opening up potential opportunities for the future in view of current tasks. He argues that this developmental competence benefits both the organisation as a whole and the individual employees personally. Going down the 'U' that Scharmer has used as a visual model for his theory, the practices of presencing are 'suspending', 'redirecting' and 'letting go'. Going up the 'U', they are 'letting come', 'enacting' and 'embodying'.[5] Scharmer claims that he has extended two previous extensions, initiated by Husserl and Heidegger respectively. According to Scharmer, who relies here on anthroposophy, the epistemological extension of explicit, context-independent knowledge with tacit, situated knowledge must itself be supplemented with self-transcending, not-yet-embodied knowledge. Similarly, the ontological extensions of simple, linear systems with autopoietic systems must be supplemented with self-transcending, emergent systems (Scharmer, 2005).

As we seek to formulate our own understanding of presence, we conclude that the concept of presencing is not useful to us. It is more akin to an observational strategy which does not make its normative components explicit. Nevertheless, we think that the practising of presence in the primary process, as we understand it, does require a particular, relational way of managing and directing.

Conclusion

As we have seen, there are many references to presence in scholarly literature on the variegated practices of nursing – a very embodied practice – and therapy – a very conversational practice (see Table 3.2). In both disciplines, presence is conceptualised at the nexus of being there with the patient or client and being effective in this interaction with the patient or client. In both disciplines, presence has been substantively fleshed out through qualitative research. We have also seen that presence is at risk of being misunderstood as a method, an intervention, a technique or a competence. What appears to be lacking is an inquiry into the institutional requirements for and impediments to presence in the primary process. The literature on missionary pastoral care in deprived urban neighbourhoods has provided us with the concept and practice of 'exposure' as a way of learning and sustaining the practice of presence. We will return to this in the following chapter, where we discuss the practice of presence as Baart found and conceptualised it.

3

Presence: the practice

Now that we have considered presence as a concept and its occurrence and use in scholarly literature, this chapter will address what we call the 'practising of presence' in caring and working with and for people. This practice was first found, systematised and theoretically substantiated in a long-term qualitative study of neighbourhood chaplaincy (*buurtpastoraat*) in the Netherlands, a form of outreach pastoral care in deprived, resource-poor urban neighbourhoods. The study involved empirical research, confrontation with the literature, theory development and ethical reflection.

Qualitative research into neighbourhood chaplaincy in the 1990s

Andries Baart, together with several co-researchers, conducted a qualitative study of the work of two neighbourhood chaplains from 1991 to 2001.[1] These chaplains were theologically educated and pastorally trained professionals, who each worked in a different neighbourhood of the Dutch city of Utrecht and who tried 'to be there' for people of all backgrounds, religions and convictions. They had not been charged or tasked to engage in church planting, and were told not to start by setting up an office or building a supportive community. The two chaplains, who were considered by residents and colleagues to be good at their profession, were interviewed every month for seven years, in lengthy and detailed interviews. Baart and his co-researchers analysed these chaplains' case descriptions, reflection reports, diary excerpts and so on and discussed these with them. This case study was embedded in a multiple case study that examined the work of several other neighbourhood chaplains. The researchers used various qualitative and induction-oriented analytical techniques to interpret and understand the professionals' meaning attribution, rule management and action dynamics. These were also analysed in the context of wider theoretical frameworks (drawn from theology, sociology and philosophy) to see how they could best be interpreted and understood. The researchers gave the two professionals whose work was their main research object the position of co-researchers.[2] On more than a hundred occasions spread across several stages of the research, they asked the chaplains for feedback on the preliminary results, which led to new data collection and corrections to their understanding and interpretation of the chaplaincy work. The whole endeavour was undertaken to develop a 'theory of practice' (*praktijktheorie*), that is, a theory derived from, developed for and belonging to a certain practice, which also contains a normative component (see the next chapter). Although it did not follow Glaser and Strauss's (1967) grounded theory method in every detail, the resulting theory was firmly anchored in social reality. The whole endeavour has been characterised as an exemplary theory-of-practice-oriented case study that combines elements of action research and qualitative inquiry (Baart, 2004c; in response to Smaling, 2004).[3]

During the course of this study, Baart had to divest himself of three mistaken assumptions about the work of the chaplains: (i) that it was only about problems – it was also about honour, desire, happiness, loyalty and so on; (ii) that it was only about working systematically – it was also about concern and solicitude (*bekommernis*) and all the doing, letting and being that give expression to this; and (iii) that it was only about looking for solutions – it was also about staying with people who have no prospect of any solution. In an attempt to let the logic and configuration of meaning of the empirical material speak for itself, Baart began to reconstruct rules and patterns. After some time, and in intense interaction with the material, he began searching for a *Gestalt*, a kind of overall picture, to understand the material in its coherence, to show the rationality behind it and comprehend its inner dynamics. Eventually, it became clear to him that what the two professionals were actually practising could best be understood as 'presence', a qualified, efficacious way of being there for others by being with them.

The so-called 'presence approach', 'practising of presence' or 'practice of presence' was discovered, not invented. It proved resistant during the process of analysis to all overly hasty attempts at theoretical reinterpretation. At the same time, it was capable of being developed as an ideal type and of being held up as a mirror to the very professionals in whose practice this practising of presence had been found. We deliberately use the term 'practising' – as in practising yoga or practising virtues – to stress that presence is something that must be constantly pursued and is never completed. Sometimes this is more successful than on other occasions, but the constant aim of the professional who seeks to practise presence is to be there for others by being there with them.

The practising of presence

The practice of presence, distilled as an ideal type from the work of outreach chaplains in deprived urban neighbourhoods (especially in Utrecht) and theoretically fleshed out and elaborated, has been succinctly described as: 'the efforts of the chaplains to be meaningful to the local residents by being there with them and thus also being there for them'

(Baart, 2001: 728). A characteristic of these professionals was that they 'were there for' others without focusing directly on solving problems. Problem solving could indeed be a result of their efforts, but it was not their primary intention. The most important thing these chaplains brought to the people they served was the faithful giving of themselves: being there, making themselves available, coming by to visit and listen, having coffee together or sharing a meal, completing small household tasks, running errands, accompanying the other on visits to the doctor, going for a walk together, visiting a grave, sending a birthday card, playing together on the street, being there when a child takes its final swimming test. Not all their activities were as rosy as the ones just described. At times, the neighbourhood chaplains were witnesses to severe poverty, domestic violence, problems stemming from addiction, and to structural problems that threatened the communities as a whole (Baart, 2003b). But their focus was primarily on cultivating caring relationships, relationships which might reveal what was morally desirable, what was feasible, what fit the specific life of the person in question and what their aspirations were. These relationships themselves were already caring and beneficial, and never purely instrumental.

Based on a survey of the inhabitants of the two neighbourhoods in Utrecht, Baart formulated the importance and significance of what the two professionals offered in the following way (Baart, 2001: 630):

> Positively responding, on the one hand, to the need of the people to whom they minister to show themselves also as persons developed in a non-problematic way, and, on the other hand, to their complex experiences of abandonment, isolation and disorientation, the chaplains offer themselves in a qualified, quasi-natural relationship, in a manner that has the underlying structure of a free gift, as stable and respectful attachment figures, to pursue the core values of the good life, which constitute the conditions of happiness, together with the people to whom they minister (and others who are involved with them). In so doing, the people to whom they minister feel seen, and engage in the hopeful experience that life can be different, and in their perception the chaplains acquire the traits of friends or dear relatives.

Since Baart (2001), the practising of presence has been studied further in different contexts, in particular in contexts with difficult circumstances. This has generally been done and is still being done together with healthcare and social work organisations and their professionals, and in a characteristic oscillating movement between critical, conceptual, hermeneutical research on the one hand and phenomenological, qualitative research on the other. Although its particulars vary in different contexts, the main feature of the practice of presence is always the same: the care provided arises from relationship-based programming. Its overall methodology includes: patience, attentiveness and receptivity, relational attunement, virtue- and competence-driven dedication and the ability to give attention even to the most severe problems in the small everyday things of life. Professionals who practise presence make free but professional use of rather loose and mixed forms of contact that are closely linked to the ordinary rhythms and patterns of daily life. They adhere to the social structures and linguistic conventions of the people they work with and for. The practice of presence requires great self-discipline, a radical form of self-emptying and restraint. It also requires that the practitioner has come to terms with their own life and is able to recognise and handle what wells up in their mind and body, and to reflect thoroughly, systematically and professionally on the things that happen. The practice of presence sometimes involves accepting major responsibilities in relatively unregulated settings.

Exposure as the beginning of presence; presence as the continuation of exposure

The neighbourhood chaplains studied started their work with some sort of exposure. Exposure as we understand it is a supervised mode of exposing oneself to life in a particular situation, context or practice through thorough, methodical and intentional immersion in the situation, context or practice in question and the lifeworld of the people involved in it. Its aim is to promote and facilitate a change of perspective by making the perspective of the persons one encounters one's own, instead of regarding everything exclusively from the perspective of one's own, outsider's frame of reference. In the practice of presence as we understand it, exposure is not only a precursor to, or a way of entering into, the practice of presence, but also a permanent, professional and basic attitude of this practice. Through constant exposure, professionals who practise presence struggle with their own ideals, intentions and aims, and their own rhythm, language and logic and so forth. They become rooted in and participate in the situation or practice in question. They gradually take on responsibility, position themselves, also in relation to other professionals, and find out, from their exposure and from the slowly developing practice of presence, and in interaction with their own personality, what they have to offer to the partakers in the situation or practice. This kind of exposure comprises a four-stage task:

1. to bracket, suppress or 'turn off' the knowledge and judgements that inhibit the practitioner from coming to know the situation or practice and the persons involved in it from within;

2. to provide scope for people and things that are different and strange by constantly unmasking and purifying oneself;
3. to permit and accept that people and things that are strange and different appeal to one's own moral intuition, responsibility and interpretation, and give rise to other moral intuitions;
4. to devote oneself to the other people in the situation or practice in question, and to what is good for them.

When it is successful, exposure produces a sustainable openness to the reality of the situation or practice in all its ambiguity and paradoxicality, and increases the professionals' tolerance for frustration (Baart, 2001). According to Baart, exposure is characterised first and foremost by an internal debate within the professionals-in-exposure themselves; it must therefore be carefully supervised. The interaction between the A world of how reality is interpreted in the institution and by the experts, and the B world of how reality is interpreted in the situation or practice and by the people involved in it, occurs in the C world of how reality is interpreted in the biography of the professional-in-exposure. The C world is the arena where the professional attempts to prioritise the B world and to bracket the A world (Figure 3.1). Successful exposure leads to a mutual opening of the A and B worlds (Baart, 2001). When understood in this way, exposure is also a spiritual practice: it promotes and facilitates a kind of conversion or, more accurately, a turnaround (*ommekeer*).

Figure 3.1: Three 'worlds' in tension with each other during exposure

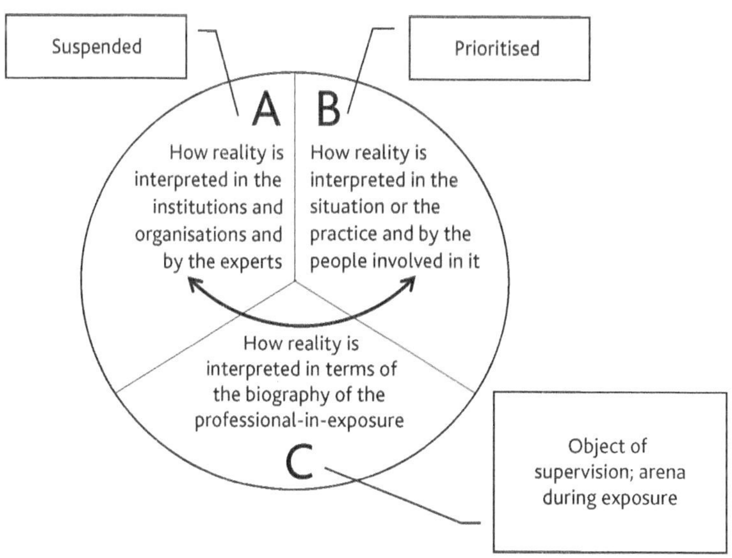

Source: Adapted from Baart, 2001: 228

The working principles of presence

Baart identified eight clusters of features of the practice of presence from the practices of the professionals studied, supported by theoretical explorations. Each one of these was formalised into a working principle, and a value implied in its realisation was identified (Baart, 2001; van Heijst, 2011). Most of these working principles of presence are characteristic not only of what professionals who practise presence do (and have to do) but also of what they allow (and have to allow) to happen to themselves (Table 3.1 provides an overview). Three dimensions have been assigned to each of these working principles. Most of the working principles can be practised in both the active and the passive mode. The term 'principle' is slightly misleading, because the working principles are not simply prescriptions. They are inductions: they were found in the practice studied, as apparently existing rules or goals. The practice of presence is not a procedure that involves the application of principles.

The *first* working principle is that professionals who practise presence free themselves and let themselves be freed by the other. Aspects of this free positioning of oneself include: working without routine, resisting the claims and demands of the employing organisation and working with an open agenda. In a sense, it is about a question of power, namely the question of whose interests take precedence in the definition of the situation, and how much of his or her power the professional yields to the other. The value involved is availability (*beschikbaarheid*).

The *next* working principle is that professionals who practise presence open themselves up and let themselves be opened up by the other. This includes dedication, the willingness to overcome one's defensive reflex and accostability. It can mean assuming the role of a symbolic, idealised neighbour or sister, that is, the neighbour or sister one would wish to have oneself. This working principle involves the value of receptiveness (*ontvankelijkheid*), especially on the part of the professionals who practise presence themselves, as well as availability. *Another* working principle is that professionals who practise presence have regard for the other, in a relationship that is shielded and intimate, on the one hand, and public, on the other, and in which the other always has the option of pulling out without explanation. In this relationship, the professional must be unbiased, open-minded and focused on the other and on how they are really doing. At the same time, the relationship is more than a context. In fact, the way it develops also shapes the professional's further practice in that relationship. This involves the value of attentive relationship (*aandachtige betrekking*). This relationship is the fulcrum: it is constitutive of what will come and it brings increasing responsibility.

The *fourth* working principle is that professionals who practise presence attune their practice to the other, and let their practice be attuned by the other to what is happening in the other's everyday life and what is important to them. The practitioner connects with what the other articulates and with the way they articulate it. They do not expropriate or disown the other's story, pain or joy, pride or sorrow, but recognise what is 'at stake' for them, and work with the other's existing networks and with their family, street or neighbourhood. This working principle incorporates the value of confirmation (*bevestiging*).

The *next* working principle is that professionals who practise presence situate themselves, and allow themselves to be situated, in the lifeworld of the other. They try to find out what the other's world revolves around, and what is at stake for the other. If this requires endless conversations, then the professional engages in endless conversations. Professionals who practise presence, on the one hand try to enter into the situation or the practice, instead of providing advice from the outside, and on the other hand they try to speak to the other about what the other longs for, positively or negatively, in such a way that the other is in fact able to articulate it. The professional who practises presence stays, even when nothing succeeds. Professionals who practise presence assume an insider's perspective, reconstruct the local logic as much as possible and place themselves on the side of the other. This working principle encompasses the value of solidarity. A basic act of recognition takes place before any care, help and support is offered: the suffering, the dignity, the desire, the anger of the other is represented as real, the appeal is accepted, reciprocity is established, the other is included in a network of relationships, a common frame of reference is created (Vosman and Baart, 2011).

After this act of recognition, the *sixth* working principle is that the other is allowed to determine the way in which the professional who practises presence helps. The professional not only offers their instrumental resources but also their social-cultural and moral capital, that is, they present themselves as an example – in word and deed – of a different way of living one's life, of handling conflicts and so on. Meaning and significance (*zin*) are the values involved. The *next* working principle is that professionals who practise presence do not hurry, but take their time and give others time. They allow time for that which may turn out to be good for the other to emerge. The other person is generally allowed to determine where things are going. The value involved is the value of the good end (*goede doel*). The *eighth* working principle is that professionals who practise presence give themselves, without self-interest, and that they are loyal and reliable. They do not run off with the other's story, and their attention does not have to be earned. In the final analysis, they would rather let themselves be deceived than do wrong to someone else. They search for the other in his or her loneliness and abandonment – according to presence theory, loneliness is at the heart of much suffering – so that he or she will overcome this or at least be able to deal with it. This working principle involves the value of loyalty (*trouw*).[4]

Since 2001, Baart has added two further working principles and their corresponding values on the basis of further research. The *ninth* working principle is that professionals who practise presence verify, and let others verify, whether the people with and for whom they care consider the professionals' activity to be good and completed care. The value at stake here is that of the experienced benefit (*ervaren baat*). The underlying idea is that care is good only when it has been beneficial to the other in their specific situation – ultimately, the standard of quality is never external. The *tenth and final* working principle is that professionals who practise presence intervene in public debate and publicly speak out about the vulnerability and resilience they have discovered, and about the good of the people with and for whom they work. This is about democracy as a practice of care, not only at the level of society (compare Tronto's 'caring democracy', Tronto, 2013) but also at the level of the group, the institution or the neighbourhood.

Practising presence and Tronto's caring process

Although this series of ten working principles should not be understood as a phased model, there is a certain sequence to the principles. The principles can be associated with the five consecutive process goals for the care professional who practises presence: becoming ready to care (*zorgbereid worden*: working principle 1–2), committing oneself to care (*zich tot zorg verbinden*: 3), identifying the care needed (according to the profession) (*de zorg identificeren*: 4–5), providing care (*de zorg geven*: 6–8) and completing care (*zorg voltooien*: 9–10). A different association is: exposure (working principle 1–2), relationship (3–4), offer (5–8), feedback (9–10). When these two sequences are compared with Berenice Fisher and Joan Tronto's five-phase model of the integrated caring process (Fisher and Tronto, 1990; Tronto, 1993; Tronto, 2013), a certain parallelism emerges, as well as a number of differences (Table 3.1). Fisher and Tronto distinguish between caring about, taking care of, care giving and care receiving. Later, Tronto has connected a particular ethical element, a virtue, to each of these stages: attentiveness, responsibility, competence and responsiveness (Tronto, 1993). Although we realise that Fisher and Tronto were reflecting on their own and their students' experience in developing their model, we believe that it is seriously deficient empirically. Our model was developed in an empirically grounded way and was theoretically systematised in the course of comprehensive, long-term research into a particular practice, which is why we believe it more adequately reflects reality. While Tronto connects only what can be called virtues to her model, our description of the practice of care comprises process goals, working principles and values. Comparing both approaches in the three shaded areas in Table 3.1, it must be noted, first, that the principle that the professionals free themselves, the first working principle, which is assigned

Table 3.1: Working principles of practising presence compared to Tronto's caring process

Baart 2001; 2003b				Tronto 1993; 2013
Phase	**Process goal**	**Working principle**	**Value**	**Phase: ethical element**
Exposure	Becoming ready to care	1 Set oneself free/let oneself be set free by the other	Availability	
		2 Open oneself/let oneself be opened up	Receptiveness	Caring about: attentiveness
Relationship	Committing oneself to care	3 Relate oneself/let oneself be related attentively to the other	Regardful involvement	(Taking care of: responsibility – as an emotional response)
	Identifying care	4 Attune one's practice/let one's practice be attuned to what is given	Confirmation	
Offer		5 Place oneself/let oneself be placed in the other's lifeworld and rhythm	Solidarity	Taking care of: responsibility – as a volitional response, enacted in a practice
	Providing care	6 Put oneself/let oneself be put at the other's disposal	Meaning	Care giving: competence
		7 Restrain oneself/let oneself be restrained by the other	Good end	
		8 Dedicate oneself	Loyalty	
Feedback	Completing care	9 Monitor oneself/let oneself be monitored	Experienced benefit	Care receiving: responsiveness
		10 Participate in public debate	Democracy as a practice of care	Caring with: caring democracy

Source: Adapted from Timmerman and Baart, 2016b: 202, based on Baart, 2001; 2003b; Tronto, 1993; 2013

Table 3.2: Caring presence and other concepts of presence

	Pastoral presence	Nursing presence	Therapeutic presence	Caring presence
Core	Being in the factory or neighbourhood that constitutes the workers' or residents' lifeworld	Being with the patient as a person	Being with and being there for the client during the therapy session	Being there for the other by being with the other in their lifeworld
Moving away from	Church planting, starting from a 'knowing' position	Being an object or a functionary to the patient	Acting on one's own ideas about the client's issues	Hyper interventionism
Warning against	An inauthentic, self-referential presence of the church	Understanding presence as an intervention or a competence	Understanding presence as a technique, specifically a mindfulness technique	Modern forms of absence: abandoning the other, leaving them to their own devices
Relationality	Manifold relationships	One-to-one relationship	One-to-one relationship	Manifold relationships, both on the side of the caregiver and care receiver
Institutional requirements	Backing from the authorities	Supportive management	None mentioned	Relational leadership and so on
Normativity	Preference for the most vulnerable people	Tacit	Tacit	Preference for people in precarious situations

to the process goal of becoming ready to care and to the phase of exposure, is missing in Fisher and Tronto's model. According to Tronto, the first phase of 'caring about' starts with 'noticing the need to care' (Tronto, 1993).[5] In the practice of presence, the professional can and should respond to the other's joy, their aspirations, their endurance of living conditions and so on – in short, to whatever is at stake for the other. Second, Fisher and Tronto's model does not explicitly consider the aspect of establising a relationship. They speak about contact, especially bodily contact, when discussing the phase of care giving. We think Fisher and Tronto take responsibility as a volitional response. But taking care starts with committing oneself to care. One could say: with recognizing and accepting responsibility, as an emotional response. Finally, Fisher and Tronto's model does not include the dedication (*trouwe toeleg*) that is the eighth working principle, while professionals in care, help and support often work with and for people whose opportunities to help themselves are permanently at risk. The practising of presence does not primarily focus on needs, problems or suffering, but on paying unconditional attention to the other person.

Conclusion

As we have seen, in Baart's long-term qualitative study of neighbourhood chaplaincy a care-ethical account of practising presence was developed. Exposure is the beginning of the presence approach as this approach is the continuation of exposure. Ten working principles were found, not as prescriptions but as apparently existing rules and goals. Compared with the other concepts and practices of presence discussed in Chapter 2 (Table 3.2) and with Fisher and Tronto's model of the caring process (Table 3.1), our care-ethical account of the presence approach is more empirical, more radically and comprehensively relational and more political. The comparison with Fisher and Tronto's model anticipates the conclusion that presence is indispensable to all good care, help and support in healthcare and social work, not just to pastoral care or care for residents in deprived urban neigbourhoods. In fact, our research shows that presence is at the heart of all good professional care, help and support. We will return to this in the following chapter, where we discuss Baart's care-ethical theory of presence.

4

Presence: the theory as originally formulated and its reception

Now that we have described the practice of presence, this chapter will present the theory of presence as it was originally formulated (Baart, 2001) and its reception. This empirically grounded, care-ethical theory of presence explains why the practice of presence works and is valuable, and specifies what particular understanding of common humanity it implies.

A theory of practice with five subtheories

The case study of the neighbourhood chaplains in Utrecht was embedded in a multiple case study and accompanied by theoretical research. The whole endeavour was aimed at developing a 'theory of practice', that is, a theory derived from, developed for and belonging to a certain practice.[1] It is *derived from* a practice, because it is based on a qualitative study of a practice, more particularly a professional practice. It was *developed for* a practice, because it is comprehensible, manageable and useful for the intended users, the practitioners. And it *belongs to* a practice, because it was developed in a research project in which the practitioners were positioned as co-researchers. Any theory of practice must include three components. First, an understanding of the logic and dynamic of the practice, including its rules of action and relationship management. Second, a normative framework, consisting of three normative moments: (a) evaluation criteria to identify good practices, (b) a description of the identity of the practice as a normative anchor point for the evaluation criteria, and (c) an implicit or explicit favoured reading of social reality. Third, a repertoire of action, consisting of tools for specific situations and an understanding of these tools and of how they are constructed. This last component of theories of practice resembles *savoir faire*, knowledge on how to do things, but it is never a recipe that must simply be followed in order to succeed.[2] From the beginning, Baart sought to ethically position the presence theory, and he found a way to do this in 1995/96 in the political-ethical ethics of care (Baart, 1997).

In developing the theory of presence, Baart first proposed five subtheories, which ultimately provided the various components of the presence theory, while a subsequently developed sixth subtheory completed it. Analysis of the empirical material resulted in a model which reflects the fact that the

Figure 4.1: Structure of the empirically grounded, care-ethical theory of presence

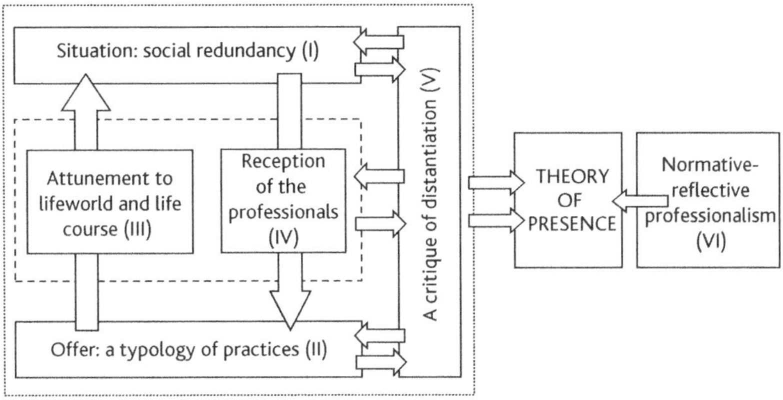

Source: Adapted from Baart, 2001: 283

practising of presence derives its effectiveness and comprehensiveness from its responsive structure (Figure 4.1). This model was discovered, not designed, much less created, prior to the empirical research (Baart, 2004c). In the next sections we will concisely present these subtheories.

Social redundancy

The first subtheory addresses the situation of the residents of the two neighbourhoods where the two professionals worked, and is founded on quantitative, qualitative and discourse analyses as well as theoretical reflections. The aim of this theory is to understand the context in which the two professionals functioned, and not, for example, to explain the situation of the residents of these two neighbourhoods, or to impute responsibility for their situation. This aim inspired the choice of 'experiential-participatory discourse', connected with the perspective of the modern welfare state, to consider and characterise the situation in question. A discourse is a combination of language and perspective. Unlike practical discourse, truth discourse or rhetorical-persuasive discourse, experiential-participatory discourse uses lifeworld language, and the perspective of a relatively unstructured, attentive, steadfast nearness. From the residents' first-person perspective, 'social redundancy' (*maatschappelijke overbodigheid*) emerges as a better, wider and deeper characterisation than, for example, poverty, marginalisation or deprivation. Social redundancy was conceptualised as consisting of six overlapping dimensions: lack of money, stunted socio-cultural participation, low-grade environment, inadequate mastery of (bureaucratic) skills, mental instability and the occurrence of a continuous assault on dignity, and their sub-dimensions (Table 4.1). In 2023, in a renewed

Table 4.1: Social redundancy: a multidimensional concept of poverty in an experiential-participatory discourse

<table>
<tr><th colspan="3">1st dimension: FINANCES > lack of money</th></tr>
<tr><td>Income</td><td>Expenses</td><td>Debts</td></tr>
<tr><th colspan="3">2nd dimension: PARTICIPATION > stunted socio-cultural participation</th></tr>
<tr><td>Work</td><td>Education</td><td>Social networks and cultural resources</td></tr>
<tr><th colspan="3">3rd dimension: HABITAT > low-grade environment</th></tr>
<tr><td>Quality of housing</td><td colspan="2">Quality of the neighbourhood</td></tr>
<tr><th colspan="3">4th dimension: SKILLS > inadequate mastery of skills</th></tr>
<tr><td colspan="3">Budgetary · Bureaucratic · Social · Health-related · Pedagogic</td></tr>
<tr><th colspan="3">5th dimension: MENTAL HEALTH > mental instability</th></tr>
<tr><td>Fickleness</td><td>Addictions</td><td>Learning disabilities</td></tr>
<tr><th colspan="3">6th dimension: DIGNITY > a continuous assault on dignity</th></tr>
<tr><td colspan="3">Hurt · Recognition · Self-image · Attachment</td></tr>
</table>

Source: Adapted from Baart, 2001: 316–17

analysis of social redundancy, Baart added a seventh dimension: physical health (Baart, 2023).

Experiencing yourself as socially redundant may mean: feeling that you and who you are and what you have to contribute to society is useless, invalid and insignificant. In fact, social redundancy is a complex, experiential concept of human suffering. It is at the centre of Baart's theory of presence.

A typology of practices

The next subtheory is about what the outreach chaplains in deprived urban neighbourhoods had to offer. It was based on the foregoing analysis and was additionally tested in five cases. The aim of this theory is to understand the rationality of what the professionals have to offer. In order to do this, Baart developed a typology of pastoral practices in deprived urban neighbourhoods. The central category of this typology is the professional's primary, relational orientation towards the other person as (a) an individual, (b) a culture bearer, (c) a member of the community or (d) a citizen. A first subcategory is the mode of working, which can be called either 'making' or 'letting', depending on who predominantly determines the goals, duration and nature of the relationship. In the 'making' mode, it is the professional who mainly determines the goal and the other aspects; in the 'letting' mode, it is the other person who does this. A second subcategory is the symbolic process role that the professional fulfils: friend, helper or moralist. When we relate

Figure 4.2: Disposition model

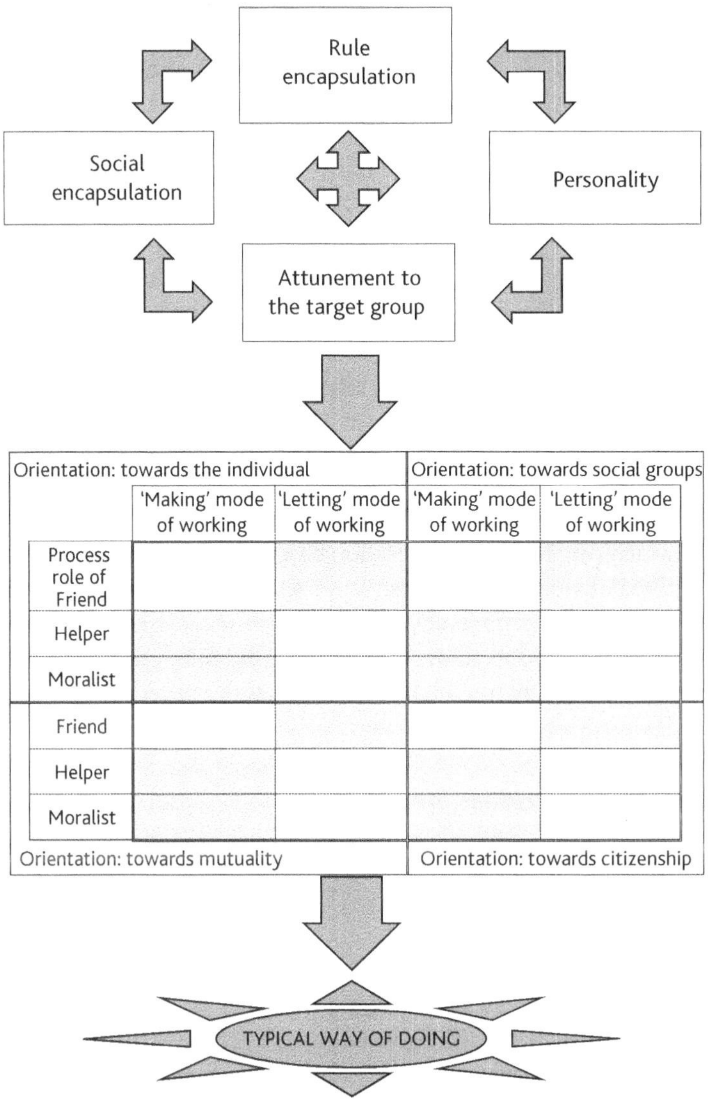

Source: Adapted from Baart, 2001: 389

these three variables – orientation, working mode and process role – to each other, the results can be displayed in a table consisting of 4 × 2 × 3 = 24 cells. The rationality of these connections can be understood through a so-called 'disposition model' (Figure 4.2), which provides an explanation in terms of the probability that the professional will engage in certain typical ways of acting; it is not a causal explanation. The four independent variables of this model are: (i) 'rule encapsulation', that is, the impact the professional permits the technical and ideological rules to have on their actual practice, (ii) 'social encapsulation', that is, the impact the professional permits the institutional context, functional relationships and groups to have on their actual practice, (iii) attunement by the professional of their practice to the target group and (iv) the personality of the professional.

Rule encapsulation (by professional standards and ideological hints) and attunement to the target group (the fine-tuning between what the professional offers and what the residents need) co-determine the orientation of the professional. Social encapsulation and the professional's personality (personal skills and identity) co-determine the working mode and the process role. When the ideology has a major influence on how the practice is organised, but the residents and their reality are approached openly and flexibly, this can be called open ideological rule encapsulation. This type of encapsulation disposes the professional to orientation towards the other as an individual or as a member of the community and to a 'letting' mode of working. Closed ideological rule encapsulation orients the professional towards the other as a culture bearer or a citizen. Both closed ideological and disciplinary technical rule encapsulation dispose the professional to the working mode of 'making'. These different forms of rule encapsulation are all compatible with the practice of presence, but the open ideological form is particularly consonant with the theory of presence and its underlying philosophy. The ideology in question is important for the way in which the practice is organised, but the approach of the persons involved and their world are open and flexible.

Attunement to lifeworld and life course

The third theory deals with the lifeworld approach of professionals who practise presence, and it was developed on the basis of a theoretical study and a trial consisting of six cases. The aim of this theory is to understand and explain why that which the professionals have to offer is welcomed to the degree it is and why it works so well in practice. The theory was developed after the professionals told the researcher they wanted to connect to the lifeworld of the residents. Further probing revealed that the professionals associated this connection with warmth, closeness and respect, that they wanted to be able to also relate to persons who were strange to them, wanted to contribute to improving the connection that the residents felt with their community and with society and wanted to find out what is good to the residents themselves. This theory was developed on the assumption that change is desirable and that developments that tend towards a more satisfying life must be promoted.

In general terms, one's lifeworld is one's self-evident understanding of reality, enshrined in contexts of meaning and images of the world, society and the self, and which also includes a time perspective (Schutz and Luckmann, 1973;

Habermas, 1981). It shows itself indirectly and always partially, through the keyhole of themes. At the centre stand experienced time, one's concrete place and the current other. In a circle around this, there are other themes, times, locations and people in increasingly receding zones of proximity. The lifeworld shows itself in stories, practices, relationships, expressions, food, clothing, inner speech and so on. It is a configuration of three structural components: shared frameworks of interpretation, an ordered social life and accountable role models.

The lifeworld is organised on the basis of six principles:

1. meaning construction by patterns of selecting, ignoring, relating and ordering aspects of reality and sharing their meaning with others;
2. becoming aware of the other person's position, perspective and perspectival bandwidth;
3. intentionality: it is aimed at something that is of value and is therefore worth pursuing;
4. temporality: it exists in different dimensions of time, each offering different orientations;
5. spatiality, which orients the gaze and limits its scope; and
6. a plausibility structure: it contains built-in protections against doubt.

Someone who wants to connect with the lifeworld without identifying with it completely will have to reconstruct these six formal aspects. Connecting with it means that one constructs meanings in the same way, takes an analogous position and a similar perspective, tries to stand in the same intentionality, tries to adopt the applicable time dimensions, maintains the same scope in one's gaze and takes thorough account of the structures that stabilise, if not freeze, the lifeworld.

Furthermore, the lifeworld is the intersection of the subjective and objective dimensions of social reproduction: it is where the perspectives of individuals and their socialisation encounter the social institutions. A lifeworld has six aspects: cognitive, affective, relational, moral, expressive and conative. These aspects are about knowledge or cognition, feelings and emotions, connections with others, representation of good and evil, expression of needs and experiences and, ultimately, also efforts to act.

This general characterisation of the lifeworld did not suffice to understand the lifeworld approach of professionals who practise presence. What was needed in addition was an understanding of 'category-specific lifeworlds': lifeworlds of certain groups or categories of people, especially of people who experience themselves as socially redundant. Moreover, a dynamic as well as a static understanding was needed. To understand category-specific lifeworlds, it has to be remembered that they are often contested due to the existence of different conceptions among various groups of what is good, worthwhile or even normal. To be able to understand a category-specific lifeworld, it is necessary to recognise patterns, types and life domains, to identify survival strategies and cultures and to reconstruct the inner rationality and logic behind it – a rationality and logic that revolve around dignity and recognition. An essential condition is that residents are considered to be competent actors.

To understand the lifeworld approach in a dynamic way, the concept of 'life course' was needed. To understand this concept, a distinction had to be made between category-specific discourse and institutional discourse, and it was recognised that there are transitions between these discourses. Additionally, development trajectories and careers, life phases and status transitions, life events and turning points had to be recognised. Moreover, it was necessary to identify perpetuation mechanisms, and to work with different kinds of capital, including social, cultural and moral capital. Connecting with someone's lifeworld and life course is about trying to understand, not about identification. It is possible to distinguish different kinds of connecting, according to the kind of understanding it pursues. The lifeworld approach of professionals who practise presence is primarily aimed at achieving a reconstructive-rational understanding from a reflective internal perspective, not just an emotional understanding or explanatory-rational understanding from an external perspective.

All these conceptualisations and distinctions led to an analysis-and-evaluation raster consisting of two main questions, which were further broken down into 40 specific questions. The first main question is what the professional observes in his or her contact with the residents with respect to their lifeworld, their available resources and the developments that are or were relevant to their lifeworld and life course. The second question inquires whether and how the professional connects with and acts upon the lifeworld of the other (Baart, 2001: 447–9).

Analysis and evaluation of six cases on the basis of this raster showed that it is possible to determine to what extent and how the process of connecting with the lifeworld was successful and how it could have been improved. They also showed what tensions this kind of lifeworld approach entails: some tensions were related to the guiding principles of this approach, others to how the problem at hand was dealt with, and still others to the professional's role. Different strategies can be chosen within the lifeworld approach, depending on a number of basic choices; for example, whether the professional focuses on individuals or on groups and communities, whether he or she uses the existing infrastructure as it is or adds new elements to it and whether the professional places themselves primarily in a category-specific or in institutional discourse.

The reception of the professionals

The fourth subtheory starts where the others end: it seeks to understand the situation of the care receiver, the nature of the offer of the professional who practises presence and how these are connected. The next question is how this offer is appreciated and why it is appreciated as much as it actually is. This subtheory addressed the reception of the professionals by the residents of the neighbourhood, and it was developed on the basis of an analysis of qualitative interviews with residents. Given the fact that this fourth subtheory clarifies what the professionals offered and how they went about doing this, the aim of this theory was to understand the significance of what they had to offer in the reception by the residents. Why did the residents appreciate these two professionals so much? The analysis of the interviews shows that what the professionals had to offer satisfies one or more unmet, but essential needs that involve either a deficit to be eliminated or a potential to be articulated or deployed. The residents experienced themselves as socially redundant, had difficulties dealing with tensions and had insufficient resources at their disposal. In offering what they offered, the professionals also offered themselves. That is why they were described in terms of images derived from intimacy. They were somewhere in between three symbolic positions: friend (or brother or sister), neighbour and social worker, with corresponding role tensions between love and meddlesomeness, availability and gossip, help and keeping distance. Residents could also show themselves to be carriers of valuable potential, and in the relationship with the professional they obtained and seized the opportunity to deploy this potential *in actu*.

In a stagnant life, self-realisation (*zelfontplooiing*) can take one of three basic forms, each with several variants: (1) strategic distancing: surmounting, avoiding or reframing difficulties (through humour), (2) affiliation: connecting with others or fulfilling another role for others (resilience) and (3) rehabilitation: enforcing respect or claiming the right to be unattuned to what is commonly considered reasonable, responsible or civilised. The professionals had three things to offer. They provoked, stimulated, encouraged and confirmed the residents in their process of becoming who they are in the community. They offered themselves as an audience so that residents could share with them what is usually not seen as valuable. And they offered themselves as a take-off platform, target, mirror or projection screen. The residents' biggest problem was loneliness, isolation or exclusion, in one or more of five (non-exclusive) domains: (a) psycho-biographical, (b) communicative-relational, (c) mental-rational, religious, (d) bureaucratic-institutional and (e) physical-material. To professionals who practise presence, this abandonment (*verlating*) and loneliness are what underlies social redundancy and they are therefore a more fundamental description of the residents' situation. In the modest and limited things they could offer, the professionals to a large degree offered themselves and their institutional, professional and experiential resources and networks. They did this in what we call a 'qualified, quasi-naturalistic relationship', which operates in a 'gift economy'. They offered themselves as attachment figures, who model ways in which the residents work towards a good life, that is, a happy life, which means being yourself in a satisfying way, belonging to significant others, seeing a meaningful future before you, having sufficient influence and rights, being sure of your life and knowing that you are beneficial to the people around you or to society.[3] Nevertheless, the way in which the professionals practised their work was unavoidably beset by interferences, tensions and risks.

A critique of distantiation

The last subtheory is a more philosophical theory about the institutionalisation of care, help and support, and it gives rise to a 'critique of distantiation', that is, a critique of the sense of being abandoned by professionals that local residents or clients have. This theory was developed to understand why abandonment had become such an important issue in the research up to that point. It also intended to discover why residents spontaneously compared presence practitioners with regular professionals, and why this comparison was often to the detriment of the regular service providers. It turns out that the regular provision of care, help and support is increasingly struggling to deal with suffering and the inevitability and insolubility of many problems. This critique of distantiation was developed by analysing engagement patterns (*patronen van betrokkenheid*, cf Blokland-Potters, 1998), requests for help, types of suffering and responses, and tragic modes of support. It implies a plea for pluriform engagement (motivated by efficaciousness, affinity and affectivity), for being sensitive to the cry for recognition that requests for help may contain, for giving people who experience themselves as socially redundant time and scope to manifest themselves in the bureaucracy of healthcare and social welfare, for focusing on the person (thinking in terms of tragic) instead of becoming obsessed with how to make the problem disappear (that is, thinking in terms of repairable fate), for being able to endure one's own powerlessness and for not abandoning the other and being near to them in consolation (*troostend nabij*) to them wherever there is loneliness behind the suffering. To console means to acknowledge suffering – however massive, enigmatic and unstoppable it is – and to include the sufferer – that is, not to ignore that this is a person who is suffering. In the regular, highly bureaucratised organisation of care, help and support, many professionals face the risk of burnout and seek refuge in self-consolation (*zelftroost*) as a coping strategy. The criticism of distantiation formulated here is directed against policy without commitment; the bureaucratic perpetuation of suffering; a 'making' manner of dealing with suffering, fate and the tragic aspects of life; systemically standardised procedure; and hyper interventionism in which interventions have become self-referential, that is, they arise from the professional's own framework, disciplinary concerns and organisational tasks, and therefore actually constitute subtle, complex and hyper-modern forms of absence.

These four subtheories and this critique of distantiation, which stand in a specific relationship to each other, were the foundation for the development of presence theory (see Figure 4.1). What the professionals have to offer is an answer to the situation of experiencing social redundancy. The aim is to ensure that the situation and offer become attuned to each other, so that the offer makes a difference to the inhabitants of the neighbourhood. This substructure, including the four subtheories, is constantly subject to challenge by the critique of distantiation.

Normative-reflective professionalism

Presence theory was completed by the formulation of a sixth subtheory, which entails a normative-reflective model of professionalism. This model is necessary because of the negative effects of the introduction of market economy principles in the human-oriented, contact-seeking professions. Regular socio-technical professionalism does not suffice. Normative-reflective professionalism is normative because it orients the professional towards a substantive concept of good care, help and support, acknowledging that all care, help and support are moral enterprises, which involve the ethos of the professional – their virtues, goods, character, courage and so forth – and that professionals are engaged in the good (*bonum*) of others. It is reflective, because it orients the professional towards the freedom to engage with this particular other in this particular situation. The professional has the intellectual and institutional freedom to come to their own situational judgements, interpretations and actions, and to justify these. The necessary reflection is personal and self-critical. A distinction can be made between methodical, hermeneutical, biographical and projecting reflection. Normative-reflective professionalism is professional because it orients the professional towards the theory, techniques, rules and guidelines of the profession, towards knowledge on how to use and apply these and towards the ability to account for their work. The work is, furthermore, carried out in a learning community which is engaged in moral deliberation.

The ninefold offer in response to social redundancy

The fundamental problem that the practice of presence answers is the experience of being socially redundant: 'I am not needed, I am of no value. The sooner I disappear, the better. I am a burden, a redundant thing.' Social redundancy is the most adequate articulation of the careful analysis of marginalised people's lived life and self-experience. This redundancy is at the forefront of the insider's perspective and can be phenomenologically reconstructed in the following request for help: 'Does it matter (1) to you (2) that this (3) always (4) happens to me (5) here (6) in this way (7), that it hurts (8) and that it should end (9)?' (Baart, 2001: 651; 2004d: 15; Baart and Vosman, 2011: 198).

The first thing is: does it matter? This is a request for recognition and relevance, a protest against loneliness. Then: does it matter – not in a general way, not to an abstract institution, but to a human being I can see, feel and address? Does 'it' matter, not as an abstract issue, or a well-categorised and bureaucratically recognised illness, defect or infringement of a right, but rather as something concrete and tangible, regardless of what it is called or how it is classified? And then the final two elements: it hurts and it should stop. This phenomenologically reconstructed question is subsequently analysed by Baart from the perspective of the tensions it entails, professional viability and so forth. The tensions that professionals who practise presence, like all professionals who work with and for people, have to navigate are: they 'must choose, act professionally, stay critical, not lose contact with the institutional discourse, be fair, simplify complexities, add instrumental capital, keep some distance, and free themselves from fixed and perspectiveless time' (Baart, 2001: 656).

In the last step of the analysis, each of these elements is matched with a specific political claim, or, to put it differently: with normative criteria for good, just and 'careful' politics and government policy. This is where this ideal-typical request for help is 'translated' into political criteria for good care. Table 4.2 summarises the request for help, the consequences for social policy if the request is answered positively and the criteria for a politics that facilitates good care. The presence practitioner answers this ideal-typical request for help affirmatively, and follows this up by nine concrete commitments, which are sustained up to the political level. Being present in the lives and lifeworld of residents is followed by presenting the residents' lives and concerns at the political level, as a witness who testifies, as an amplifier of the voice of people who cannot speak easily and whose voice is seldom heard at that level, and as an advocate of their cause.

Premises, underlying philosophy and its relation to care ethics

The practice of presence can be understood as resulting from a return, at a weakly institutional level, to the purpose of caring with and for people, and a radical turn towards those aspects of being human that are currently being oppressed. It presupposes four assumptions about reality:

1. Humans are reasonable beings and are answerable for their actions (even when they do stupid things).
2. The good always coexists with the tragic aspects of life.

3. What matters to people reveals itself in the situation, and can be found only by committing oneself to their lives and to their living together.
4. People can flourish even in very unfavourable situations, provided their dignity is maintained or restored.

Table 4.2: Request for help and responses on the political level

Elements of the request for help	An affirmative answer entails that social policies must recognise, respect, make room for ...	Good social policies give, respect and safeguard the care receiver's ...
Does it matter	The care receivers and their concerns	Right(s)
To you	A fellow human being who is approachable to the care receivers	Access to normative-reflective caregivers
That this	The care receivers' experience as it is	Identity (singularity)
Always	The comprehensiveness of the context in which it occurs and the care receivers live	Lived coherence of life
Happens to me	The care receivers' dignity and subjectivity	Political power and influence
Here	The care receivers' own perspective	Situatedness (framework)
In this way	The care receivers' experience of tragedy and contingency	Means, facilities and knowledge
That it hurts	The care receivers' own logic and the ways they express themselves	Voice and language
And that it should end?	The substance or time that makes sense to the care receivers	Time, rhythm and meaning

Note: The left and right column also appear in Baart, 2004d: 15 and Baart and Vosman, 2011: 198–9.
Source: Adapted from Baart, 2001: 662–3

The practising of presence prefers an experiential-participatory discourse about poverty and social redundancy (see earlier in this chapter, 'A theory of practice with five subtheories'). This practice is informed by at least seven moral guidelines:

1. It addresses the basic human desire to be included in a meaningful commonality.
2. Access to the desires and potential of the other can be achieved through sustained exposure.
3. Presence practitioners seek, protect and nourish the good life, but do not create it.
4. Time and space are understood as being meaningful and essential.
5. The commitment to rights is oriented to care that is understood as attentive engagement with needs, accepted responsibility, skilled help and responsiveness.

6. In complex situations, professionals who practise presence would rather be deceived by the other than do wrong to them.
7. Attention to the person is more important than attention to the problem.

The practice of presence is strengthened by the criticism of distantiation described earlier. Baart positioned the practice and theory of presence within the political-ethical framework of care ethics (Baart, 1997).[4] Ultimately, the practice and theory of presence are about a good life with and for others in just institutions (Ricœur, 1992) and in a sustainable world – and a good life is not necessarily the same as a successful life (Vosman, 2023).

Our care-ethical presence theory differs from other presence theories in several respects (see also Table 3.2). First, it was developed on the basis of empirical studies of skilled and advanced professionals, who were seeking to connect with the lifeworld, life course and biography not only of individual people, but also of larger social units, such as families and neighbourhoods. Second, it deals with literature not only about pastoral care and healthcare but also about social work and management. Third, it is topic driven – 'How can we contact people who live in poverty and experience themselves as socially redundant?' – it positions presence in the context of a political take on care ethics and it acknowledges that care is a socio-political practice which realises goods, but can also aggravate the situation of the people affected, and which in any case focuses on particular issues while considering anything else of little or no relevance. Fourth, it contrasts presence with hyper interventionism and is nourished by a critique of distantiation. Fifth, through interaction between empirical studies and conceptual-theoretical explorations, and to a greater degree than other theories, it methodically elaborates presence in a 'letting' – but not passive – mode, in which the other person predominantly determines the goals, duration and nature of the relationship, while remaining alive to the tragic aspects of life and refusing to slide into quietism or yield to the temptation of doing nothing. Sixth, it connects presence with normative-reflective professionalism and with practical wisdom (Vosman and Baart, 2008). Last, it is a full-blown theory, not an individual theorem.

The relationship between presence theory and care ethics is complicated. Care ethics, as we understand it, makes explicit and explains the moral tenor of the presence approach and places it within a theoretical framework. The practice of presence, however, should not be conceived as a method of 'applying' care ethics. Presence theory is an empirically grounded, care-ethical theory of the heart of all good professional care in the areas of healthcare, social welfare and a hospitable society – in fact, of all forms of working with and for people. As such, the theory of presence is also involved in a critical dialogue with care ethics. It draws attention to something that is – or, rather, persons who are – neglected in the usual way of thinking about care, help and support, even in the context of care ethics. The persons in question are the professionals who give good professional care, help and guidance on the basis of the perspective and the findings of care ethics. Presence theory also demands a more empirically grounded, accurate and verifiable determination of care-ethical concepts such as relationality, corporeality, vulnerability, dependency and practices.

The care ethicist Annelies van Heijst acknowledged at an early stage that the practice of presence and what she called the 'presence relationship' have an important ethical relevance in the context of late modernity (van Heijst, 2011). The turn to radical particularity that the practice of presence effects creates new insights that are also ethically relevant to other situations and practices. The presence relationship is a relationship in which the other can be both unequal and equivalent in the presence of the professional, in which the latter draws attention to the moral significance of the relationship, even when nothing changes, and in which the other is helpful in transforming the professional caring relationship between strangers into a 'professional loving care relationship' (*menslievende zorgrelatie*). Van Heijst has recognised several ethically very relevant anthropological intuitions in Baart's theory of presence: people are essentially connected with other people in many ways; asymmetry between people, that is, inequality, dependency and neediness, is part of life and does not necessarily have to be eradicated; the other's acute need is part of his or her life; at a deeper layer, both the professional and the other share the same condition of need; it is impossible to know with certainty in advance what is good for the other; people's dignity is not separate from their dependency on others, nor does it stand in opposition to this (van Heijst, 2008; 2011).

Appreciation and criticism

Since the publication of Baart (2001), the practice and theory of presence have been received positively, including in sectors far outside the realm of pastoral care. The vocabulary of the practising of presence has come to be appreciated by social workers, nurses, youth workers, professionals in addiction care, general practitioners and so forth, because it helped them articulate their own motivation and aims, and their frustrations with the way they were increasingly being trained, assessed and managed.

There has also been criticism. It has been argued, for example, that the practice of presence is viable only for virtuosi (Bootsma, 2008), that it cannot be controlled, is difficult to assess for quality by employers and sponsors and is too dependent on latitude and understanding in the organisation. It has been contended, moreover, that the theory of presence is unclear about the exact relation between the practice of presence and interventionism, that it inadequately addresses presence practitioners' own institutional, ethnic and gender-related position of power (Schilder, 2003) and that it is itself not sufficiently open to new insights (Harry Kunneman, personal communication).

In response to the criticism that the practising of presence cannot be controlled and is viable only for virtuosi, we would point out that the practice of presence was *discovered*, not invented or designed. It was discovered, and can still be discovered, in the work of professionals who were, admittedly, skilled and advanced. However, during many years of training experience since 2001, we have discovered that the practice of presence can be learned, although not by everyone (see Chapter 13). The criticism that the practice of presence cannot be assessed for quality is undoubtedly true if quality is understood as something that can be measured from the outside by applying external criteria. But good care must always be validated on the ground and, if possible, together with the care receivers, and this local validation is liable to be revised at any time (Baart, 2004d; 2018c; Vosman and Baart, 2011). We have been developing, together with Jan den Bakker, a Care-Ethical Model of Quality Enquiry (CEMQUE, see Chapter 12) since 2001. It is also true that the practice of presence is dependent on organisational and institutional circumstances. That is why we are currently researching relational ways of managing practitioners of presence, and are offering training courses for managers.

It is more difficult to respond to the criticism that the oppositional relation between the practice of presence and interventionism is unclear. The relation between presence and interventionism was not meant to represent a contrast between 'just being there, doing nothing' and 'being effective, doing something'. In the way we understand it, presence is not the opposite of absence, but of interventionism, of intervening from a particular frame of reference, with a particular purpose, in a particular way. We define interventionism – or, more accurately, hyper interventionism – as: following an elaborated algorithm that runs from a theory-guided diagnosis up to the implementation of a remedy that is derived quasi-automatically from the diagnosis (Baart, 2003b). It is a symptom of the impoverishment of the domains of healthcare and social work, an impoverishment which often paradoxically manifests itself in the multiplication of facilities and services, and which clients experience as the expropriation of their stories about what is at stake. In this paradigm, interventions are largely self-referential, that is, they pursue their own goals and are led by their own coordinates, which are different from those given by the people involved in the situation, and they keep their distance from the chaotic, incorrigible, tragic aspects of their clients' lived lives. Such interventions can actually be considered subtle, complex and hyper-modern forms of absence. We do not think that practising presence and carrying out interventions are mutually exclusive. But the exact nature of the relationship between the two is difficult to define precisely. We think it is a reciprocal and internal interrelationship which has to be elaborated in a discipline-specific way (Baart, 2003b; 2025).

One aspect of the criticism is directed at the idea that presence practitioners are expected to just be there and do nothing. This perception of inaction and passivity possibly results from a number of essential features of the practice of presence, particularly the crucial role of exposure, the importance of the 'letting mode'[5] in addition to the 'making mode', the methodical feature of being unhurried and accostable and the dedication to what is there, to what happens here and now. But these features, which are aimed at creating room for the other person and for what is at stake for him or her, so as to prevent a mismatch, do not mean that the professional who practises presence is passive. On the contrary, each one of these features requires considerable effort and skill (Baart, 2003b).

According to the care ethicist Annelies van Heijst, the repertoire of the presence approach 'is not easily transferable to the professional repertoires of cure and care that largely focus on the sick and needy body' and where, in addition to the patient and the professional, 'medical-technical devices' fulfil an independent role (van Heijst, 2008: 166–7). This is essentially the question of how and to what degree the practising of presence can be transferred to other professional disciplines in healthcare and social work. In reply to this question, we wish to note here that we think that the practising of presence can be theoretically and empirically 'mixed' into a person's profession only if, and to the extent that, the practitioner realises and acknowledges that their profession is principally a conjectural approach, not an effective procedure. Even if it has a well-stocked toolkit of methods that can be used, a profession that works with and for people is never a 'poietic' or effective procedure that can achieve the goal with any degree of certainty by taking certain steps. Instead, it is a 'stochastic' or conjectural approach, in which the practitioner must do everything possible to achieve the goal, but can never be sure in advance that they will succeed.[6] The goal of every human-related profession is unstable and is more about going in the right direction (*doelrichting*) than a fixed good that can be produced mechanically. Once this is realised, it is possible, useful and worthwhile to transfer the presence approach to the profession in question, even if it may not always be easy. We have seen this happen in many domains since 2001.

The presence theory has been developed further since Baart (2001) first proposed it. New insights, theoretical concepts and subtheories have been developed and added on the basis of a significant number of empirical studies in many disciplines – not just in pastoral care (see Chapter 7).

Conclusion

As we have seen, the theory of presence explains why the practising of presence works and is beneficial to care receivers. Both the practice and the theory of presence have been received positively by social workers, nurses, youth workers, professionals in addiction care, general practitioners and so forth. As soon as professionals realise and acknowledge that their own caring, helping or supporting profession constitutes a conjectural approach, they will be able to acknowledge that it is relevant to their profession to practise presence. However, the relationship between the practice of presence in its various manifestations, on the one hand, and care, help and support, on the other, is complicated – if only because both the practice of presence, and care, help and support can be regarded as simultaneously empirical and normative. We will nevertheless explore four possible ways of opening up this relationship, without claiming that this constitutes a definitive and unequivocal answer.

Presence deals with *the core or heart* of all good professional care, help and support in the areas of health and welfare and, more widely, in a hospitable society. Care, help and support fundamentally cannot exist if the professional does not connect with and relationally attune their practice to the vulnerable and needy other, who always co-determines what is good for him or her. Where else do purpose, direction, criteria and so on in care, help and support come from? Being carefully attentive, trying to radically connect with and attune one's practice to the lifeworld, life course, concerns, turning points, rhythm and logic of the other, and letting oneself be affected by the desire and the appeal that emerge from the other – these are all necessary requirements. It is also indispensable that professionals are always accessible and responsive, even when the task at hand involves only a simple technical intervention.

The practising of presence is not the only *condition or criterion* for good professional care, help and support, but it is certainly an *important one*. Not all care, help and support are good care. Not all care helps or supports and not all help is caring. There is such a thing as non-caring care. But the minimum expectation should be that caregivers do not add to the suffering of the care receiver, nor leave them in distress. This means that it is necessary to be relationally attuned to the needy and already-wounded other, who always co-determines what is good for him or her.

Presence is *a wake-up call*, which opens our eyes and our critical memory. Wherever presence is radically exercised, facilitated, supported and strengthened within cure, care, help, support and management, we have seen something happen that is distinct from what can be observed in present-day healthcare, social work and education: much less orientation towards pre-planned results, much less bureaucratic logic and routine professionalism, much less desire to innovate constantly, much less professional perpetuation of neediness, much less 'creaming' or 'skimming' of care receivers who are likely to offer the best opportunities and neglect of those who are unable to keep up with a society that is changing ever more quickly and is becoming more and more complex. And much more cure, care, support and management that is attuned to persons; to patients, clients, residents, citizens and professionals who know that they have been seen; and to professionals and managers who are able to manifest themselves as dedicated, people-oriented professionals.

In sum, above all, presence *addresses the desire*, the enthusiasm and the original passion of many people who work in care, help and support. It empowers them: it articulates and legitimises their already existing practices of presence. And empowerment is also a political programme.

5

Constructing knowledge (1): care ethics and the empirical turn

In the previous chapters we have concisely presented presence theory – its content, its groundedness in the practising of presence and its reception. This and the following chapter contain a more general discussion of the construction of knowledge. Presence theory was developed as a means of understanding and accounting for the practising of presence and why it works so well. While developing this theory, we dealt with a multitude of empirical, theoretical and methodological issues. These issues merit a separate discussion which places them in the general framework of how knowledge is constructed within empirical ethics, especially empirical care ethics, and which develops them further, in interaction with developments in other disciplines. The objective of academic research – whether conceptual, empirical or both – is to gain understanding that enables us to come to terms with reality, to act in cases where it is not obvious how we should act, to account for what has been done and to discard ideas that are less helpful. This chapter deals with care ethics, empirical research in ethics, theory development and knowledge construction; the following chapter deals with complex theorising, practice theory and, again, knowledge construction. These two chapters are the preliminary result of a process of thinking about empirical ethics of care that we engaged in together with Frans Vosman, who, unfortunately, died in June 2020; and it is the basis of what we call 'empirically grounded (normative) ethics of care' (Timmerman, 2010; Timmerman and Vosman, 2014; Vosman et al, 2018; Timmerman, 2018; Vosman, 2018; Timmerman et al, 2019; Baart, 2020; Timmerman and Baart, 2021). These two chapters lay the groundwork for the presentation, in Chapter 7, of what we call 'the presence-theoretical perspective' and its theorems, a further development of the presence theory, which transcends it without replacing it.

The turn to everyday life

An essential element of the practising of presence is a radical turn to particularity. This turn is motivated by two concerns. First, it matters to the professional who practises presence that the care receiver is this particular person, in this particular relational network, in this particular situation, in this particular period of their lives, in this particular context. Meeting the other in their everyday life gives the professional more knowledge, both explicit and tacit, about this person and their network, situation, phase of life and context than meeting them in an arranged situation. Second, and even more important, everyday life, the availability it affords to acquire different kinds of knowledge, and the formal and informal care that is given and received in everyday life, offers more possibilities to humanise care more permanently than incidental interventions do (cf Kolen, 2017; Schmidt, J., 2022; van der Geest, 2024).

This turn to everyday life connects the theory and practice of presence with several other 'turns': the empirical turn in bioethics (Wangmo et al, 2018), the practice turn in philosophy and sociology (Schatzki et al, 2001), the relational turn in the social sciences (Selg and Ventsel, 2020a) and the everyday turn in sociology (Sztompka, 2008). Notwithstanding the historiographical reductionism of so-called 'turn talk' (Surkis, 2012), we think it is helpful to discuss these turns in relation to the presence-theoretical perspective. This chapter engages with the empirical turn, the next chapter with the practice turn, and Chapter 9 with the relational turn. A few words are in order here about the turn to everyday life. As the sociologist Piotr Sztompka has written, the everyday turn in sociology is the turn to 'the everyday life of people amongst other people, together with them, side by side with them, in cooperation, competition, conflict, or struggle with them, in love or hatred, but never alone, in isolation' (2008: 24).

In the research project on which *A Theory of Presence* (Baart, 2001) is based, it was noticed that the chaplains turned to the residents' lifeworld, participated in their everyday life, performed everyday activities, talked about everyday things. They created, maintained, refreshed and celebrated relationships using the ordinary things and routines that are at hand in the lifeworld. All these everyday activities were done for their own sake but, at the same time, they were more than just everyday activities. They have a surplus of meaning and a mediating character. In performing these activities, the professionals conveyed recognition, they consoled and empowered, and remained alert to signals of aspects that were vulnerable or under threat. Everyday life was a source of knowledge to them (Baart, 2001: 137–9, 737–8).

In care ethics, as in other forms of ethics, care is acknowledged to be an eminently quotidian activity – certainly not something that is exclusively linked to the domains of healthcare and social work[1] – an activity that makes the world go round, keeps it liveable and prevents it from decaying. Everyday life is not simple; it is messy, complex and ambiguous. On the one hand, everyday life is where people live together and find possibilities to live a good life. On the other, it is a trivial, grey and insignificant element of life that must be endured. On the one hand, everyday life is where ordinary people are subjugated to routines, to the strategies of those in power. On the other, it is where ordinary people employ tactics as a creative, opportunistic defence against power structures (de Certeau, 1984). According to Dorfman, in Chouraqui's words, the everyday 'is spent neither in the fantastical everyday, nor in eventfulness, but in an in-between space structured by the repulsion towards the former and the projection towards the latter, a projection that endlessly fails (making any idealised notion of eventful time just as fantastical as the false idea of the everyday)' (Chouraqui, 2016: 260). In addition to being ambiguous, everyday life is shot through with tragedy. For people in precarious situations – especially those whom Vosman calls 'survivors' – it is often accompanied by uncertainty, discontent and 'emerging steepness' (Vosman, 2023: 41). Survivors carry on within four kinds of tension: (1) the tension between 'passibility and steepness'; (2) between 'everyday persistence and resistance against being annexed by someone else's "progressive" project'; (3) between 'irreversibility of what was undergone and done' and 'surprise arising from misunderstanding'; and (4) between 'the fictional representation of a successful life' and 'carrying on when that representation breaks down' (p 48).

Like the practice turn and the relational turn, the everyday turn addresses the issues of institutions versus individuals, of systemic context versus individual actions, of structure versus agency. In focusing on social practices, relationality or everyday life, they try to mediate between the two terms in each binary pair. People are 'neither completely determined nor completely free' (Sztompka, 2008: 3). The everyday turn gives special attention to what really matters to ordinary people in their everyday activities (Sayer, 2011; Olthuis et al, 2014b; Laugier, 2018), as signalled by emotions (Nussbaum, 2004; Baart, 2013).

Care ethics as a political, intradisciplinary ethics

As we have said in the preceding chapters, Baart placed the practice of presence within the framework of care ethics, while it simultaneously transcended and challenged care ethics. Care ethics, as we understand it,

1. is a political-ethical practice that understands care as a culture-specific, everyday practice that is socially and institutionally embedded, and is broader than healthcare;
2. focuses on relational interaction as a (contested) locus of knowing, a restrictive framework for the coordination of care, the place where people can receive recognition and attention, a source of legitimacy and a stage on which people can appear;
3. acknowledges that good care, help and support are always context bound and situation specific, and can be validated only locally – that is, through the experience of the care receiver; and

4. studies practices of care, help and support in an oscillating movement between critical, conceptual, hermeneutic theoretical work, on the one hand, and phenomenological, qualitative research, on the other.

As a discipline in its own right, with its own history (Vosman, 2020), care ethics works together with other disciplines in a intradisciplinary way, making critical use of the knowledge, theories and methods of those other disciplines, probing them for coherence and consistency according to the criteria mentioned earlier. This cooperation with fellow travellers also represents an opportunity to criticise, amend and further develop the knowledge, theories and methods of care ethics (Baart, 2020).

Our position on empirical research in care ethics is characterised by several insights, developed through both political and theoretical considerations and long-term experience with qualitative-empirical, care-ethical research (Klaver et al, 2014; Leget et al, 2017; Vosman et al, 2018; Timmerman et al, 2019; Baart, 2020). The first is that normativity and morality are part and parcel of every practice. It is never a matter of imposing these upon the practice, nor can they be avoided. 'Ethos' (Kluxen, 1974) or 'intra-normativity' (Pols, 2015) can be found *in* the practising of the practitioners, including criticism of their own acting. In fact, recognising this is to take professionals seriously as moral actors or 'strong evaluators', who are able to articulate their motivations, preferences and reasons in substantive, and not only in procedural moral terms (Taylor, 1985; Timmerman, 2018; cf Webb, 2015).

A second insight that underlies our form of empirical research is that not only is good theory very 'practical' (Lewin, 1951: 169) but it is necessary to perceive well in the first place. First you have to perceive carefully, accurately and in detail, before you can judge. And it is not possible to perceive well without good concepts and theories. In addition to the original theory of presence (Baart, 2001; Baart, 2018c), the concepts and theories that can help might be those on practice (Nicolini, 2012; Schmidt, R., 2012; Nicolini and Monteiro, 2017), attentiveness (Arvidson, 2006), embodiment (Slatman, 2014), vulnerability/precarity (Lorey, 2015), relationality (Slife, 2004; Burkitt, 2016; Selg and Ventsel, 2020a; 2020b), goods/values (Sayer, 2011) and phenomenology (Waldenfels, 2004; 2011; 2015). Many of these concepts have since been incorporated into the theory of presence. Other relevant concepts and theories are on time, responsibility, class, intersectionality and so on.

A third insight is that perceiving well, accurately and in detail also includes 'zooming out': investigating how other practices interfere with the practice you are investigating; not only other caring practices, but also technological, bureaucratic-systemic, legal and political practices. We believe that researchers should be involved in analysing the effects of neoliberalisation and precarisation (Vosman and Niemeijer, 2017; Biroli, 2020; Baart, 2021a). That, too, is about taking the professionals who do the work seriously; about not ascribing to them what is not their doing and what they do no control.

Our fourth insight is that what qualitative-empirical normative-ethical research can and should do for practitioners, besides developing empirically grounded theory, is, at most, supplying 'stepping stones'; not instructions in the sense of 'this is how you should always do it', but in the sense of 'this-or-that has proven to be good to others in such-and-such situations and contexts; it may help you too, under such-and-such conditions, with moral issues that you encounter in your practice'. Not prescriptions, but relational 'soft suggestions' (Pols, 2015).

Empirical research

We are convinced that empirical research is indispensable to care ethics. Without empirical research, there is a risk that ethicists will reflect only on their own assumptions, perceptions and experiences (Walker, 1998), that situations and practices are perceived, analysed and interpreted without adequate theoretical concepts, and inappropriate modes of action are promoted, or even that the situation is completely misunderstood. In other words, the purely epistemological theories that many theorists propose run the risk of being epistemically paternalistic, insofar as they claim to be able to determine what constitutes the well-being of vulnerable and injured people and what benefits them, without interacting with these people themselves, or with the professionals who work with and for them, professionals who are able to discover, together with these people, what would actually be good for them (Fricker, 2007). We have to add, though, that empirical research can be faulty, too, if inadequate, misguided or prejudiced questions are asked or the empirical material is selected or constructed in an inadequate way. We therefore advocate engaging in a process of qualitative empirical research oriented to theory development, which is informed by state-of-the-art knowledge of empirical research and appropriate theoretical concepts and theories, and which is accompanied by ethical reflection.

We want to contribute to the maintaining, promoting and strengthening of practices of good care by identifying such practices, analysing why participants evaluate these practices as good care and discovering how such practices can be facilitated. We seek to gain an understanding that can help participants in practices of care to come to terms with reality, to act in situations where it is not obvious what the right way to act is, to account for what is done and to reject ideas that are not helpful. In this book, we concentrate on care professionals, but we think that our proposition is valid for caring practices in general. We realise that, in late modern society, professional practices take place in highly complex organisations (Vosman et al, 2016). This insight makes it possible to acknowledge the paradoxes that impose themselves upon practices in late modernity, and to avoid thinking in terms of people as individual actors supposedly conscious of and responsible for their doings and in command of the circumstances. It also means recognising the complex entanglement of doings and sayings, rather than assuming that human actions are normally free and unfettered. The qualitative research that we have conducted therefore (i) acknowledges the internal morality of practices, (ii) uncovers deeper influences and structures that are not immediately obvious but nevertheless have a bearing on the care practices in question, and (iii) delivers theoretical concepts and theories that are conducive to good care and are not just descriptive.

Empirically grounded normative ethics of care is what we call the specific combination of qualitative empirical research, theory development and ethical reflection that we espouse. The term 'grounded' expresses our aim to develop concepts, insights and theories that do justice to – are 'grounded' in – concrete practices of care and the tacit knowing and situational practical wisdom of participants in those practices, as they appear – and are concealed – in our construction and analysis of empirical material. To undergird this proposal, we must methodologically account for the complex intersecting relationships between empirical research and ethics (side I of an imaginary triangle – Figure 5.1), between empirical research and theory development (side II), and between social and political theory and ethics (side III). We believe that these three sides must be considered in their interconnectedness.

Figure 5.1: Constructing knowledge: an oscillating movement

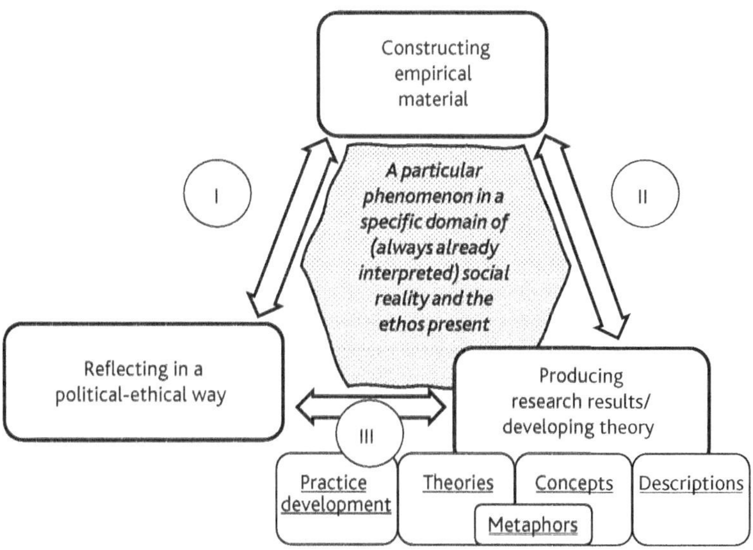

Empirical research and ethical reflection

An intensive debate is ongoing in empirical bioethics about this discipline's methodology and standards (Christen et al, 2014; Davies et al, 2015; Ives et al, 2017; Ives et al, 2018; Wangmo et al, 2018). Although this debate is almost exclusively focused on the relationship between empirical research and ethics, and thus ignores the other two sides and their mutual connectedness, it has a bearing in care ethics on the development of different approaches to empirical research. This is especially the case in the Netherlands and Flanders because of certain specific developments in empirical research in bioethics there, most of which has been undertaken as part of government-funded medical research programmes. Our interest in care ethics as a form of normative political theory means that we conceive of situations and practices as sites where normative and ethical (that is, theorising) insights can be found, and not primarily as areas where normative and ethical insights should be applied. Two varieties of bioethics can be distinguished that take a similar position: 'critical applied ethics' and 'integrated empirical ethics' (Molewijk et al, 2004). In critical applied ethics, empirical and normative views on reality are complementary; in integrated empirical ethics, the empirical and the normative view are understood as mutually dependent.

But empirically grounded care ethics as we conceptualise and practise it differs fundamentally from both critical applied ethics and integrated empirical ethics (Baart and Timmerman, 2016; Timmerman, 2018; Vosman et al, 2018; Baart, 2020). Unlike critical applied ethics, we aim to integrate empirical and ethical methods, and not to resort to a two-phased model of first doing empirical research and then reflecting ethically upon it. However, unlike integrated empirical ethics, we retain a distinction between empirical research methods and ethical reflection, given the risk of 'smuggling' morality into seemingly neutral descriptions (for example, the equivocal term 'resilience'). In contrast to critical applied ethics, we are concerned with discerning and promoting practices of good care and not with establishing and describing moral problems, nor with analysing alternative solutions to problems and their consequences and affording these solutions normative weight by giving moral theory authority over the empirical material. Contrary to what integrated empirical ethics argues, intuitions, judgments and responses to vignettes or fragments of cases are not the loci of normative-ethical insights. Concrete practice, moral experience and the situational practical wisdom of the participants in this practice are, however.

In empirically grounded normative ethics and care ethics, empirical research goes hand in hand with ethical reflection from the outset. Normativity emerges from three sources: 'the positioning of acting and its internal goals as central, the elaboration of the critical correctives that can be found in the practices researched and the ethical reflection by the ethicists who carry out the empirical research' (Timmerman, 2018: 51). The practical knowledge and wisdom of participants in the practice that is being studied, and the proper empirical, theoretical and ethical capacities of the researcher are both essential if the research is to perceive and discern what is morally relevant, address what theoretical 'veil' is alienating or obfuscating what is at stake, and come up with feasible proposals for the people who participate in that practice.

Essential aspects of our position are:

a. the assumption that social reality (and not just care) is morally laden, not neutral (Taylor, 1989; Timmerman, 2018) and
b. a kind of political-ethical reflection that helps to articulate this moral ladenness.

Conversely, empirical research raises ethical issues. For example about the ownership of the participants' bodies, lives, experiences, stories and views (usually captured by 'informed consent'), the participants' privacy (usually captured by the requirements of confidentiality, especially pseudonymisation) and the consequences for the participants, both beneficial and adverse, both during the study itself and after the publication of the results, for both individuals and groups or communities (cf Doody and Noonan, 2016). Researchers who engage in qualitative research must be committed to adhering to the usual procedures, to the extent that these are sensitive to the ethically relevant characteristics of qualitative research. Qualitative research often deals with complicated and unexplored situations or practices, and/or sensitive topics. The researcher is the main instrument in qualitative research. Moreover, qualitative research often starts with a provisional formulation of the problem that becomes definite only later and that undergoes cycles of construction and analysis of empirical material. One of the consequences of this is that research ethics procedures can give rise to ethical issues, for example, in situations where written forms of informed consent cannot be safely kept by participants (González-López, 2011) or where pseudonymising participants' testimonies undermines their dignity (Einwohner, 2011). To be able to deal with unexpected ethical issues, researchers need to be present with and for the participants in their research (González-López, 2011), to be reflexive throughout every phase of the study (Guillemin and Gillam, 2004; Subramani, 2019) and to exercise practical wisdom.

But there is more to research ethics. Researchers always have particular moral preferences. We are interested in the predicament of the people in the most precarious situations, both professionals and clients. We want to help make their voices heard, their knowledge acknowledged and their concerns alleviated (cf Baart and Hoffman, 2021). When confronted with concrete ethical dilemmas while in the field, we ask ourselves:

- What is morally at stake here? And for whom?
- How do the process and possible findings of our research affect different people with different positions, interests and ideas about the good life?
- What responsibilities do our different relationships with these different people entail for us as researchers?

We try to answer these questions with a view to the people in the most precarious situation, while staying connected with and attuned to, that is, deliberating with, all participants in the study.

Empirical research and theory development

The German sociologist Gesa Lindemann has mapped the interconnectedness of empirical research and theory development (see Figure 5.1, side II), in connection with the other two sides. She has pointed out that data collection and analysis are not free of theoretical assumptions. According to her, these assumptions cannot be falsified by empirical data and cannot thus be further developed. Drawing on Georg Simmel, she has proposed a distinction between three levels of sociological theory development (Lindemann, 2008; 2009). The first level encompasses 'social theories', which contain the theoretical and methodological assumptions about what a social phenomenon is and what concepts are crucial to studying it. The second level consists of 'limited range theories', theories about specific social phenomena, including 'grounded (substantial and formal) theories' and 'middle-range theories'. The third level consists of 'theories of society', that is, 'theories about large historical formations such as modern society, capitalist society, or functionally differentiated society' (Lindemann, 2009: 6).[2] Lindemann has further shown that the relationship between theory and empirical research has to be conceptualised differently on each of these levels. Thinking in terms of verification and falsification is adequate only on the second level, that of limited range theories. She has proposed that the empirical basis of theories about society (level three) should be investigated with the help of the difference between plausible and implausible *Gestalt* extrapolation (Lindemann, 2008: 124; 2009: 10), and that of first-level theories with the help of the 'precise/troubled distinction' (Lindemann, 2008: 124; 2009: 14). But we think there is an ambiguity in how Lindemann explains these social theory levels. On the one hand, she seems to understand social theory as one single paradigm within which researchers think, observe and do research. On the other, she understands social theories as heuristic devices (*Sehinstrumente*, Lindemann, 2008: 114): they do not define or interpret what is perceived but make it possible to disclose what presents itself. The researcher's troubling experience (*Irritation*) that these devices are incapable of capturing reality precisely enough can become a motivation to develop them further (cf Baart and Timmerman, 2016; Vosman and Niemeijer, 2017). Our inquiries concern the second level, but also, and substantially, the first level, that of concepts and theories as heuristic devices to perceive well.

The empirically grounded ethics of care that we are proposing also involves an intertwining of empirical research, on the one hand, and concept and theory development, on the other. Theoretical and conceptual reflections are used to recognise details that are particularly relevant and are saturated by complexity, to perceive more closely, to perceive what was not perceived before and to give a plausible account of what has been discerned. Empirical research is carried out to operationalise and differentiate abstract concepts (relationality, vulnerability, corporeality) and to repair or broaden deficient concepts (autonomy, self-reliance, co-creation, shared decision making). Empirical research makes it possible to 'talk back' to theory and to ask questions that stimulate further, relevant theory development. This sometimes also implies showing how the use of a particular theory, for example on vulnerability or power, has become shallow or uninformative. Going beyond mere descriptions of experiences, our aim is to develop concepts and theories grounded in our empirical research. We propose that there should be an 'oscillating' movement between empirical work and theory development, one which commits these two to each other. 'Oscillating' here means 'swinging in an intended, methodological way, detecting what questions the observed practice raises, as well as what questions the theoretical notions used raise, rigorously inquiring into these questions, and updating the preliminary findings' (Vosman et al, 2018: 413).

In this oscillating movement between empirical work and theory development, research carried out by other scholars in ethics, philosophy and social science who are working with the same intuitions is important, both for empirical work and for theory development. The empirical and theoretical research findings of these 'fellow travellers' can broaden our knowledge, raise questions or offer concepts that support and maintain the oscillating movement. Researchers can thus gradually gain a deeper understanding of the situation or the practice, develop clearer theoretical concepts and avoid both empirical naivety and fact-free reasoning. Such an inquiry is fuelled by observations that do not make sense, and it prepares the way for a different perspective, possibly also a different theoretical take on the practice, if the theory used does not fit or ignores the fine fabric of the care practice. The focus is always on a practice (Nicolini, 2012; Schmidt, R., 2012), and primarily on acting and undergoing (or, to put it in phenomenological terms: the *passibilité*) of living beings (Vosman et al, 2016), and on the tacit knowing and practical wisdom of the persons who offer care and help, in this case professionals. At the same time, theoretical understanding is developed further, from concepts to grounded theories to more comprehensive theories that point beyond the concrete situation or practice. This reciprocal approach focuses primarily on theory development at the first two levels that Lindemann distinguishes ('social theories' and 'limited range theories').

Our proposal has two prerequisites:

a. the assumption that every perception and experience is theory laden (cf Hirschauer, 2008) and
b. a procedure that helps to articulate the theoretical implications of the practice rather than distort them or even replace them with inappropriate theoretical concepts.

The connection: political phenomenology

As care ethicists concerned with political ethical theory, we argue that the connection of the three sides between empirical research, theory development and ethical reflection lies in a phenomenological inquiry into the lived experience of the persons who act and undergo (care receivers and caregivers), and their first-person perspectives. In our empirical research, we use instruments and approaches from the traditions of ethnography, phenomenology, discourse analysis, visual data analysis, narrative analysis, auto-ethnography, ethnomethodology, conversational analysis, institutional ethnography, document analysis and many other traditions, depending on the concrete practice, the situation and the specific research interest. However, the actual experience of the persons who act and undergo, and their first-person perspective, always take precedence. Whatever concrete methods or approaches we use, we always do this with a certain phenomenological interest, not in the tradition of the epistemological-egological phenomenology of Edmund Husserl and Alfred Schütz (see Aspers and Kohl, 2013), but in that of the interpretive phenomenology of Martin Heidegger, Hans-Georg Gadamer and Charles Taylor (see Benner, 1994) and the political phenomenology of Hannah Arendt, Maurice Merleau-Ponty and Paul Ricœur, in particular Bernhard Waldenfels's 'responsive phenomenology of the alien' (Waldenfels, 2011; 2015). We espouse a phenomenology that is political, that really attends to concrete practices and that confronts and reflects on its own morality in relation to the presuppositions of modernity (Vosman, 2018; Vosman et al, 2018). A person's bodily experience of themselves, the seemingly purely intimate experience between two persons and their experience with third persons are also political in nature. Political-ethical care ethics must always be alert to these layers of organised sociality.

Phenomenological, theory-oriented 'N=N case studies'

Care ethics began with the empirical research conducted by the moral psychologist Carol Gilligan and her colleagues. In her famous book *In a*

Different Voice, Gilligan relates an observation she made halfway through a decade of research into how people talk about morality and about themselves (1982). She began to hear two ways of speaking about moral problems and about the relationship between the other and the self. One of these two ways was familiar to researchers who worked in the line of Lawrence Kohlberg, Gilligan's mentor and colleague. But there was also another, different voice. A voice that spoke of interconnection instead of equality, relationships instead of rules, attachment instead of separation, care instead of fairness, conflicting responsibilities instead of competing rights. Gilligan had the intuition that it was important to discern this voice further and strengthen it in order to correct moral psychological theory, and to do justice especially to the experience of many women. She decided to study not only how people think about problems that are presented to them for resolution (Kohlberg's *modus operandi*) but also how they define moral problems and how they talk about real moral conflicts in their own lives. Her argument in the book, which was based on three empirical studies, was criticised because she could not substantiate the claim that there were gender differences between men and women (for example, Luria, 1986). But her argument was not about statistics. It was based on a sufficient number of exemplary cases, but with a certain comprehensiveness – not on the representativeness of the samples studied. Her argument 'was interpretive and hinged on the demonstration that the examples presented illustrated a different way of seeing' (Gilligan, 1986: 326). Gilligan's book provoked many responses, including much affirmation, leading to the rise of what is now called 'ethics of care' or 'care ethics' (Dingler, 2016).

Four formal characteristics of Gilligan's study have inspired us in particular:

1. It started with an observation and an intuition.
2. The argument was based on just enough exemplary cases, with a certain comprehensiveness.
3. The theoretical concepts developed were innovative and offered a new and productive moral vision.
4. In addition to criticism and even rejection, it received much affirmation in response.

Our own research has two additional features:

5. We study what participants in practices of care do and refrain from doing, and what they undergo.
6. We position professionals as co-researchers with their own responsibilities.

All six characteristics apply to the research of neighbourhood pastoral care that resulted in presence theory (Baart, 2001). It started with a strong intuition: that sound and thorough qualitative research would be able to deliver insight into neighbourhood pastoral care that was substantially different from, and better than, the insight that was then current. Two comprehensive cases were studied in the context of a multiple case study. The central focus in these cases was how the practitioners acted and how and what they perceived, considered, assessed, weighted and evaluated – rather than their beliefs, opinions or responses to prefabricated vignettes. A lot of qualitative subanalyses were carried out in the analysis of the cases. And a lot of conceptual and theoretical work was done so as to observe well and accurately name what was observed. The resulting reconstruction was then presented to the practitioners who participated in the study, and they supplemented, corrected and ultimately generally confirmed it. Of course, the researchers were responsible for the detailed outcomes and their wording. The study resulted in the reconstruction of what was called the 'practice of presence'. An important criterion of the quality of the study was the nature and extent of the approval these reconstructions received from the practitioners involved. Although critical during the process of constructing and analysing the empirical material, their acknowledgement and approval of the ultimate findings were great, often in the form of recognition: 'Yes, that's how we do that! Yes, that's how it is for us!' Contrary to common expectations, the study showed that neighbourhood chaplains are not systematically involved in solving problems.

As our aim is to study the real-life complexity of inevitably morally imprinted care processes, our empirical material typically consists of extensive and comprehensive case descriptions. We therefore characterise our inquiries as 'case studies'. Given the goal of our inquiries, the number of cases included (N) is not decisive for their quality, as long as the analysis of these cases provides sufficiently profound theoretical insight into the practice studied. Neither the requirements of statistical generalisation nor data, code, meaning or theoretical saturation (Hennink et al, 2017) determine the number – although saturation can have a function in the analysis. What is essential is the information richness or 'information power' of the case descriptions (Malterud et al, 2016). Together with Frans Vosman, we called our kind of inquiry a 'phenomenological, theory-oriented N=N case study' (Timmerman et al, 2019).[3] The validity, trustworthiness and transferability (or aptness for 'heuristic generalisations', Tsoukas, 2009) of the findings of an N=N case study are based on the exemplariness and extensiveness of the case descriptions, the rigour of the analysis, the innovative power of the empirically grounded theoretical concepts that are developed and the approval the findings receive from the participants in the practice. We will now clarify each of these four criteria, although they deserve a more detailed discussion.

The first criterion concerns the choice of cases. These should be exemplary, that is, they should be derived mostly from the practice of practitioners who are recognised as good practitioners by colleagues or residents, clients, pupils or patients (cf Bronk, 2012). These cases should be reconstructed benevolently and critically, in all their relevant dimensions. The case descriptions should be extensive and comprehensive, written after in-depth, semi-structured interviews of the participants – possibly preceded by or embedded in some form of observation, document study or group interaction. Describing exemplary cases extensively and comprehensively using newly developed theoretical concepts also means constructing exemplars that can be used to clarify other cases and can be transferred easily to other contexts and practices.

The second criterion concerns the rigour of the analysis, which is determined mainly by construct and process validity, many criteria for which can be found in the methodological literature. Which of these are applicable depends on the research aim and the empirical material that is at hand or can be constructed.

The third criterion concerns the concepts, metaphors and theories that are developed. These should be innovative, that is, they should contribute to new and productive ways of perceiving, understanding and acting. Judgement on whether these concepts are innovative belongs first and foremost to the researchers and secondly to the practitioners who can judge their usability. In our search for good care, we are especially interested in theoretical concepts that can help professionals to act in cases where there is no obviously right way to act, to account for their actions and to reject anything that serves goals other than contributing to good care.

The last criterion is 'resonance validity', the approval the findings receive from participants in the practice studied (cf Anderson, 2004; Charmaz, 2006). This is not the same thing as the extent to which participants in the research believe the findings represent them. Resonance validity involves a judgement about the response that partakers in the practice give to the findings, about how and to what extent they understand, confirm and criticise it and explain how it helps them to act. These four criteria are not like binary electrical switches that are either on or off, but they are like the strands of a rope – they all contribute together to the overall strength of the argument.

Conclusion

Constructing knowledge about the complex, dynamic and emergent everyday world of care and caring requires a complex, dynamic and emergent conception of doing research, developing theories, reflecting on moral and ethical issues and the ways these practices interact with each other. Without empirical research, ethicists run the risk of completely misunderstanding the situation or the practice. But also with empirical research but without theory development and ethical reflection, situations and practices can be completely misunderstood. Essential to our position are the assumptions that social reality is morally laden and experience is theory laden. Concerning the quality of our research findings, resonance validity, the approval they receive from participants in the practice studied, is important to us. In the next chapter we will return to the issue of constructing knowledge, from the perspective of complexity thinking and practice theory.

6

Constructing knowledge (2): complex theorising and the practice turn

After having considered questions about empirical research in care ethics, we now turn to issues about theorising in care ethics. We seek to gain an understanding, also on a theoretical level, that can help participants in practices of care – professionals, informal caregivers and those who benefit from the care provided – to come to terms with reality, to act in situations where it is not obvious how best to act, to account for what they have done, to reject ideas that are less helpful and to develop the practice further to make it more conducive to good care, help and support.

Evaluative social science

In Chapter 5, we discussed sides I and II of the triangle that is constituted by empirical research, theory and ethics (see Figure 5.1). Here, we will address side III, the relationship between theory and ethics. Mainstream social science has invested much in being 'objective', wishing to free itself from what the sociologist Andrew Sayer has called 'a kind of dogmatism which would foreclose debate on normative matters by claiming a scientific warrant for some conceptions of the good over others' (Sayer, 2011: 57). This tendency likes to quote Max Weber's advocacy of 'value-free' social science, David Hume's warning against unwarranted transitions 'from is to ought' and George Edward Moore's exposure of the 'naturalistic fallacy'.

'Objective' social science has relegated morality to a separate realm, that of 'values'. The concept of values originates in the economy, where it means the purchase price: the amount of money needed to buy a product or a service. This meaning is reflected in the idea of 'value-based healthcare', or, better still, 'value-based competition on results in healthcare', where 'value' means the health outcomes achieved per dollar of cost compared to peers (Porter and Teisberg, 2006).

The term 'value' was introduced in sociology and philosophy at the turn of the 20th century. Over the course of that century, values came to be conceptualised as implying 'free-floating, seemingly arbitrary ideas about what is good or what one ought to do that can be left to individuals to choose as they see fit' (Sayer, 2011: 28). Sayer has drawn attention to the consequences of this quest for objectivity: a kind of social science that finds it difficult to acknowledge that our relationship to the world is marked by concern. Concerns have to do with the fact that we can be 'well-fed or malnourished, healthy or sick, respected or despised and humiliated, powerful or powerless, supported or exploited, and loved or unloved; we can have a sense of self-worth or worthlessness, be stimulated or bored, happy or depressed, and so on' (Sayer, 2011: 5). Human beings are evaluative beings, beings to whom things matter. They can thrive and flourish, but also suffer. Conceptualising values as 'free-floating, seemingly arbitrary ideas' is not helpful when doing empirical ethical research into the lived experience of evaluative beings. Social scientists must acknowledge that values are always about things in reality and that they can be rationally discussed and evaluated. According to Sayer, social scientists need to learn to be connected participants in the social reality they study rather than its detached spectators.

Sayer has suggested an alternative conception of values: as ' "sedimented" valuations that have become attitudes or dispositions, which we come to regard as justified' (Sayer, 2011: 25). We continuously evaluate things, people, situations, actions and so on. These particular, concrete evaluations contribute to attitudes and dispositions which in turn influence the evaluations we make. We reflect to some degree on our values, although they are usually not articulated unless they are challenged. We use our values as criteria to evaluate not only others, but ourselves too. Our ' "professed values" may differ from our "values in use" ' (Sayer, 2011: 26), due to lack of reflection and self-knowledge. The underlying social ontology views 'actors not only as causal agents and as self-interpreting meaning-makers, but as needy and dependent, having an orientation of care and concern about some things, and capable of flourishing or suffering' (Sayer, 2011: 139–40).

In our empirical research, we are more interested in values-in-use than in professed values. But even then, values remain dependent on human acts of ascription and evaluation. They can be ascribed and taken away. We are interested in what *shows* itself as good or bad, right or wrong in our acting and reacting in particular situations or practices. To mark the fact that we have a different approach to values than that of mainstream social science, we prefer to use the expression 'emerging "goods" (*bona*)' (Timmerman, 2018).

If social science is to do justice to the lived experience of evaluative, sentient, embodied beings, it will have to work with 'thick ethical concepts' (a term of Bernard Williams), concepts that contain descriptive and evaluative elements that cannot be separated. 'Care' itself is a thick ethical concept, for it cannot be distinguished from other behaviour without some evaluative content as to what is good for those concerned (Sayer, 2011; 2016).

Constructing knowledge

As we said in Chapter 5, the core of our research consists of an oscillating movement between three poles: (a) the construction of empirical material,

(b) the production of research results – descriptions, concepts, metaphors, theories and/or practice development – including theory development, and (c) political-ethical reflection.

Empirical material

In our research we are interested in care practices, located in care organisations that are part of society. Our concrete studies inquire into a particular phenomenon in a specific domain in social reality. A phenomenon can be a concrete event, situation, action or interaction, process, innovation, transition, practice, discourse, network, form of life, organisation, institution or society. It is always located in a specific domain of social reality: healthcare, youth care, social work, care for older persons, care for the mentally disabled and so on. Social reality, unlike physical reality, is always already interpreted. We therefore always need a 'double hermeneutics' (a term of Anthony Giddens): lay concepts intrude into academic discourse, but academic concepts similarly intrude into everyday discourse. Social reality, therefore, consists of objects, bodies, human and non-human actors, situations, processes, discourses and practices – and interpretations thereof.

There is always some reason why we are interested in a particular phenomenon: it might be a burning issue, or something that is at stake for professionals working with and for people who are experiencing a difficult time, either temporarily or permanently, or we might have an intuition about what kind of research outcome could be relevant to them. For example, the research into neighbourhood pastoral care that resulted in the presence theory started with the strong intuition that sound and thorough qualitative research would be able to deliver insight into neighbourhood pastoral care that is substantially different from – and more conducive to good care than – the insight that was then current.

To study the particular phenomenon we are interested in at any given point, we need to construct empirical material. The term usually used in empirical research is 'to gather empirical data', but we think that empirical data is never simply given, and gathering empirical data is never an objective, neutral procedure. We therefore use the expression 'empirical material', which we have adopted from Mats Alvesson and Dan Kärreman (Alvesson and Kärreman, 2007; 2011), to express that what is often called 'empirical data' is always co-constructed, generated by particular methods. Because of these methods, which are usually derived from the social and behavioural sciences, and because empirical material is always generated from a domain of social reality which is already interpreted and therefore theory-laden and morality-laden, empirical material is never free of theory and concepts or free of morality and ethics.

Research results

Research is about more than gathering data or constructing empirical material. The research question requires an answer, the research aim requires results, funding bodies require outcomes. Research results in general are descriptions and comparisons, theoretical concepts, models, analogies and metaphors, full-blown or partial theories and/or practice development. Pieter van Strien has distinguished between 'theory as the final *product* of scientific inquiry, and theory as a *tool* that is used in the process of theory formation' (van Strien, 1993: 150). If we extend this distinction further, it can be said that concepts, models, analogies, metaphors and theories are not only research outcomes, but also heuristic devices with which to look at other phenomena, and construct and analyse empirical material. We take 'heuristic device' to mean a concept, model, analogy, metaphor or theory that we use with the purpose of perceiving more and better, and of analysing more profoundly what actually happens in practices (Vosman and Niemeijer, 2017).[1] In grounded theory studies in particular, but also in other kinds of qualitative research, the analysis begins as soon as the gathering of data starts. There is constant interaction between gathering and analysis, between constructing empirical material and producing research results. Our heuristic devices are often clarified and improved during this process. If they are understood as heuristic devices, the concepts and theories that are developed or empirically enriched in our research can be helpful for looking at other phenomena in subsequent research.

Ethical reflection

In addition to the construction of empirical material and the production of research outcomes, there is a third pole of our research: ethical reflection. This is part and parcel of the kind of care-ethical empirical research we espouse. As we outlined in greater detail in Chapter 5, we reject the idea that ethical reflection is a second phase, conducted after the first phase which consists of empirical research. Our ethical reflection is political care-ethical reflection, and is guided by what we call, in Frans Vosman's words, 'critical insights'. Critical insights are developing ethical insights that were gained from previous care-ethical empirical research and that are indispensable to care ethics. Examples are insights into the relevance and meaning of relationships, contextuality, positions and empirical groundedness. These critical insights also fulfil a role in constructing empirical material and in producing research outcomes. This pole of ethical reflection is not the most important one – nor is it the ultimate purpose of our research – but it is nonetheless an indispensable pole.

We have summarised our ideas on the process of constructing knowledge in Figure 6.1.

Figure 6.1: Constructing knowledge from a presence-theoretical perspective

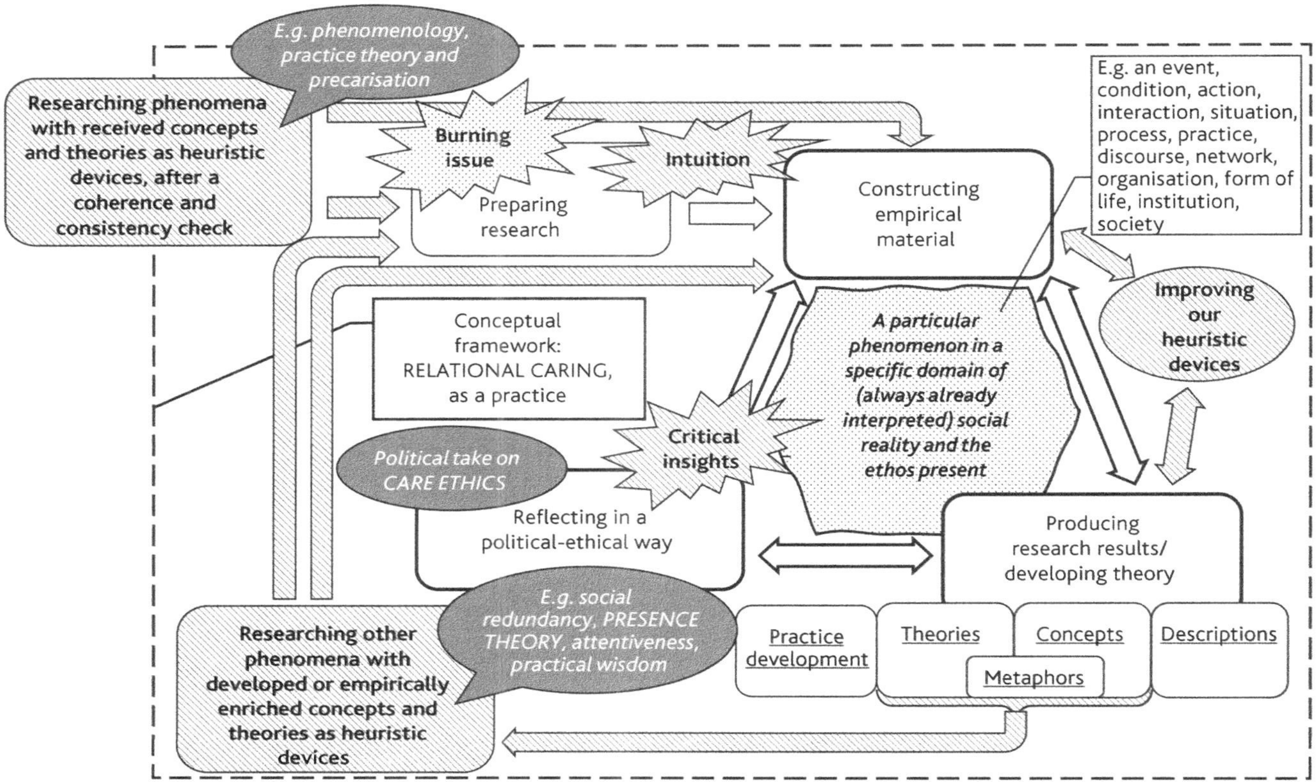

Source: Adapted from Timmerman and Baart, 2021: 130

Conceptual framework

One more element in Figure 6.1 requires further explanation: the conceptual framework. This was not adequately explained before (especially in Baart, 2001). But it is essential to the presence-theoretical perspective we are presenting in this book to recognise, understand and acknowledge that care is always (a) relational caring and (b) a practice. Care is always 'done' within the context of a relationship between caregiver and care receiver. This relationship should not be misunderstood as a self-contained one-to-one relationship. There are almost always others involved, both on the care receiver's side (relatives and friends) and on the caregiver's side (colleagues). Professional caring relationships are always embedded in an organisation as the embodiment of an institution in society (see Chapter 9). And this 'doing of care' – not only by the caregiver, but also by the care receiver – should be understood as a practice, an interplay of the doings, sayings, refrainings, undergoings, relatings and the artefacts used by a multitude of human and non-human actors. It is also always co-determined by the rules and messages of the embedding organisation, including various kinds of systemic influences.

Practices and practice theory

In general, we conceptualise care as a practice and use practice theory as a heuristic device in our inquiry into care practices (Reckwitz, 2002; Schmidt, R., 2012; Nicolini and Monteiro, 2017). It has already been noted by Sara Ruddick and, subsequently, by Joan Tronto that it is possible to avoid idealising, sentimentalising and romanticising care by thinking about it in terms of a practice (Ruddick, 1989; Tronto, 1993). A practice is a more or less ordered interplay of materially meditated 'doings and sayings' (Schatzki, 1996), refrainings and 'undergoings' (Vosman et al, 2016) and 'relatings' (Kemmis and Grootenboer, 2008), with a history, with virtuoso practitioners, with a community of participants and with a *telos* (Ruddick, 1989; Tronto, 1993; MacIntyre, 2007; Vosman and Baart, 2008; Jaeggi, 2015; Nicolini and Monteiro, 2017). A practice always happens in time and space, and includes objects, bodies, machines, artefacts, buildings and spaces (Nicolini and Monteiro, 2017). Furthermore, a practice is often supported by institutions (Ricœur, 1992; MacIntyre, 2007; Vosman, 2008), navigated by practical wisdom (Vosman and Baart, 2008; Bontemps-Hommen, 2020; den Uijl, 2022) and accompanied by a discourse which produces and reproduces, and is produced and reproduced, by the practice (Graham, 2002). A practice and its accompanying discourse always entail certain 'configurations of privilege and subordination' (Graham, 2002), but are also open to (immanent and external) criticism and transformation (Ruddick, 1989; Frazer and

Lacey, 1994; Jaeggi, 2015). Supporting institutions can become sources of corrupting power, which can be resisted by practising virtues such as justice, courage and truthfulness (MacIntyre, 2007).

The concept of practice can be traced back to Ludwig Wittgenstein and has been discussed by many contemporary thinkers, such as Alisdair MacIntyre, Paul Ricœur and Theodor Schatzki. However, thinking about practices is much broader and is known as 'practice theory'. Practice theory is a type of social theory as outlined by authors such as Anthony Giddens, Pierre Bourdieu, Bruno Latour, Theodor Schatzki, Robert Schmidt, Andreas Reckwitz and Davide Nicolini. According to Reckwitz, the 'turn to practices seems to be tied to an interest in the "everyday" and "lifeworld"' (Reckwitz, 2002: 244). Within the main social theories, practice theory belongs to what Reckwitz calls 'cultural theories'. Whereas the 'social' in the social theories of *homo economicus* and *homo sociologicus* consists of 'the intended or unintended product of subjective interests' or 'a consensus of norms and roles', in cultural theories it consists of 'symbolic and cognitive structures of knowledge' (Reckwitz, 2002: 246–7). *Homo economicus* is a self-interested and calculating individual and *homo sociologicus* a norm-following and role-playing member of society, but in practice theory, agents are 'body/minds who "carry" and "carry out" social practices' (p 256). Within cultural theories, practice theory is a conceptual alternative to mentalism, textualism and intersubjectivism. The 'smallest unit' of the social in these other cultural theories refers to the mind, discourses or interactions, but in practice theory the smallest unit consists of practices. Reckwitz understands practice theory as a heuristic device, 'a sensitizing "framework" for empirical research in the social sciences' (p 257).

Given, on the one hand, the broad variety of practice theories and the advantages and limitations of each of them and, on the other, their family resemblances, Davide Nicolini proposes what he has called a toolkit approach. He approaches practice theory as a 'package of theory, method and vocabulary' (Nicolini, 2017). Because good science should make us more articulate, he proposes to use the different practice theories as various theoretical sensitivities, as various conceptual lenses, in two alternating movements: zooming in and zooming out. Zooming in means using different conceptual lenses to study the practice as it is discursively, socially and materially practised, and its accomplishments. It entails focusing on sayings and doings; interactional order (positions); timing and tempo; bodily choreography; tools, artefacts and mediation work; practical concerns; tensions between creativity and normativity and processes of legitimation and stabilisation (Nicolini, 2012: 220). Zooming out means discerning the relationships of the practice under consideration with other practices, trailing these connections in space and time by following the intermediaries (people, artefacts and inscriptions), and thus investigating the texture of associated practices, in order to understand and describe the wider picture. Zooming out also investigates how connections between practices are kept in place, and how practices constitute identities and hierarchical power relationships (p 230). Nicolini's notion of zooming out criticises the 'eliminativist' idea of differentiating between micro, meso and macro levels, or between a practice and its 'context' (p 234).

Discussing practices, Nicolini has emphasised their processual and performative nature and has described them as 'regimes of a mediated object-oriented performance of organised set of doings and sayings' that 'have a history, social constituency and hence, a perceivable normative dimension'. Part of this normative dimension is that practices are 'always oriented and organised around a telic dimension' that 'is partly given and partly emergent, continuously changing, and always subject to negotiation and contestation (which makes it impossible to fully articulate in language)'. Nicolini's key point here is that this *telos* is 'carried by the practice, not by individuals' (Nicolini, 2017: 22). This is not unlike our ideas about finality as outlined in Chapter 10.

Nicolini has also stressed that practice theory is 'a theoretical orientation towards the study of the social where the methodological element remains central' (Nicolini, 2017: 19). It is geared towards generating questions, not providing answers. He has distinguished four research strategies. The first is situational research, in which the 'concerted accomplishment of orderly scenes of action' (Nicolini, 2017: 26) is analysed. To Nicolini, this should be the logically and methodologically predominant approach. The second is genealogical research, in which the historical dynamics of individual practices are studied. The third is configurational research, zooming out, in which is studied how 'concerted accomplishments and performances are connected and hang together to form constellations or larger assemblages' (Nicolini, 2017: 30). The fourth is dialectic or conflict-sensitive research, in which the co-evolution of and the conflict and interference between two or more practices are examined (Nicolini, 2017; Nicolini and Monteiro, 2017).

Nicolini writes about associations and networks of practices; Rahel Jaeggi has taken 'forms of life' – that is, inert ensembles or bundles of social practices that form instances of problem solving – as her object of study (Jaeggi, 2015; 2019). Just like practices, forms of life are to a certain extent inert, and are materialised in institutions and in buildings and spaces, artefacts and tools, bodies and material structures. They enable us to do things in a certain way and set limits to what we can do. They are given as well as created. Jaeggi has described forms of life as 'instances of problem-solving'. They respond to second-order problems and are claimed to be the best possible solutions to those problems. The problems that forms of life attempt to solve are always second-order problems, problems that concern 'the conceptual-cultural resources that a form of life has at its disposal in order to solve first-order problems' (2015: 22–3). They never address 'pure facts', even if they result from a first-order problem. Second-order problems are both encountered and, in a particular way, created by the existing form of life itself. Each form of life that solves problems also creates new ones. Forms of life can be criticised from within, starting from the problems, crises and conflicts that arise within that form of life.

Complexities and complex theorising

Practices of care, help and support are usually complex, dynamic and emergent (Greve and Schnabel, 2011). On the ladder of degrees of complexity, from simple to difficult, wrapped and complicated, to wicked and complex, one crosses an epistemic threshold when one arrives in the category of wicked and certainly complex issues. Then, the usual ways of conceptualising, knowing, ordering, predicting, acting and so forth fall short. This is when advanced modes of muddling through, of incremental learning, of moral imagination combined with a focus on the finality of the institution involved tend to be more helpful. We have to find ways to think about complexity without simplifying, that is, reducing, complexity too much in the way we think, and we must acknowledge what we lose whenever complexity is reduced. Tsoukas has even advocated 'complexifying' our describing, thinking and theorising, because ' "simplified" theories come with a heavy price: they miss the "understanding backwards–living forward" dialectic that critically permeates the lives of those management scholars study' (Tsoukas, 2017: 134). Complex practices, processes and organisations must be thought about in complex ways, ways that give scope to uncertainty, dynamics and emergence. We need concepts and theories that are sensitive to complexity.

Many interdependent factors are often involved in how a patient, client, neighbourhood is doing, in how a physical condition, mental illness, social problem occurs and develops (and sometimes disappears). Cause–effect relationships are often unclear and ambiguous. All kinds of feedback processes are at work. Unexpected developments occur that often cannot be understood and explained as the result of the individual action of an individual factor, nor even as the sum of all the actions or all factors. When the focus shifts in clinical medicine from one-size-fits-all medicine to personalised medicine, or from acute illness to chronic disease, the concept of complexity becomes more necessary and promising (Zimmerman, 2011).

In complex, dynamic and emergent processes, we see good, practically wise professionals handle these processes in such a way that the existing complexity, dynamics and emergence are accounted for and not reduced. In our study of end-of-life care by general practitioners in the Netherlands, we reconstructed that particular practice in such a way as to retain rather than reduce and unduly simplify its complex, dynamic and emergent character (Timmerman and Baart, 2016a) (see also Chapter 11). We saw that general practitioners (GPs) continuously interpret the current situation of the patient through images and stories, recursions to lived reality, and through an imagined synthesis. They perceive the patient's physical situation and complaints, the suffering of the patient and of their relatives. They also perceive themselves, including their emotions. They move with the dynamics of the process and respond to what presents itself. We also saw that GPs do their utmost to anticipate unexpected developments. They have the courage to change course, and sometimes make a leap by deciding to act in a specific way. They remain very close to the moment both in the way they act and in the way they recount how they acted, but they do this without losing sight of the entire process – including everything that has already happened and the point they and their patient are trying to reach.

In order to reconstruct the whole process of end-of-life care by GPs, we had to develop our own vocabulary, grammar and syntax. Central in this reconstruction was the idea that the GP configures, deconfigures and reconfigures the approach they take. They do this on the basis of how they continuously assesses and reassess the nine components in order to be situationally adequate. These configurations are context-, patient- and situation-specific (and GP-dependent) and dynamic. They are accompanied by a process of interpretation through images and narratives, while the GP continuously makes imaginary syntheses: where does this lead and do I evaluate that as something good? GPs regularly make a leap to another configuration or reconfiguration. The configurations are shaped in interaction with the GP's working style, and together they form a trajectory through an imaginary configuration space. This trajectory represents the GP's policy in this particular case.

Professional caring practices are always embedded in caring organisations, which does not mean, however, that professional caregivers do not sometimes have to violate the norms and practices of their organisation to deliver good care. Anyway, in late modernity, caring organisations have become increasingly complex organisations. One of the most complex organisations is probably the hospital (Georgopoulos and Matejko, 1967). Vosman, den Bakker and Weenink have mentioned a

> range of factors that bring about complexity in hospital care. Ongoing specialization is one. […] The upswing of technology in care is a second factor of increasing complexity. […] There is another source of complexity growth […]: societal pressure […] to ensure patient safety, […] to increase transparency of hospital outcomes, […] towards austerity measures. (2016: 119–20)

Vosman and Niemeijer have mentioned 'many kinds of (social) technological systems [that] have been introduced into health care because of the (perceived) demands of society, such as the demand for (more) transparency; but also the demands springing from developments in medicine and demands from patient organizations' (Vosman and Niemeijer, 2017: 471; cf van Heijst, 2011: 172). They point to the caregiver's complex task of what they call 'knitting': the process of sharing information with colleagues with a view to subsequent action (p 470). Managers have the important task to reduce this complexity, but, paradoxically, they also contribute to complexity 'by increasing the pace of work, movements and fluidity in organizational processes' (p 471). Consequently, caregivers and other professionals start 'surfing', 'remain[ing] at surface level, refraining from diving in too deeply into anything, instead preferring to resort to short description(s) and quick solutions, trying to stay on top of things' (p 471). Drawing on scholars such as Schmidt, T. (2017), Vosman and Niemeijer have provided a heuristic working definition of complexity: 'the ongoing confluence of different strivings, governed by different reasonings, all aiming at the sustainment of the organization by permanently changing it' (Vosman and Niemeijer, 2017: 470).

Complexity is also the subject of the so-called 'complexity sciences', a family of theories and theoretical approaches that have been developed since the 1940s and 1950s in five major intellectual traditions.[2] The 'hard science' core of the complexity sciences is made up of mathematical complexity theories, applied and further developed in physics, chemistry and biology. These complexity theories inspired new, complexity-sensitive approaches to medicine, public health, sociology, economics, management studies, psychology, philosophy, education and even morality and ethics. Often, these complexity-sensitive approaches consider their object of study – for example the living body, the living together of human and non-human bodies, healthcare, a care organisation, a population – as complex systems.

Complexity is a real-life phenomenon, but it is also a theoretical concept and an 'ideal of contemporary science' (Le Moigne, in Alhadeff-Jones, 2008: 68). According to Alhadeff-Jones, three generations of theories have emerged since the 1940s, moving from organised complexity to 'organising complexity' (Le Moigne). He has discerned two different paths in the third generation of theories that have emerged since the 1980s: the study of 'complex adaptive systems' and epistemological reflections on the concept of complexity.

Edgar Morin's work on 'complex thought' belongs to the second path. It questions 'the limitations of contemporary processes of knowledge production. [...] [C]omplex thought involves the integration of both the complexity of our identity as human beings ... and the complexity of ethical issues generated by a conception of science understood through its own uncertainty' (Alhadeff-Jones, 2008: 75–6). Instead of disjunction and reduction, complex thought relies on distinction, conjunction and implication. It acknowledges that the interaction between order and disorder is essential to organisation, the interaction between knower and known is essential to knowledge and knowledge construction and the interaction between observation and intervention is essential to research. Complex thought embraces plurality, uncertainty, complexity and ambiguity (Montuori, 2008). According to Tsoukas, complex thought requires an 'open-world ontology' which assumes that the world is always in a process of becoming, a 'performative epistemology' which assumes that knowing is action and a 'poetic praxeology' which sees the practitioner as 'inevitably shaped by the discursive practices he/she is thrown into' and, at the same time, as necessarily shaping 'them back by taking a stand on his/her experience through undertaking purposive action that is relatively opaque in its consequences, variably clear in its motives and desires, and contextually situated' (Tsoukas, 2017: 148). Consequently, conjunctive theorising develops open-ended concepts, sees concepts as being partly defined through practice and looks for 'conceptual novelty spurred by empirical specificity' (p 149).

With regard to the socio-cultural world, complexity as the complexity sciences understand it may be considered an ontological dimension of the object of study, whether in a reductionist sense or in the sense that concepts associated with complexity are considered metaphors or analogies between different levels of organisations. Rosenhead has explored the usefulness of complexity theory as a metaphor, rather than an analogy, for management and leadership (Rosenhead, 1998; Rosenhead et al, 2019). However, complexity can also be considered 'a characteristic attributed by the observer to a phenomenon' in order to deal with the fact that it is impossible to give a complete description of a process or organisation (Alhadeff-Jones, 2008: 77). Finally, complexity can be considered an attribute of collective – as opposed to individual – thinking, especially of the organisation of our thinking. Tsoukas and Hatch (2001) have called this 'second order complexity', and have proposed a narrative approach to organisational complexity, which they have claimed follows the logic of complexity theory itself.

None of these perspectives is free of ambiguities and uncertainties in the definition of complexity, and this is due to the historical development of complexity theories. In addition to this epistemological ambiguity, there is also a socio-cultural ambivalence. On the one hand, complexity-inspired theories have an emancipatory potential, for example because they are critical of traditional modes of organising knowledge (Morin, 2008). On the other hand, such theories also 'carry the potential of perpetuating new forms of intellectual and social alienation' (Lafontaine, in Alhadeff-Jones, 2008: 78) by uncritically applying concepts developed for technological developments to the socio-cultural world. Or by supporting neoliberal ideas of self-organisation and governmental non-interference (Rosenhead, 1998).

Does practice theory suffice or do we need complexity theory?

Care is a complex practice, often performed in complex organisations, and always in a complex world. Complex processes must be conceived in a complex way, and undue simplification must be avoided. If necessary, reductions must not only be judged on their conceptual and practical returns, but also on their costs. So we need practice theory, and we need complexity-sensitive concepts and theories. But do we need complexity theory? What can we understand or do with complexity theory that we cannot understand or do with practice theory? What can we understand or do better with complexity theory than we can with practice theory? And what new problems does using complexity theory cause? Vosman, den Bakker and Weenink, and Bontemps-Hommen, Baart and Vosman prefer practice theory to complexity theory, because the former can 'help to dig up matters of concern to those working and being ill in the hospital organization and … is also capable of capturing issues of complexity and normativity' (Vosman et al, 2016: 118), whereas the latter will not 'help health care professionals, managers and policymakers sufficiently with the moral question […] we have raised, because [it] ignore[s] the moral purpose of medical practices' (Bontemps-Hommen et al, 2019: 96).

In addition to the questions of normativity and morality, there are other issues, of which we will here mention two. The first is addressed by Nicolini when he criticises using the notion of context instead of making 'a more detailed analysis of how the conditions for actions came about' (2012: 234). Instead of talking about a practice and its context, or, for that matter, a system and its environment, he advocates zooming out: 'studying analytically and processually how different practices are associated, and what are the practical implications of their relationships for the practice at hand' (p 234). The second issue is addressed by Vosman when he criticises what he calls 'biolayering' (a term borrowed from Thrift, 2004), buttressing an ethical proposition by referring to the biological constitution of being and of the human being in particular, because it 'distracts from the political, that is, from the actual gathering, chafing, caring and clashing of people' (Vosman, 2023: 36). For these reasons, we prefer practice theory to theories inspired by complexity sciences.

Conclusion

Constructing knowledge is an oscillating movement between doing qualitative research, developing and using theory and reflecting in a care-ethical manner. The conceptual framework in which this is conducted is that of relational caring as a practice. Although we acknowledge the complexities of care and caring, we prefer practice theories to theories inspired by complexity science. We can now continue and present, in Chapter 7, what we call 'the presence-theoretical perspective' and its theorems. It is a further development of the original care-ethical presence theory, which it transcends without replacing the original theory.

7

Presence: the presence-theoretical perspective on relational caring

This last chapter of Part I deals with the care-ethical theory of presence as it has developed since 2001. Before going into the major topics in relational caring that are discussed in the chapters of Part II, we present the presence theory as a presence-theoretical perspective on relational caring, a configuration of diverse 'lenses' with which to look at care practices in healthcare and social work. This configuration and the lenses with which it is configured are flexible, complex heuristic devices that are put together on the spot, as it were.

Qualitative presence-theoretical research since 2001

Since the publication of *A Theory of Presence* (Baart, 2001), the description, analysis, theoretical elaboration and justification of the practice of presence have been received quite positively, including in fields far beyond the realm of pastoral care. The vocabulary of presence has come to be appreciated by social workers, nurses, youth workers, professionals in addiction care, general practitioners, educators and so forth, because it helps them to articulate their own motivation and aims, as well as their frustrations at the way they are increasingly being trained, assessed and managed, and to think and deliberate with colleagues about their work and the issues they face. Since 2001, the practising of presence has been developed horizontally – to other professional domains, situations and issues – and vertically – to leadership, quality of care, the formation of professionals and transitional processes. This was done in concrete, specific practices and in many qualitative studies, both by Andries Baart, his PhD students and others.

Relational caring and its prerequisites were studied in the care of people with a psychiatric background, relating it to such concepts as 'paving the way', 'recovery' and 'contact after treatment'. In her PhD study, 'Paving the way: Making scope for people with a psychiatric background' (in Dutch), Doortje Kal answered the question of how to work on the hospitable reception in community centres and voluntary work of people with psychiatric disabilities. She makes it clear that what appears to be an individual problem is in fact a problem of how we organise society. If we want someone with a psychiatric background to participate in society, then we will have to accommodate, to give in (Kal, 2001). In his PhD study, 'Recovering care: A contribution to a theory and practice of good care', Jean Pierre Wilken analysed narratives of people who had experienced or were still experiencing serious mental health problems. In these narratives, recovery is characterised by instability, moving back and forth, with ups and downs. Two sub-processes constitute recovery. The first is recovery of the self, resulting in awareness of personal assets and competences to take care of personal vulnerability. The second sub-process is social recovery, resulting in participation, valued social roles and meaningful activities. In the stories, associated with good care were the following themes: connecting, understanding, affirming, securing and strengthening. Good care promotes autonomy, by helping the person to become stronger and restoring the ability to exercise control as much as possible, and social inclusion (Wilken, 2010). In her PhD study, 'Aiming at contact: Relational caring and everyday interaction as effective principles in clinical forensic care' (in Dutch), Petra Schaftenaar used qualitative and quantitative methods to study the value and meaning of relational caring in forensic psychiatry. It showed the relevance and value of maintaining contact after treatment and how this as well as relational caring can contribute to reducing criminal recidivism (Schaftenaar, 2018).

Relational caring was also studied in hospital care, relating it to 'attentiveness' and 'practical wisdom'. In her PhD study, 'Dynamics of attentiveness: In care practices at a Dutch oncology ward', Klaartje Klaver developed a grounded theory of caregivers' attentiveness in hospital oncology care. She found nine types of attentiveness, which are characterised by a certain goal and a strategy to achieve that goal. Two factors are decisive to explain the occurrence of the different types of attentiveness: first, is the attentiveness person-oriented or task-oriented? Second, is attentiveness making care possible, organising care, complicating care or making care impossible? Klaver found three cultures of care: self-absorbed, open and relational. The socio-institutional enclosure of the caregiver – the space they experience to break free from the preponderant institutional orientation towards the physical body of the patient – turned out to be significant (Klaver, 2016). In 'The comeback of the patient: Working on professional loving care in hospitals' (in Dutch), various authors report on a transition and research project in a general hospital in the Netherlands (2009–14). The main goal was to observe, interview and converse in groups about how both patients and caregivers conceive of good care and what kind of behaviours may be considered good care. Letters of complaint, learning communities, vulnerability of older patients, a difficult family, concerns, attentiveness were studied (Baart and Vosman, 2015b; see also Vosman and Niemeijer, 2017: 470; Timmerman et al, 2019: 577–8). In her PhD study 'Practical wisdom: The vital core of professionalism in medical practices', Marij Bontemps-Hommen studied the practical wisdom of medical specialists in their everyday practice in a general hospital. The dissertation comprises four qualitative studies, including one of 100 multidisciplinary sessions. This last study shows that medical specialists in hospitals can acquire and develop practical wisdom in their practices through regular, learning-oriented case discussions (Bontemps-Hommen, 2020).

Also in nursing and general practice, relational caring and its prerequisites were studied. In *Nursing and presence: A search in dialogue for the meaning of presence for nursing* (in Dutch), Mieke Grypdonck and Andries Baart investigate what presence practice and theory can mean for nursing and for various nursing specialisms. The common ground of nursing and the practising of presence by outreach chaplains is that they are both about suffering. Attuning one's practice to the care receiver is important not only in palliative care, nursing care for psychiatric patients and care for diabetes patients, for example, but also in emergency care. Even if immediate action is required, starting from the perspective of the care receiver will not only contribute to the lived experience of that care, but also to its medical effectiveness (Baart and Grypdonck, 2008). *Unregulated good: The general practitioner at the bedside of their sick and dying patients* (in Dutch) reports on our research into end-of-life care by general practitioners (GPs) in the Netherlands. We were interested in what GPs perceive and in the things they reflect upon, and how they assess and weigh things, how they act and how they evaluate the process at the bedside of their sick and dying patients. A heuristic use of the concept of 'practical wisdom' turned out to be helpful. Our conviction grew that complex matters should be thought of as complex. So we reconstructed the process of perceiving and so forth of the GPs in a complex way and empirically enriched the concept of practical wisdom (Timmerman and Baart, 2016a; see also Timmerman, Baart and Vosman, 2019: 578 and Chapter 11).

Relational caring was also studied in social work, for example relating it to 'tumpling sensibly'. *Tumpling sensibly: The complex practice of social workers* (in Dutch) reports on a study of the practice of two teams of social professionals in two neighbourhoods in the city of Utrecht. After the decentralisation effected by the Social Support Act in 2015, professionals and clients tried to draw up a profile of the 'new social professional': who are they? What should they be able to do? What do they need? A 'lifeworld team' of professionals from different organisations was set up, and its lifeworld-oriented work was the subject of extensive study. In this study the metaphor of tumpling as a roly-poly toy that rights itself emerges for the social worker who has to be able to give in to all kinds of influences and powers, but also return to their own position and what their profession is about. An awareness of what the finality of your profession is helps to resist everything that pulls and drags on you as a professional (Leest et al, 2018).

Relational caring and its prerequisites were studied in youth care, care for teenage mothers and care for multi-problem families. The research report

Vulnerable but not only vulnerable: About accessing and supporting multi-problem families, vulnerable children and teenage mothers (in Dutch) is based on three pilot studies: (1) a study of how multi-problem families and vulnerable children are reached by professionals who practise presence, (2) a study of how vulnerable children and youth are reached by professionals who practise presence, and (3) a study of the situation of teenage mothers. These studies, especially the first two, show that the practising of presence, when correctly understood, does indeed help to reach people in precarious situations. This requires a professionalism and a management that gives space to relational caring (Baart et al, 2007). In the PhD study 'Honourable young motherhood: A study on the lives of adolescent mothers' (in Dutch), Sabrina Keinemans reports on a qualitative study of the lifeworld of adolescent mothers. Their experiences with pregnancy, motherhood and their relationships with people from their network are described from an inside perspective. In order to theoretically deepen this description, three themes are elaborated: the difficulties young mothers struggle with, the help and support they receive and the lack of recognition they experience. The difficulties faced by these young mothers are not described as problems, but conceptualised as 'ordeals'. Ordeals are accompanied by discrepancies and frictions, characterised by a complex and layered neediness, and experienced as burdensome and heavy (Keinemans, 2010).

Relational caring was also studied in nursing homes, especially in the care for people with dementia, and in a study about how it is to be someone with advanced dementia. In her study 'Relational attunement: With presence enriched nursing home care for people with dementia' (in Dutch), Madeleine Timmermann investigates how the presence approach can enrich care for patients with dementia in nursing homes. The starting point for her reflection was troublesome situations of caregiving, recorded in a nursing home in the context of the Video Interaction Supervision method. Timmermann concludes that looking from a presence perspective draws attention to the fact that care for people with dementia is about standing near to someone and not about treatment, is a continuous search for fine-tuning and is about dealing with suffering in a differentiated way. She also formulates some conceptual recommendations towards presence theory because of what she calls the pathology of dementia. As a consequence, a more momentaneous and more modest in content notion of relationship should be considered. The central location of relational fine-tuning is the body of the person with dementia and in need of care (Timmermann, 2010). *Dementia from within: A search for what it is like to be someone with advanced dementia* (in Dutch) is based on a phenomenological study of what it is like to be someone with advanced dementia who is dependent on residential care. Six residents of two nursing homes were intensively followed for a period of time. Being a person with advanced dementia means both suffering and zest for life, both having a lot of time and not enough time, an outside world that enters the inside world both too much and too little. To navigate this heightened ambiguity for the care receiver as well as the caregiver, more radical relational caring is required. In the care for people with advanced dementia, this means continuing to search together for meaning in the behaviour of the other, realising that information about someone with advanced dementia is always a story told by someone about the person with dementia and the one who is telling the story, and being oneself together in the most familiar way (Leest, Timmerman et al, 2021; cf Timmerman and Leest, 2022).

Relational caring and its prerequisites were also studied in everyday care for people with mental disabilities. In his PhD study, 'The unknown potential of the everyday', Michael Kolen examines the everyday interaction between youths with a mild intellectual disability and the attending care professionals. His empirical research resulted in a typology of that everyday interaction, containing 'broken game' in which the interplay between actors is stifled, 'regulated game', in which the everyday interaction proceeds according to the norms set by the institutional context and 'new game', in which what is at stake for all actors is curated and the interplay of actors results in a new game. Here, the actors together discover new possibilities for good care (Kolen, 2017). In her book *They Can't Say it: About Autonomy and Dependence in Everyday Support for Persons with Severe Intellectual Disability and Behaviour which is Difficult to Understand* (in Dutch), Geertje van der Geest examines everyday care for people with severe intellectual disabilities and behaviour which is difficult to understand and often difficult to handle. In the practice studied, caregivers were always busy interpreting behaviour, 'reading' the person. What do they need now? What do they ask of us? The caregivers tried to find out what the person's interests and capabilities were and to look at the situation from the perspective of the person involved, in order to attune their practice to that person. In everyday practice, van der Geest observed attention to autonomy in many different forms: offering choices, allowing people to experience influence, examining what they want, expanding their lifeworld, promoting ownership of their own body. To make the promotion of relational autonomy possible, two conditions stood out: relational security and knowing the person – as well as possible (van der Geest, 2024).

In these studies, there were always theoretical, conceptual and research methodological issues at stake. For example, about the concepts of attentiveness (Baart, 2004a; Klaver, 2016; Timmerman and Baart, 2016a), concern (Keinemans, 2010; Baart and Vosman, 2015b), autonomy (Wilken, 2010; Timmerman, 2011; van der Geest, 2024; Baart, 2024), practical wisdom (Timmerman and Baart, 2016a; Bontemps-Hommen, 2020) and muddling through (Baart and Carbo, 2013; Leest et al, 2018). Baart's essay *Attentiveness: Studies in presence* (in Dutch) was about attentiveness: what it is, what it does and what it perceives. At its core, it is about the mode of perceiving that is essential to the practising of presence. That mode is determined by being interested, not by being concentrated or focused: can I let it get through to me? (Baart, 2004a). The concept of 'ordeal' (*opgave*) in Keinemans' study is further developed into the concept of 'concern' (*opgave*) (Baart and Vosman, 2015b; see also Olthuis et al, 2014b). In his PhD study, 'With regard to the other: Respect for autonomy and authenticity in pastoral care' (in Dutch), Guus Timmerman reported a case study into personal pastoral care by chaplains working in a parish. It showed how autonomy and authenticity are related and that both are relational concepts. A typology of steersmanship as a metaphor for co-navigating the pastoral process, perceiving the freedom, mobility and self-course of the care receiver, was developed (Timmerman, 2011). The short book *The Care Trap* (in Dutch) explores the phenomenon of the 'care trap': care often does not work properly, goes awry, perpetuates problems and unintentionally makes people go from bad to worse. Three functions of relationality in relational caring are added: the place where the power of professionals is bridled, the continuation of meaningless treatment and intervention is restrained and the perpetuation of need is countered. In the context of how the cultural perpetuation of need and neediness can be countered, Baart introduces the concept of muddling through and the distinction between sentiments, emotions and affects (Baart and Carbo, 2013).

In these studies, also, the theory and practice of qualitative research into relational care was further developed. We especially mention the PhD studies by Timmerman (2011) and Schaftenaar (2018). Timmerman's dissertation contained an analysis of how empirical research, ethical reflections and theory development interact. This analysis has been further developed in later publications (among others, Timmerman and Baart, 2021; see also Chapter 5 of this book). Schaftenaar's dissertation contained a mixed-method study. It showed that patients who received relational care and subsequently were provided with voluntary contact after treatment recidivated later and at a lower rate than patients from two control groups receiving care as usual (Schaftenaar et al, 2018).

Finally, practical issues were also studied, for example relating to transition, formation and quality of care. *Flexible care in an inflexible world: Presence as a strength for transition* (in Dutch) is a study of presence as a transitional power. The project of which it is the result initiated, facilitated and studied a transition trajectory in four locations run by three organisations in long-term care. It concerned a youth healthcare institution, ambulatory counselling of people with cognitive and psychiatric problems, a shelter for homeless families and small-scale housing for people with dementia. The study showed that the practice of presence can be initiated in a structured way. It can be learned, and for professionals exposure is the way of learning it

(Baart et al, 2011). *The comeback of the patient: Working on professional loving care in hospitals* (in Dutch) reports on a transition and research project in a general hospital in the Netherlands (2009–14). In the epilogue, attention is drawn to the separate spheres that caregivers have to deal with, to the phenomenon of repulsive learning in which caregivers absorb new insights and skills but thereby forget older ones, and to the supporting story (about patient-centredness for example) that in fact does not support (Baart, Vosman and others, 2015). *Good care is movement, good care requires movement: Realising, organising and justifying good care at De Hagert* (in Dutch), contains a study by Jan den Bakker of a care facility run by two organisations, one that provides care to people with dementia and one that provides care to people with intellectual disabilities. The care provided at this facility is highly valued. At the same time tensions exist between the daily realisation of good care and its organisation and accountability for it. Relational caring must be supplemented with relational collaboration, relational leadership, relational management and relational design. If simply following rules does not lead to good care, then space can be sought in the rules themselves. Den Bakker distinguishes three interacting main processes in good care: realising, organising and accounting-for. Accounting-for is about providing insight into the care provided by caregivers and forming an image of the care provided by managers, directors, administrators and others (den Bakker, 2018).

Presence-theoretical theorems as heuristic devices

Practices of care, help and support are complex, dynamic and emergent. We have to find ways to think about real-life complexity without reducing this unnecessarily and while acknowledging what we lose due to reduction. We must think about complex processes, practices and organisations in complex ways. One way to bring complexity into our theoretical reflection on professional practices of care, help and support, and indeed on other relational activities in civil society, is to speak not of subtheories, but of critical insights, theoretical concepts or 'theorems'. We use the term theorem as denoting theoretical configurations which mediate between theory and practice and which also serve a heuristic purpose. Theorems articulate something about good care, help and support, they help to perceive and inquire into care and so forth, they contribute to the promotion of good care and so on, and they are themselves supplemented, criticised, adapted and further developed in the process. In sum, they are heuristic devices (Vosman and Niemeijer, 2017).

We present seven such theorems in this chapter, describing them briefly so as to emphasise that they are flexible, complex heuristic tools that are put together on the spot, as it were. They should not be regarded as the topics of the following chapters, in Part II. They are operative in each of these chapters, but in some more so than in others.

These theorems demonstrate that relational caring is not just about knowing how to act, but above all about founding, maintaining and managing a practice. Together, they form a larger theoretical configuration that offers a presence-theoretical perspective on relational caring. This presence-theoretical perspective is a 'sensorium', consisting of different heuristic devices, which can be adjusted to what the issue or research at hand needs. Using the metaphor of sight, it could be called a set of binoculars or a microscope that is fitted with various lenses and lens systems that are assembled in the field, as the needs and possibilities of the issue, the field and the interests at hand dictate.

Unbiased, careful perception

The theorem of unbiased, careful perception is based on hermeneutic benevolence. It has a critical wonder as its main characteristic, a conscious and reflexive change of perspective and the willingness to 'expose' oneself to the lifeworld and the lives of those concerned.

Relational handling

The theorem of relational handling accounts for the double character of relationships: founding and maintaining a relationship are instrumental, but they are also an 'expressionate act'. It is essential to connect with, and attune your practice to, the lifeworld, the life course, the longing and the 'concerns' of the other. Otherwise, the caregiver and care receiver are likely to be a mismatch. The relationship must honour, acknowledge and confirm the vulnerable other. This theorem can be considered a specific operationalisation of the more generic conceptual framework of relational caring as a practice.

Staying-with

The theorem of staying-with stipulates that the other must never be left to their own devices, even when their suffering or situation is hopeless, even when they prove difficult to access or are violent. Staying-with is essential, since the person who leaves the other prematurely adds to the suffering; and what is 'premature' is determined by the feedback of the other. It is also essential because, in complex situations, it is often the case that nothing can be done other than lean back and try to understand, in the hope of finding new possibilities.

Restraint

The theorem of restraint states that the professional can be moved, physically, mentally and socially, by the movements of the other person. It is about the ability to be attentive and sensitive to serious problems within small everyday activities (Baart and Vosman, 2011: 187).

Attentiveness

The theorem of attentiveness stresses the importance of genuine interest in the other, a sensitivity not only to the other person's request for help and to the 'request behind the request', but also to the other person's longing and to their tacit appeal embodied by the other The professional also takes a metaphorical position in the informal network of the other person (for example, as a friend), and reacts to their own emotional and moral involvement with self-care and reflection.

Professional power or powerlessness

The theorem of professional power or powerlessness is about a powerlessness that must sometimes be endured, and a power that must never be exercised in a manner that maintains or perpetuates the neediness of the other (Baart and Carbo, 2013). It must always be exercised as a 'sensible and loving muddling through', in the perspective of the 'broken good'.

Quality awareness

The theorem of quality awareness states that professionals must always ask themselves the following questions, both privately and in the context of small learning communities: what is the purpose or the tenor of what we are doing here and now? This question as to the finality of the practice must be answered by proposing not only an idea of 'accountable care', but also an idea of good care that is determined in qualitative terms, for example by narrative methods and by carefully 'perceiving in detail' (*klein kijken*). Navigating in complex practices requires practical wisdom.

Conclusion

The presence-theoretical perspective is a flexible, emergent, dynamic configuration of presence-theoretical theorems, which themselves are flexible, emergent, dynamic configurations of empirically grounded theoretical concepts, within the conceptual framework of relational caring as a practice (Figure 7.1). Depending on the situation, the issue and the persons, and their relationships and mutual responsibilities and what is at stake for each of them, one or more theorems will be more to the fore than the others. They all apply at all times, however, and sometimes it is helpful to bring certain theorems that are in the background to the fore

Figure 7.1: Presence-theoretical perspective on the practising of presence

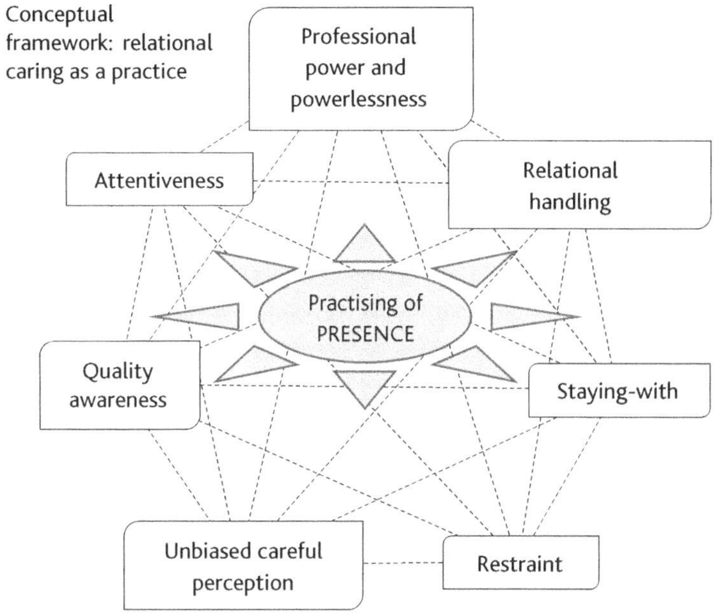

again. Depending on the issue, the situation and so on, these theorems emerge and interact with each other in different configurations. In a way, this configuration is the more complex, more dynamic and more emergent variant of the 2001 theory of presence presented in Chapter 4 (compare Figure 7.1 with Figure 4.1).

PART II

Major topics in relational caring

PART II

Major topics in relational caring

8

The socio-political consequences of relational caring

Motto

In healthcare and social work, the political issue of the formal and informal organisation of our society is always also involved.

CASE FRAGMENT 8.1

The crossbowman

On 17 September 2021, K. stabs two people to death. With the same knife with which he previously attempted suicide during a psychotic episode, he violently kills his 70-year-old downstairs neighbour in her apartment. He also kills her 52-year-old cousin. A nurse, who had just put an infusion on the elderly woman, manages to flee via the balcony. Back in his apartment, K. shoots at the police, who have now been summoned, with a crossbow. He misses. A police officer shoots him down. K. survives and has been imprisoned in a prison psychiatric ward ever since. A court declares him completely insane and imposes a TBS (Hospital Order) with compulsory treatment. The Public Prosecutor is appealing.

Less than three weeks earlier, K. had been arrested by police after taking cat food from a supermarket without paying for it, making a fuss, wrestling with officers and yelling 'I'm from hell' and 'My soldiers will sort it out'.

In his file, the police read that K. had attempted suicide on New Year's Eve that year. He had been under the influence of LSD and alcohol and had been in a psychotic state, it was later determined. The police, alerted by a report, had found all kinds of weaponry in K.'s apartment. Possession in itself was not an offence. The officers had handed him over to the paramedics and left it at that.

At the police station, police officers try to communicate with K. He's on his knees in the cell, his face against the floor, his hands out in front of him. He doesn't respond to anything. Inquiries at the hospital where he was taken after his suicide attempt yield no information about aftercare. Although he had been seen once by the hospital psychiatrist during his admission, his rehabilitation had consisted only of physiotherapy. The next day, new police officers are briefed about K. One of the officers is an old acquaintance of K. He once received martial arts training from him and tells his colleagues that he was always a normal nice guy who never got involved. K. is called 'psychotic' and 'extremely dangerous'.

That same day, a psychiatrist and a psychiatric nurse from the crisis service visit. They also do not manage to communicate with K., who only makes some hand gestures. They let the police know that K. is too erratic and too violent to place him in their mental health institution. Because K. has no criminal record and has committed only a minor crime, the police let him go. He receives no advice. Police officers try to make contact with K. in the days that follow, but they fail. One time, local residents see him walking naked in the park at night. Another time, he is seen on all fours, barking at a dog.

Until that fatal day.[1]

This was not the first time someone has died from the 'misunderstood behaviour' of a 'confused person'. In 2014, U. murdered former Minister of Health Els Borst. In 2015, an investigative report by the Hoekstra Committee in response to that case concluded that mental healthcare institutions had been forced by the government between conflicting demands: providing more safety with less money and fewer resources. In 2008, the mandatory risk excess was introduced in the healthcare sector, raising the threshold for requesting or accepting help. Care institutions that do try to offer unsolicited help are often not reimbursed for this. In 2015, far-reaching decentralisations were implemented, and at the same time cutbacks were made. Many shelters were closed, while at the same time less money was spent on ambulatory care. Since those decentralisations, the ministries involved no longer know how many shelters there are for people with complex disorders and for confused people. There are many agencies involved in the care of these people. They are all responsible for a small part, but there is no overview. The current government places the full responsibility for the number of shelters with the market. Interference care has deteriorated to such an extent that it often fails to materialise. Until the patient – whom one can call 'confused', but who has actually become 'lost' – has become a perpetrator.

What does it mean for society if presence and relational caring are acknowledged and promoted as the core of professional care, help and support? And how does this influence the demands on politics? We will first discuss care ethics as the background of presence and relational caring. Taken as a political theory, care ethics supports the political implications of presence and relational caring. Then we will discuss how presence theory extends the concrete involvement of the professional who practises presence to the political level. Next, we will address presence as a political counter-programme and the political task of relationally caring professionals and organisations. We will conclude the chapter by addressing a crucial element in presence theory, the experience of social redundancy, and connecting it with the concept of precarisation.

Background: care ethics as political theory

Presence is at the core of good care in healthcare and social care. Care ethics – at least the political take on care ethics that we endorse – regards care as a political category (Brugère, 2019). Care is political in the sense of 'the political' – the actual, formal and informal organisation of society and the determination of what happens or does not happen, in cooperation, friction and struggle – not necessarily, and in fact mostly not, in the sense of 'politics' – party politics and the formal practices of representative democracy (cf Mouffe, 2005). Care is 'about living together, as hard as it becomes, in concrete caring practices that are nested into political contexts' (den Uijl, 2022: 201). First-wave feminism took a stand against the exclusive association of women with insignificant care work, and second-wave feminism attempted to make the economic value of care visible, but care ethics started by rehabilitating care as a moral category. First-generation care ethicists such as Carol Gilligan, Nel Noddings and Sara Ruddick associated care with relational work in the lives of women and men, foregrounding vulnerability, dependence and interdependence into consideration (Gilligan, 1982; Noddings, 1984; Ruddick, 1989). The catchwords of this first wave of care ethics were relationship, vulnerability, emotion and context. From the start, care ethics was also an epistemology, which asked what and whose knowledge counts (Vosman, 2016). Second-generation care ethicists, especially the political theorist Joan Tronto but also Marian Barnes and Selma Sevenhuijsen, started to develop a concept of care as a political category and of care ethics as a political theory (Tronto, 1993; Barnes, 1997; Sevenhuijsen, 1998). Care ethicists began to recognise and acknowledge that caring and receiving care are constitutive to society. Furthermore, care began to be regarded as a practice more than as a principle or disposition or emotion. And, as a practice, care is embedded in and intersected by other practices, and entails conflict, requires all kinds of resources and is both particular and universal. In her book *Moral Boundaries*, Tronto explained that care ethics transcends the boundaries between morality and politics, between detached and relational ways of moral judgement, between private and public life. According to her, good care requires an 'integrated' care process (Tronto, 1993; Olthuis et al, 2014a).

Regarding care ethics as a political ethics means recognising and acknowledging that care practices shore up, bear, shape and support the lives of people and their living and working together – society, in one word. The way society is organised both facilitates and fails to facilitate caring practices. Caring practices can contribute to humanising the way society is organised and managed. In her book *Caring Democracy*, Tronto developed a conception of democracy in which all voices are brought to the table to assign and negotiate caring responsibilities (Tronto, 2013). Tronto has been criticised for being too idealistic, for failing to face complex, ambiguous and messy reality, for being too normative about responsibility, for limiting her understanding of power to the Weberian concept of domination and for not sufficiently taking conflict and struggle into consideration (including by van Heijst, 2011; Engster and Hamington, 2015; Vosman, 2020; den Uijl, 2022). Building on Tronto, Daniel Engster has pointed out that care ethics still has to transcend the boundary between in-groups and out-groups, between 'us' and 'them' (Engster, 2018). And Tiina Vaittinen has directed the attention of care ethics to the political meaning of the 'vulnerable body', especially that of the marginalised care receiver (Vaittinen, 2015).

A political interpretation of care ethics takes a special interest in ordinary, everyday practices of care and in how these are embedded in political practices of domination, action in concert, power structures and hegemony. Much of the care provided in society takes place in everyday life and must benefit the care receiver in their everyday life. What good care is, is discovered in ordinary, everyday practices of care, including in hospital and residential care (Laugier, 2009; Barnes, 2012).

Inspired by the thinking of our late colleague Frans Vosman, we espouse a political interpretation of care ethics. For Vosman, care ethics is bound by the anguish of the world, by the trials and tribulations of groups of people, organisations, national and supranational institutions, by their burning issues. In care ethics, attention for the relational aspects of care should be complemented by the notion of 'position', which is related to 'honour' (with regard to very old persons: Vosman and Baart, 2010). In caring and receiving care, people find themselves in relationships, they enter into relationships, or refuse to do so. But they also find themselves in positions, they assign positions to others and positions are assigned to them. Any attempt to stress responsibility as a duty should critically reflect on the fact that it is liable to become intersected by a neoliberal discourse of responsibilisation. Beyond criticising neoliberalism (Biebricher, 2021) and its use of care (Tronto, 2017; Brugère, 2019: 68–74), care ethicists have to look at how concepts and ideas derived from neoliberalism have an effect on actual practices of care in healthcare and social welfare. This helps to clarify issues that professionals and their managers encounter in the practices in which they work, which they manage and for which they make policies (Vosman and Baart, 2017; Timmerman, 2019; Baart, 2021a).

According to Vosman, caring and receiving care are much more ambiguous than is often realised, including by care ethicists. Care must be perceived as 'a mixed practice, marked from the start not only by moral aspects and the directly physical, technical, material, and institutional aspects, but also by violence' (Vosman, 2020: 36). Giving and undergoing care involve potential conflict. While it should postpone any moralising, care ethics should attend to the layer that underlies actual caring and receiving of care, that is, the layer of encountering one another as embodied people, and of starting to relate to one another and of ordering these relationships in various ways. This layer includes 'bearings ranging from understanding and love via the central uncertainty and the opaque to chafing, struggle, battle and war' (Vosman et al, 2018: 414). This is an argument for connecting care ethics with political phenomenology (Vosman, 2018) and for doing political-phenomenological empirical research. In his valedictory lecture, Vosman invited care ethics to orient itself to 'surviving' as a form of life rather than to the pursuit of a 'successful' life, which is the late modern, bourgeois version of 'the good life'. Surviving is about people who have to endure permanent 'steepness', difficulty and heaviness in everyday life (Vosman, 2023). It relates to the notion of experiencing social redundancy, a topic to which we will return later in this chapter.

From concrete involvement to policy and politics

In the original study in which presence theory was developed, the basic problem to which the practice in question was responding was the experience of social redundancy: 'I am not needed, I am of no value. The sooner I disappear, the better. I am a burden, a redundant thing.' As explained in Chapter 4, social redundancy is a multidimensional concept of poverty in an experiential-participatory discourse (see Table 4.1). This redundancy was phenomenologically reconstructed in the following request for help: 'Does it matter (1) to you (2) that this (3) always (4) happens to me (5) here (6) in this way (7); that it hurts (8) and that it should end (9)?' (see Chapter 4). This phenomenologically reconstructed question was subsequently analysed from the perspective of the tensions it entails, professional viability and so forth. In the last step of the analysis, each of these elements was matched with a specific political claim or, to put it differently: with normative criteria for good, just and 'careful' politics and government policy. This ideal-typical request for help was thus 'translated' into political criteria for good care. Politics should enable, respect and safeguard care receivers' rights, their access to phronetic professionals, their unique identity, lived coherence of life, political power and influence, their situatedness, means, facilities and knowledge, their voice and language, and their time, rhythm and meaning (see Table 4.2).

The professional who practices presence responds affirmatively to the ideal-typical request for help mentioned earlier, and follows it up by making nine concrete commitments, which are sustained up to the political level. Being present (*present zijn*) in the lifeworld and lives of residents, clients, patients and pupils must be followed up by presenting (*present stellen*) the care receivers' lives and concerns at the political level, with the professional acting as a witness who testifies, an amplifier of the voice of people who do not speak easily and whose voice is seldom heard at that level, and as an advocate of their cause.

Policy making requires translation. The experience of care receivers and caregivers, the care receivers' concerns and the 'front-line' caregivers' concrete involvement have to be translated if policy is to make a difference in the lives of care receivers and caregivers. Translation involves, for example, removing local characteristics, generalising, positioning a case in a larger whole, reducing it to an assumed, preferably simple and unambiguous core, relating it to other things that require attention, and bringing it within a hierarchy, removing unreasonableness and emotionality, and assigning it to specific disciplines. Whenever this process threatens to do injustice to the residents, clients, patients or pupils with and for whom the professionals who practise presence work, then they must oppose this translation by presenting their clients' lives and concerns at the level of the policy makers.

Presence as a counter-programme

Presence is a form of cultural critique. It is a political, moral and epistemological counter-programme that contributes to the empowerment of those who care for others, as well as those who are cared for. And it can also act as a motor for organisational transitions (Baart et al, 2011). The presence-theoretical perspective criticises an ideology that contends that the world is malleable, that frailty and vulnerability can be removed and that care and help can ignore tragedy. Presence and relational caring oppose hyper interventionism: 'Many are busy with you, but few are looking after you' (Baart, 2011),[2] and help to prevent the bureaucratic perpetuation of suffering (Baart, 2013). Presence theory also stresses the importance of addressing the finality or inherent end of the practice on which the care, help and support are based (see Chapter 10). In youth work, for example, it would make a huge difference if 'being able to flourish' were to be acknowledged as its finality, instead of safety, as is now often the case. Although we do not espouse teleology, we consider the question of the *telos* of a caring practice as essential and argue that it should be answered in terms of solicitude and not solely or preferably in terms of problem solving.

Presence theory considers the caring relationship to be a steering principle. It invites professionals to use their person, knowledge and practical wisdom critically, including their ability to navigate powerlessness. To counterbalance the increasingly methodological orientation, standardisation and protocolisation of the way professionals act, the differentiation of work and the bureaucratisation of the organisation, presence theory suggests focusing on integrated, relational work. This means, for instance, that skilled professionals must navigate their own emotions, engage in normative, reflexive self-control and moral deliberation, and it also includes development and use of the knowledge that the persons who are being cared for and their relatives have. Incorporating patient and family knowledge curbs the 'epistemic paternalism' of the professional, diminishes 'epistemic injustice' and promotes a more just distribution of 'epistemic authority' (Fricker, 2007; Brister, 2012; Dotson, 2012). Being aware of cultural differences is conducive to promoting 'cognitive justice' (de Sousa Santos, 2018).

This requires professionals to engage in a process of continuing formation in communities of practice, in which they learn to observe openly, unbiasedly and attentively, to receive education, to undergo exposure, to critically examine and strengthen their knowledge, to complement it and develop it further (see Chapter 13). Their task is also political, as it requires contributing to and criticising both formally and informally organised society. This task includes making one's own professional logic accessible for citizens, understanding the implications of and criticising government policy, opposing the individualisation of societal issues, giving residents, patients, clients and pupils a voice, also within the professionals' own organisation, presenting the care receivers' lives and concerns, including in public debate, and developing professional alternatives. This should be done not only by individual professionals but also by teams, organisations and the profession at large (cf de Jonge, 2015; 2018).

However, if presence and relational caring are to stand a chance within any organisation, this requires management that leaves the professionals both discretionary and systemic 'space to try things out' (*scharrelruimte*), including room for relationship-oriented, loving and reasonable 'muddling through' (Baart, 2013). Also, it means that persons who work in management, sit on the board, work in supervisory authorities or as financiers must undergo a deep learning process. Care organisations also have the political task to criticise governmental policies that subvert presence and relational caring, even 'if some things appear […] inevitable from the perspective of the individual organization' (den Uijl, 2022: 297).

Our political take on care ethics and political phenomenology informs our awareness of power, not only as domination (Weber) but also as action in concert (Arendt), as power structures (Foucault) and hegemony (Gramsci) (den Uijl, 2022). Deeply rooted powers are always already ensconced in every concrete care practice, disciplining the way participants act, both caregivers and care receivers. These powers consist of people in positions and unequal relationships, of groups of people working together, of compulsory procedures, rules and routines, and also of discourses about care, care receivers and about what is 'normal'. The distribution of care and caring responsibilities reproduces an unequal society in which certain categories of people deserve care and others do not, and certain categories of people are predominantly the carers while others claim to be shielded from the responsibilities of caring ('privileged irresponsibility', Tronto, 2013: 103–6).

This distribution of care and caring responsibilities is internally connected with the distribution of power, of precarity and of recognition. To counteract these connections and to reach the people in need who rarely receive care or are reluctant to receive care, it is wise to have 'presence workers' in neighbourhoods, residential care homes and other places where people live together, that is, professionals who practise presence and who have no other task than to connect with and attune their practice to residents, clients, patients and pupils, build relationships with and between them, and discover, together with them, what can and must be done.

Social redundancy and precarisation

The presence-theoretical perspective addresses social redundancy and precarity, and criticises neoliberalisation practices, the entanglement of discourses about care with neoliberal ideas, and precarisation and its normalisation as an instrument of governance (Vosman and Baart, 2017; Baart, 2021a).

As we have already discussed in this chapter, presence is a response to the experience of social redundancy. This experience is the subjective, phenomenological side of the phenomena designated by concepts such as vulnerability, dependency, poverty, marginalisation, exclusion, injustice and indigence. We have noted earlier that this experiential concept is also political. On the basis of a vast amount of literature (including Bourdieu, 1998; Castel, 2003; Standing, 2011; Marchart, 2013; Lorey, 2015), we conceptualise the objective, analytical aspect of these phenomena as 'precarity'. Talking about precarity means talking about negative circumstances, about 'problems'. Talking about the experience of social redundancy means talking about negative experiences, about 'sufferings'. Precarity is related to a lack of economic and social security, and the experience of social redundancy is related to a lack of social and political recognition. It is helpful for care ethics to complement the concept of precarity with that of the experience of social redundancy, because it makes clear what is at stake and embodies an appeal to which care is the appropriate response (Baart, 2021a). This focus on the experience of social redundancy signifies an ideological critique of a political theory or a care ethics in which the situation of people in precarious conditions is perceived only externally, in terms of problems rather than sufferings.

Precarity and the experience of social redundancy are related to the concepts of 'precariousness' and 'precarisation'. Precariousness is the ordinary, inevitable human vulnerability that is inescapably embedded in social arrangements (Butler, 2004). When a political community constructs this precariousness as a threat against which it wants to be 'immunised', it attempts to 'compensate' for it, resulting in the precarity of particular groups within this community (Lorey, 2015). This production of precarity is called precarisation. It is mediated by processes of 'othering', in which members of groups that do not meet the norm begin to be perceived and treated as abnormal, threatening 'others'. When this precarisation becomes a constant, broadly accepted, culturally supported, pervasive and self-extending process that has no other purpose than to govern, it becomes normalised. Precarisation as an effective mechanism to discipline and govern others and oneself then becomes a normal political instrument (Lorey, 2015). The normalisation of precarisation is caused by various destabilising processes: deregulation of the economy on the national, supranational and global levels, flexibilisation of the labour market, individualisation and de-traditionalisation of society and culture, climate change, social acceleration (Rosa, 2013). Its consequences for the lived lives of people are that it increases social insecurity (Wacquant, 2009), liquifies social arrangements (Bauman, 2007) and gives rise to a risk society (Beck, 1992).

In late modern Western societies (not in the Global South, see Millar, 2017; Baart, 2018a), the powerful forces of precarisation are, at least partially, compensated by the provisions of the so-called welfare state. By providing, augmenting and facilitating different forms of 'capital' – economic, social, cultural and personal (Bourdieu, 1983; 1986) – the welfare society helps precarious people to survive and, hopefully, improve their conditions of life. But these different forms of capital offer opportunities for a good life only to people who have the capabilities required to seize these opportunities, to do and be what they have reason to value (Sen, 1985).

The problem with the welfare state's compensating mechanisms is that they are characterised by the same conditions that they try to compensate. Organisations that provide care, help and support tend to reproduce the same rationality that is dominant in the legitimisation of neoliberalisation processes: self-government, competition, transparency on expected outcomes, responsibilisation, self-improvement (Bröckling, 2007; Leibfried and Mau, 2008). This reproduction of precarisation is enabled by the ambiguity of many ideologically motivated compensation mechanisms. For example, the late modern ideal of self-reliance, self-government and self-care involves emancipation and diminishing paternalism, on the one hand, but the dismantling of solidarity and the introduction of new forms of privileged carelessness, on the other. To give another example: stimulating participation, informal care and volunteering means empowering people and strengthening civil society, on the one hand, and withdrawing professional care and help, on the other, instead utilising volunteers as free labour forces, often straitjacketing professionals and sometimes penalising those who do not assume their share of informal care. Presence and relational caring, when informed by a critical analysis of neoliberalisation

Figure 8.1: Overview of relevant concepts relating to precarity

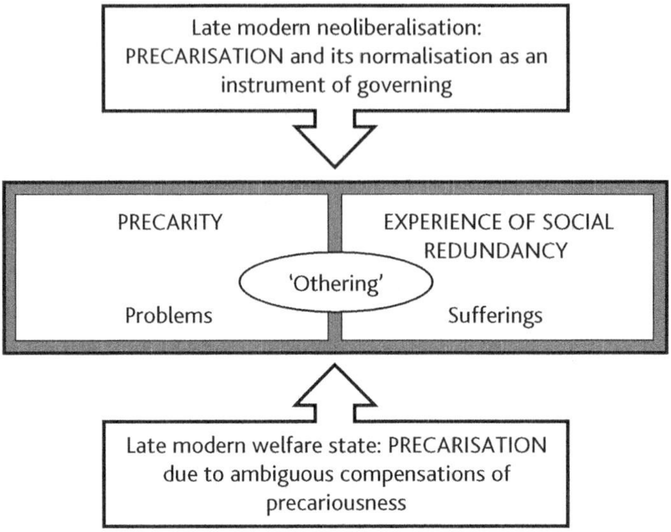

Source: Adapted from Baart, 2021a: 103

and precarisation, try to evade or subvert this mechanism (Baart, 2017; Timmerman, 2019).

Figure 8.1 summarises the discussion up to now in a map in which ontological and empirical terms – precariousness and precarity – static and dynamic concepts – precarity and precarisation – and two balancing powers that both produce precarity – neoliberalisation and the welfare state – are related to one another.

Conclusion

The political purport of presence and relational caring is strengthened by a political take on care ethics and political phenomenology, one that is interested in ordinary, everyday practices that are embedded in political practices of domination, action in concert, power structures and hegemony. The concrete involvement of professionals who practise presence has consequences all the way up to the political level. Relationally caring professionals and organisations have a political task, in the first place to present their care receivers' lives and concerns at the political level. Presence and relational caring are a counter-programme that opposes hyper interventionism and offers an alternative to ignoring tragedy. We argue that presence workers should be sent to neighbourhoods, residential care homes and other places where people live together. Focusing on the experience of social redundancy makes it possible to perceive the situation, or people in precarious conditions, not only from the outside, in terms of problems, but also from the inside, in terms of sufferings. All this requires a broad, public and political debate about good care, help and support, about what is conducive to a 'decent society', understood as a society whose institutions do not humiliate citizens (Margalit, 1996), and about how that can be financed.

9

Opening oneself up and staying open to the other or others

Motto

The other is a human being who has to be recognised and acknowledged as a member of the human family, who therefore deserves relational and social inclusion.

CASE FRAGMENT 9.1

'Listen, observe and shut your mouth!'

In the 1940s, the Brazilian psychiatrist Nise da Silveira (1905–99) returned to work in a psychiatric hospital in the outskirts of Rio de Janeiro. She refused to work with the – at the time – innovative methods of electroshocks and lobotomy for the treatment of schizophrenics. As a consequence, her colleagues left her to do occupational therapy, where she started a revolution by inviting the patients to draw, paint and interact with pets. Roberto Berliner made a docudrama about her called *Nise: The Heart of Madness* (2015). In this film, we see Da Silveira, played by Glória Pires, welcoming her new patients in a spacious room. The two nurses assisting her seem confused by Da Silveira's approach. Da Silveira says to one of them, a man, 'Ouça, observe, cale a boca! O que eles falam aqui tèm que ser uma educação. É a nossa matèria prima. Ouça, observe, cale a sua boca! (Listen, observe and be quiet. What they say is meaningful. It is the start of our work. Listen, observe and shut your mouth)'.

A central presupposition of the presence-theoretical perspective on relational caring – one that it has in common with care ethics in general[1] – is that no one should be left to their own devices, especially when they are in need. The other is *a* human being who must be recognised and acknowledged as a member of the one human family and who therefore deserves relational and social inclusion. However, the other is also *another* human being: like me but also different from me. The similarities between the other and me enable me to do something meaningful with and for the other. But the differences mean that I cannot take for granted that what I do will indeed be meaningful and helpful to the other, even if it would be meaningful and helpful to me. In one way or another, and to the extent that this is possible, I must see and try to understand the other *in their otherness*. But this otherness may, and in fact to some degree always will, escape my understanding. There will always be a surplus of meaning in my understanding of what the other experiences, does, undergoes, says, shows, indicates. 'In their otherness' means that the other is always beyond what I allow them to be. The other is not an extension of my own categories. 'In their otherness' also means: however sick, mentally ill, deformed, dirty, foul-smelling, unattainable, aggressive or violent the other may be, they are worthy to be seen and relationally and socially included.

Because I must try to understand the other in their otherness and, at the same time, this otherness will always to some degree escape my understanding, we regard the following points as essential to our presence-theoretical perspective. Relational caring fundamentally starts with and permanently revolves around:

1. unbiased, open, careful perceiving of the other in their own relational network, in their contact with other professionals, in their situation and context, including the institutional context;
2. faithfully staying-with the other in their relational network, both literally and metaphorically;
3. regardful attentiveness towards the other and their concerns;
4. permanent inquiry; and
5. the 'letting' mode.

We consider open perception, staying-with, attentiveness and permanent inquiry to be related prerequisites for good care, help and support because the bottom line of these things is that the other is not left alone, but included, both relationally and socially. I can still stay with the other – both literally and metaphorically – even if their problem cannot be solved, their illness cured, their health restored, their need alleviated or their situation improved, and even if the other is inaccessible. Turning away from the other means 'adding further suffering' (van Heijst, 2011: 9–11). Relational caring begins, continues and ends with perceiving, staying-with, attentiveness and inquiry. Extending this openness into the practising of relational caring is what the 'letting' mode is about. These five aspects are the subjects of this chapter, which has multiple connections with and references to other chapters, especially the next one, about relationality and finality (Chapter 10). This chapter addresses a fundamental moral conviction that underlies relational caring: the other in their unique otherness really matters. In a sense, this chapter lays the moral foundation for the following chapters.

In this chapter, as in subsequent chapters, we will say a lot about what professionals should do or should not do. This is not because the theory says so. Basically, we pass on what we have seen in the practices of professionals who are seen as good professionals by clients and colleagues. We know of the struggles that front-line professionals currently endure in the Global North, and their frustrations about not having enough time to attend to each of their clients, patients or pupils as they think necessary (see Chapter 8). However, we have seen the value of the stepping stones we offer in this and subsequent chapters in concrete practices.

Perceiving and imagining – for a purpose

I must see and try to understand the other in their otherness if I am to be meaningful and helpful to them. This requires that I perceive the other, in their relational network, as openly, attentively and carefully as possible, and as free of bias and prejudice and of my own personal concerns as I possibly can. It requires that I perceive the other and their situation with my complete sensorium, with all my senses. Seeing not only the other's behaviour, sitting in a chair and drinking coffee, but also their non-verbal responses, including muscular tension. Hearing not only what the other is saying, but also the unconscious sounds they make, and the noise from the street. Smelling not only what is dominant, but also the subtler scents of body odour, good or spoiled food, fresh coffee or coffee that has been simmering for hours. Feeling not only whether it is hot or cold in the room, but also that the chair is hard or soft, what texture something has, whether it is sticky and so on. Sensing not only how the other is feeling but also the awkwardness of a situation, the alienation of holding a formal meeting, or the expropriation of the other's story by the person who does the intake. All these senses must be used simultaneously, so that I notice, for example, that 'the chocolate offered to you is of high quality, despite being served on a grubby plate pulled out from under a chair' (Beurskens et al, 2019: 57).

If I must see and understand the other in their otherness, I must use my imagination: what would it be like for this particular human being to experience this or that (not to be noticed, or to be abandoned by someone, for example), to be treated in this or that way, to have to do this or that by themselves? This is what I must do as a professional: use my imagination, in the context of my profession and team, of the organisation and the institution in which I work, of the available time and budget. Perceiving and imagining are always situated: they always happen in a specific interaction, practice, situation, organisation, institution and society. There are many circumstances and influences that keep professionals from perceiving the other without bias; circumstances and influences that necessarily have to do not only with who I have become as an embodied, gendered person, but also with professional, organisational and institutional requirements – and even with the dominant discourse in our society about care, help and support. Perceiving in a way that is as free of bias, as open and as careful as possible is an ability that has to be learned, trained, developed and maintained – and enabled, facilitated and protected by the organisation and its management. It also requires courage. Nevertheless, however unbiased, open and careful I may be, the other in their otherness will always to some degree escape my perception and understanding. I can only do my best and keep trying. Dedication is key in this context.

CASE FRAGMENT 9.2

'Who is this?'

A team of professionals work for an organisation that cares for the homeless. The homeless they deal with often avoid care, are generally addicted to substance abuse and often suffer from psychiatric disorders. The team have gathered today in what they call a 'practice meeting' to reflect on their work. One of the team members, Annemiek, asks permission to introduce a case, and Dick, a social-psychiatric nurse who is chairing the meetings, agrees.

Dick:	Go ahead.
Annemiek:	Well, it's about a 69-year-old paranoid alcoholic, with an IQ of 75, probably addicted to illegally obtained Tramazole, Oxazepam, Zopiclone and ...
Dick:	Who is this?
Annemiek:	Um, I thought we weren't going to mention names here?
Dick:	I'm not interested in their name, I'm just asking: who is this?
Annemiek:	That's what I'm trying to say ... a 69-year-old paranoid alcoholic, with an IQ of 75, probably addicted to illegally ...
Dick:	Who is this?
Annemiek:	Sorry, I don't get you ... a 69-year-old paranoid alcoholic, with an IQ of 75, probably addicted to illegally ...
Dick:	My question is: who is this?
Annemiek:	You don't mean: what's wrong? Well, his name is Roel, he is Amira's grandfather and he's very fond of her ...
Dick:	Go on![2]

Because the other, as another human being, is worthy of being included, relationally and socially, and helped, they have to be perceived, metaphorically speaking, in their depth, length and height: not only the explicit request for help, but also what is often called 'the request behind the request': the other's implicit needs and desires, their longing, which is often not so easily articulated. But also their pride, resilience and strength, their knowing how to live (*savoir vivre*) and survive – even in difficult situations in which I would probably not survive (see Case fragment 9.2). To prevent reducing the other to the self, the other must be perceived in their otherness and, as much as possible, from their own perspective. To prevent self-referentiality – the tendency to refer only to my own framework, intentions, disciplinary approaches and so on – while assuming that the other is a competent meaning-giving actor, I must reconstruct and understand the other's lifeworld, situation, fears and concerns, longings and prospects, and the meanings these have for them, in their own logic. Perceiving in this sense is not the same thing as sorting and categorising – 'physically sick', 'mentally ill', 'socially deviant' – or diagnosing in the sense of classifying into predetermined categories – however helpful classifications such as those of the DSM (*Diagnostic and Statistical Manual of Mental Disorders*) and ICF (*International Classification of Functioning, Disability and Health*) may be. It is also different from simply noticing and acknowledging the stories and narratives the other tells.

In our study into the end-of-life care by general practitioners (GPs), we discovered that the GPs have different, complementary ways of determining the pain and suffering of their patients. They not only categorise cognitively, based on a taxonomy of physical, mental, social and existential suffering. They also perceive positionally, based on their social and physical nearness to the patient. They not only see and hear the patient, they experience through all their senses. They also have to deal with culturally determined expectations about what they have to do – relieving all the suffering, for example. And the GPs, in the context of the requirements for euthanasia by a physician not to be a criminal offence, have to relate what they perceive and experience to what the patient communicates about the unbearableness of their suffering (Timmerman and Baart, 2016a).

Perceiving in a way that is as unbiased, open and careful as possible requires regardfulness, attentiveness and wonder. Regardfulness – regarding the other as someone who is worthy to be perceived, understood and relationally and socially included – enables the other to come forward and show themselves. Regardfulness in this sense requires self-examination and dedication. Attentiveness – being interested in the other, in their smallness and greatness, in how they appear and in their concerns – enables the professional to become aware of the other in their otherness. This goes beyond 'instrumental' attention, and it requires a genuine interest in the other. Wonder – wondering critically but benevolently about the other in their situation and given their prospects – enables the professional to be surprised by the otherness of the other, their pride and strength as well as their weakness and frailty. Wonder is also a critique of the idea that I already know what is the case, who the other is and what should be done. In this sense, wonder is both an invitation and a critique at the same time (Verhoeven, 1972).

Several mechanisms can make it difficult to perceive in a manner that is as unbiased, open and careful as possible. I perceive the other while I am on a specific assignment. I perceive the other from my own cultural standards, with my professional and experiential knowledge or on the basis of a diagnostic label. Or I perceive the other through the lens of my expectations, or of the assumption that the other 'is not willing'. My perception of the other may also be influenced by psychological mechanisms, by what society expects from professionals, or by themes that play a role in public and political debate, such as 'participation' and 'safety' (Beurskens et al, 2019: 63–7).

As a professional, my ability to perceive the other openly and unbiasedly can be promoted by continuously practising changes of perspective, and by the presence-theoretical version of exposure. Practising changes of perspective is not the same thing as being empathic and identifying with the other's perspective. It means, first, putting myself in the other person's position in my imagination (putting myself in the other person's shoes, Chavel, 2011); second, perceiving and imagining the situation at hand, or the treatment the other is receiving, or their prospects, from the other person's perspective (looking through the other person's eyes – more precisely: looking from the other person's position); third, returning in my imagination to my own position and, finally, realising or finding out what I have to do or refrain from doing in response to what I have understood about the other's predicament. Or, at least, understanding that it is different from what I thought before the exercise.

Exposure is a supervised exercise in which I immerse myself thoroughly, methodically and intentionally in the situation, context or practice in question and the lifeworld of the persons involved in these, by taking up a position close to their position. The aim of exposure is to experience a radical change of perspective, to become sensitive to and able to tolerate what is different and strange in the situation, context or practice, to reflectively struggle with my own ideals, intentions and aims, on the one hand, and my pre-understandings, misconceptions and intuitions, on the other, and to acquire tacit knowing of the situation, practice or context. Exposure may result in a different moral view, because I have come to better understand the meaning and significance of what the people involved experience in everyday life, and their needs and concerns. As a formational resource, exposure may contribute to a wider range of registers: not only to professional competences but also to attitudinal aspects, different approaches, different views on how to do something and different perspectives (see Chapter 13). In the practice of relational caring as we understand it, exposure is not only a precursor to, or a way of entering into, this practice but it is also the permanent, professional and basic attitude of the relational caring professional (Baart, 2001: 209–82; Baart et al, 2011: 138–46; Vanlaere et al, 2012, 2016; Beurskens et al, 2019: 163–5; du Plessis and Beurskens, 2021).

Faithfully staying with the other

To be there *for* the other presupposes being *with* the other, which is a central insight of the presence approach as presented in Chapter 3. Or, as Mahatma

Gandhi once put it, 'Whatever you do for me but without me, you do against me'. If another human being is in need, leaving them alone means extending suffering and adding harm. Suffering – the inside perspective of having physical, mental or social troubles – often has a kernel of loneliness,[3] and abandonment would add to that suffering. If someone experiences social redundancy, abandonment by those from whom they expect care, help, support or protection (or effective policy) would add to their suffering. Being responsive to the situation and to the needs, concerns and longings of the other starts with being with the other, and continues with staying with the other, physically and mentally, literally and metaphorically. 'Physically and literally' means: near the other, in their proximity, touchable, addressable. 'Mentally and metaphorically' means: accessible, concerned with the other, connected with and attuned to their lifeworld (see Chapter 10). Being with the other also means: not objectifying the other, treating them as 'types' or 'cases'.[4] Furthermore, the other is not required to meet additional criteria to receive care, such as that their need must not have been caused by their own actions, or that they must adhere to agreements made, even if that is part of their problem. We reject the old Malthusian idea that those who need government aid to survive are in some way responsible for their own plight (Dean, 2013). We are concerned about what action researcher and public administration scholar Albert-Jan Kruiter has called the 'entry-exit paradox': precisely what gives someone access to care – certain behaviour, a disorder or illness – causes the necessary treatment or facility to be stopped.

Being and staying with the other in this sense is more than forming the initial intention not to leave the other. It is an attitude that is maintained throughout, a continuous activity of commitment – some would call it a virtue. Being faithful is the basis for being reliable. It presupposes that I do not consider vulnerability a disvalue, a condition that must be made to disappear, and regard suffering as something that should be ended or, if that is impossible or too expensive in terms of time and budget, ignored. Even if suffering continues and hope ceases, this does not end the need for care, in whatever form. Even then, it is necessary to stay with the other and accept tragedy as part of life. Life is not malleable. Staying with the other is a matter of decency; it is a decent response to need – 'decent' in the sense of not humiliating (Margalit, 1996). Annelies van Heijst has used a term coined by Ginters to describe staying with the other as an 'expressionate act' (*Ausdruckshandlung*). It expresses the 'dedicated connectedness' with the other and the other's worth. Expressionate acts are valuable in themselves, their value lies in what is expressed and in the person who does the expressing (van Heijst, 2011: 119–23). In essence, staying with the other belongs to the economy of the gift, in which both the professional and the resident, client or patient give freely; the professional's giving sometimes awakens certain needs for the first time (Baart, 2001: 628; cf Yan, 2005).

Staying with the other comes in various forms. It starts, even in strictly arranged situations with clearly defined roles and responsibilities, with just being around physically, familiarising myself with the lifeworld of the other and offering companionship. This can take hours, or just a few minutes, for example during consultation with a doctor.[5] If the offer of companionship is accepted, or at least not rejected, staying-with can take several forms, depending on situation, interaction, profession, organisation and so forth. Staying-with becomes even more essential if the other's situation cannot be improved, which is more often the case than many professionals in care, help and support like to think (Case fragment 9.3). Even if nothing can be done, it is still possible to keep the other person company, to console them and abide with them, to help them endure suffering. It starts with enduring the sight of the other person's suffering and seeing the work the other does to obtain care, help or support, witnessing it. This can also entail sending a postcard or a text message showing interest and compassion. If the other shows behaviour that cannot be tolerated, especially when it harms other people, staying-with means: rejecting that behaviour, but never rejecting the person. It may be necessary to educate the other.

CASE FRAGMENT 9.3

Again and again

Church and community worker Ellen repeatedly accompanies local resident Roosje to the police to report various instances of assault and rape. But Roosje habitually invites complete strangers to her home because she is lonely and just wants to have some fun. In these moments, she seems to forget completely what happened the previous time. Yet Ellen continues to stay with her, talk to her, offer her comfort. It is Roosje's life, even if it is sometimes incomprehensible to Ellen and she just thinks it is stupid.[6]

Staying with the other also means that care, help and support cannot be terminated unilaterally. Of course, budgets and time are always limited and people should not become alienated from their own lifeworld by an unnecessarily long stay in an institution, but self-referentially terminating care adds harm. Care has to be faithfully completed.[7] Completing care means, first of all: checking the benefit experienced by asking feedback from the other and their relatives. Second, it means: verifying if, and, if so, under what conditions, handing back care and caring responsibilities to the other and to their network is possible. This is not the place to critically discuss the current societal discourse of 'self-care' and 'informal care' in relation to governmental budget cuts in the Netherlands (see Chapter 8), but perpetuating need by prematurely ending care adds suffering and harm. Third, completing care also means: building networks in which people care for each other, and building communities that organise and support care for themselves and for others. Fourth, completing care means: contributing to an inclusive society in which there is room and scope for people who are not very independent and self-reliant and, more generally, for people who do not meet the criteria of what is currently considered 'normal'. Finally, completing care also means: presenting the lives and concerns of care receivers at the political level, if they cannot do this themselves; putting responsibility where it belongs.

Regardful attentiveness

In our presence-theoretical perspective, care is about the other human being and about a caring relationship with them, and for this reason perceiving and staying-with have a specific quality. One way to thematise this quality is to think about and study attentiveness (Baart, 2004a; Klaver, 2016; Timmerman and Baart, 2016a).[8] Much research is being done in psychology and cognitive science, but this is mostly limited to selective, focused and often short-term attention. There are, however, many other kinds of attentiveness that each have their own merits: open, unfocused attention, sustained, long-term attention, divided attention, dwelling attention, vigilant attention and so forth (Baart, 2004a). In fact, attentiveness has many layers and, in order to contribute to good care, the attentive professional must navigate many tensions, such as that between a narrow focus on the problem and a broad interest in the person, between attention as instrumental to good care and attention as something that is in itself beneficial to the other, or between concentration that must not be broken and the fact that the other may point the attention to something different than the professional had in mind. There are also modes of attentiveness that a relationally caring professional must avoid; for example, attentiveness that has the intention to pin the other down or manipulate them, attentiveness that the other must earn and can subsequently lose, and attentiveness without taking responsibility.

Klaartje Klaver's participant observation study of attentiveness in an oncology ward produced many insights about attentiveness that are also relevant to other contexts (Klaver, 2016). We will mention three of them here. The first is that attentiveness is something that happens between caregiver and care receiver in their context. The caregiver may help the care receiver by being open and transparent about what they perceive, what issue they are focused on at the time and the possible gap between the two. But the momentary connection between caregiver and care receiver also determines whether there can be an attentiveness that is conducive to good care for them (Klaver and Baart, 2011). The second is that being attentive in a hospital is strongly influenced by the culture of caring in that hospital. If caregivers are to be attentive, rather than just 'produce attention', they must manage what Klaver calls their 'socio-institutional enclosure' (Klaver and Baart, 2016b: Timmerman and Baart, 2016b: 141–3). Modern hospitals tend to see the biological, physical side of their patients as their core business. The extent to which caregivers are either locked into the logic of these hospitals or feel free to look beyond it largely determines how attentive they are (Klaver and Baart, 2016a). The third insight we wish to mention is that attentiveness is not about understanding the other completely, because the other always escapes our understanding to some degree.

Our study on end-of-life care by GPs similarly taught us a number of things about attentiveness (Timmerman and Baart, 2016a). The distinction between 'focus' and 'margin' is well known in the literature on the phenomenology of consciousness and attentiveness. Attentiveness is seen as a kind of spotlight. We found that we needed to distinguish between what we called 'focus', 'scopus' and the 'wider context' (cf Arvidson's distinction between 'theme', 'thematic context' and 'margin', Arvidson, 2006). If we use the theatre as a metaphor, the focus is what is in the spotlights, and the scopus is everything else on stage that is relevant to perceiving, understanding and doing justice to that which is in the spotlights. The stage itself, the backdrop, the wings, the curtain and the spotlights themselves, the people backstage, as well as the auditorium and the audience form the wider context. It is important to understand that there is no focus without scopus. For a caregiver, the care receiver and the care receiver's concerns are in what we call their 'focus'. But other people and their concerns can be in the focus too. People and issues that are first in the caregiver's scopus can, so to say, migrate to the focus and vice versa. Relational caring implies that the caregiver also explores and maps the people around the care receiver to find out what is and should be in their focus and scopus (Case fragment 9.4).

CASE FRAGMENT 9.4

Children who are minors

A GP based in the urbanised countryside of the Netherlands is asked to take care of a woman who is terminally ill and has been transferred to a hospice in the GP's town. At the first meeting she is told that the patient wants euthanasia. The GP is prepared to perform euthanasia, but discovers that the patient has children who are minors. Their father passed away a year earlier. The patient also has a mother and a brother. The patient does not want her mother to visit to say goodbye to her, and her brother does not want to come if his mother is not allowed to. The GP, who is of the same age as the patient and is also a mother, decides not to perform euthanasia, for the sake of the children. For the same reason, she also decides to let the children's grandmother visit to say goodbye to their mother, but without disturbing the patient. The GP feels responsibility for the children because they are minors. She does not feel responsibility for the patient's mother or brother. The GP's decisions regarding her responsibilities towards different

> people are at odds with the emphasis in Dutch law, which is that the physician has a responsibility to one person only, the patient.[9]

In addition to focus and scopus, the wider context is important too, the wider context not just of the care receiver and the people around them, but also of the caregivers themselves: their colleagues, the agreements and rules of their organisation and profession, legal provisions and the requirement of public accountability. The caregivers themselves are also present in the wider context. For example, their memories about other situations and other care receivers are part of this context. In this sense, the subject of attentiveness is not the opposite of the object of attentiveness – as the metaphor of attentiveness as a spotlight illustrates.

The focus, the scopus and the relationship between them are not fixed. They are found iteratively and tentatively, and they can change. The caregiver can broaden or narrow the focus. The scopus can become more or less relevant. The distinction between focus, scopus and the wider context is not only relevant to the question of who and what receives the caregiver's attention. Our study on end-of-life care by GPs taught us that this distinction is also relevant to the following questions: (a) for whom does the caregiver feel responsible, (b) for whom do they take responsibility, (c) who is actually receiving their care, (d) whom do they involve in their deliberations and (e) to whom are they willing to be accountable (see Case fragment 9.4). This means that normative and moral elements must be added to the concept of attentiveness (Timmerman and Baart, 2016a).

The core of careful attentiveness is regardfulness, a genuine interest in the other as a worthy and valuable human being. Being attentive means not only being responsive to the request for help that they articulate, but also being sensitive to the other's implicit needs and desires, concerns and longings, the appeal that proceeds from them. Receiving this kind of attentiveness is in itself beneficent: it means relational inclusion, recognition and consolation. Being attentive in this sense is also an expressionate act, an act that expresses dedicated connectedness with the other and the other's worth. Acting and relationality coincide. This dimension is what makes regardful attentiveness more than attentively perceiving the other. The professional not only perceives the other but, by perceiving them, also, so to speak, 'elects' them to be recognised, relationally included and consoled. It counteracts the experience of being socially redundant.

Attentiveness is a relational concept. Trying to be attentive to someone who does not come forward and show themselves is not enough. We discovered in our research that what the professional can do is to position themselves 'metaphorically', that is, to position themselves in the informal relational network of the other, fulfilling a specific metaphorical role. Or, to put it differently, to allow themselves to be metaphorically positioned in the other's informal relational network. This means becoming *like* a friend, a neighbour, a sister, a father, a counsellor and so on, without actually becoming a friend, neighbour, sister, father, counsellor and so on. This is possible because the professional is 'inscribable', so that the care receiver can project their needs onto that position. Metaphorical positioning is related to, but different from, transference and countertransference. The professional who occupies a metaphorical position enables the other to show themselves, with their requests, concerns, longings and appeal, and enables the professional to perceive and understand what the other is showing and articulating about themselves and their requests, longings and appeal. At some point, this metaphorical position is abandoned and handed back to the other person's relational network.

Instead of exercising 'professional distance', as professionals are often advised or even required to do, we suggest that they should practise professionally committed nearness. Professionally committed nearness means working 'with distance', not 'at a distance', to borrow a distinction made by Stoopendaal (2008) regarding the daily work of healthcare executives. To prevent identification with the other and their predicament, professionals must navigate both distance and involvement, not avoid emotional involvement at any costs. If the professional is to avoid ultimately abandoning the other, their professionally committed nearness must be accompanied by reflection and self-reflection, and they must attend to taking care of themselves also within the caring relationship itself (see Chapter 11).

Permanent inquiry

Relational caring permanently requires 'inquiry'. A relational caring professional starts from the position of not-knowing. They must find out who the other is today, what their needs, concerns and longings are today, what their relational network looks like today, what the institution and the organisation want them to do or to refrain from doing today, and, given their own condition and actual possibilities, who they themselves can be to the other today. This requires unconditional willingness to explore and, in consequence, open and unbiased perceiving of, faithfully staying with and regardful attentiveness to the other. Inquiry is a process of continuous exploratory investigation in practice, an undertaking which is at the same time a continuous learning process. It is different from scholarly research, to the extent that research is associated with certain subject–object presuppositions. By contrast, in inquiry the inquirer is personally implicated. Inquiry is embedded in what John Dewey called a 'community of inquiry' (Lipman, 2003).

Inquiry as we espouse it is marked by attentiveness, wonder, criticism and self-reflection. It requires interested attentiveness, which itself depends on both personal qualities and institutional arrangements. It also requires openness and a welcoming receptivity to what is new and unexpected, including aspects that are strange or that bother or even threaten the inquirer. Inquiry also needs curiosity and inquisitiveness (Berlyne, 1960). Finally, inquiry cannot be exercised without an attitude of wonder which is critical of received concepts, categories and names (Verhoeven, 1972). Inquiry is focused on practical wisdom, and is fuelled by recurrent exposure.

Inquiry combines elements of inquiry-based learning (Pedaste et al, 2015), heuristic inquiry (Moustakas, 1990; Kenny, 2012), appreciative inquiry (Cooperrider, 2013), therapeutic inquiry (van der Hart et al, 2006) and moral inquiry (Johnson, 1993; Kekes, 2006; Chavel, 2011). It is driven by the inquirer's own questions and its aim is for the inquirer to learn by trying to answer these. But it is also critical of the inquirer's capabilities and the quality of their sources. Inquiry is inspired by the phenomenological tradition of research of lived experience. It starts with a personal interest in the other and in what their situation means to them, a meaning that can be found only if the inquirer immerses themselves in the situation. Inquiry does not necessarily start with problems and difficulties and is not satisfied with the other person saying: 'I'm not able to do that'. It is primarily interested in the strengths, potentialities and resources of people and the possibilities of change for the better. But it is also realistic. One of the aims of inquiry is that the inquirer may open themselves up to what is at stake and to what is new and unexpected. Finally, inquiry means contributing to a repertoire of possibilities for thinking and acting from which those can draw who practise moral imagination, the 'ability to imaginatively discern various possibilities for acting in a given situation and to envision the potential help and harm that are likely to result from a given action' (Johnson, 1993: 202). Moral imagination requires the ability to see the other as myself and myself as the other, to practise a change of perspective, to imagine the other and their situation as constituting an appeal to me, to morally reflect on my own actions and decisions (including decisions to refrain from acting) and to cultivate my sources of moral capital. Moral imagination can be cultivated especially by art and literature.

The letting mode

Unbiased perceiving, faithfully staying-with, regardful attentiveness and permanent inquiry give the other scope in their otherness. This openness is not abandoned when the relationally caring professional starts to act. It is extended, so to say, into the practice of presence and relational caring itself. That is what the 'letting' mode is about: leaving the initiative to the other, letting oneself be moved by the other, moving along with the other (see 'A typology of practices' in Chapter 4). The acting of the relational caring professional is guided by the other and by how they move, both physically, mentally and socially. This letting mode is not the same as inactivity and passivity. The opposite of letting is not acting, but 'making'. The 'making' mode is a way of acting in which the professional is the main person who determines when and how to act, what the operational goals, duration and nature of the relationship will be and what the outcome should be. The professional steers and takes the lead. In the letting mode, it is mainly the other who determines the direction, nature and duration of the relationship. The professional may offer a possible perspective or an alternative, but does not pursue their own goals. Far from sitting on their hands, professionals who practise the letting mode are usually very active (Case fragment 9.5).

CASE FRAGMENT 9.5

'Sitting on my hands'

'Last week my 80-year-old neighbour spontaneously knocked on my door. We've known each other for 15 years. She came in and we talked. I could see it did her good; but that hasn't always been the case. In the 15 years that we have known each other, I always felt very sorry for my neighbour. I tried everything: I wanted to arrange help for her, or take her somewhere so she could meet others. So that she would be less lonely. But she didn't want any of that: she didn't trust help and other people might judge her because her stepson had done things that made her look bad. I cared about the situation. It frustrated me, but I also noticed that I kept coming up with solutions, which caused the contact to run aground: an uncomfortable situation. Then I started sitting on my hands more. I found that she preferred me to listen and ask questions than to solve her problems. For example, she would tell me proudly how she manages the household alone. I now understand that the problems as I saw them are different for her. I am only now getting to know my neighbour, because I am with her without an agenda, I listen more and connect with what she says. She talks about her childhood and I see her beaming more after every visit. I notice what it is like to just be there: that also gives me peace. Every time I visit her now, I notice that the contact is deeper. The contact is equal, and the mutual trust feels good. I like it that I now feel like I can do more for her.'[10]

There are different modes of acting in the letting mode; we will mention five (Leest, 2016a; 2016b; Beurskens et al, 2019: 103–5). The first is *to watch over the other*, for example when the professional cannot do much to solve the problem because it would jeopardise the relationship, while deterioration, abuse or getting stuck are real risks. Another mode is *to be a witness to the life of the other* and thereby to confirm, to the other or to third parties, what happens in that life, both the things that are going well and the things that are going badly, both successes and injustices. This can be beneficial to the other, as it can be helpful in contacts with authorities. A third mode of acting in the letting mode is *to give in, to accommodate* in order to give the other scope. This allows the other to come forward, show themselves, take the stage. A fourth and fifth mode are *to accompany the other* wherever they go and *to undergo what they undergo*. For example, to accompany the other in their journey past various authorities and to undergo the long wait, the being sent from pillar to post, the difficulty of getting to places for those who are physically handicapped, the humiliation at the counter. It may move the professional to address the troubles they experienced when being present in the other's life at a higher level: in the organisation involved or at the municipality. This may be difficult, near to impossible, for many professionals, but we have seen how it prevents mismatches (as in Case fragment 9.5). And it enables professionals to stay near in such a way that potential turning points in the other person's life can be developed.

The letting mode is a conscious, morally reasoned form of giving scope to the other by giving in, in order to understand better what the good is that should be pursued. But it is always open to the transition, for a purpose, to the making mode.

Conclusion

Our moral conviction is that the other must be recognised and acknowledged as a member of the one human family and therefore deserves to be included both relationally and socially. Abandoning and leaving the other, literally or metaphorically, especially those in need of care, prolongs suffering and adds harm. But, as another human being, the other will always to some degree escape my understanding. Therefore, good care requires professionals to open themselves up and stay open to the other through perceiving as unbiasedly, as openly and as carefully as possible, through faithfully staying with them, through regardful attentiveness to them and through permanent inquiry. Relational caring starts, continues and ends with these interconnected activities. They in turn require what we have described earlier as metaphorical positioning, the use of the professional's complete sensorium, their moral imagination, their dedication and regardfulness, faithfulness and wonder. Recurrent exposure fuels this attitude of opening oneself up and staying open. This openness serves a purpose: good care. And it must be extended into the practising of presence and relational caring through the letting mode, through giving the other scope in the way the professional acts.

10

Relational caring: relationality and finality

Motto

In – the regularly occurring – case that the professional does not immediately know what to do, they should start to work relationally. When new ground has to be broken, professionals would do well to think collectively about what their practice is about, what it is ultimately aimed at.

CASE FRAGMENT 10.1

Different from mere custodial work

Luke works as a custodian in a major teaching hospital. One time, he cleaned a comatose young patient's room. The patient's father, who had been keeping a vigil for months, had gone out to smoke a cigarette and hadn't seen Luke cleaning the room. When he came back he snapped at Luke and accused him of not cleaning the room. At first, Luke got defensive, and was going to argue with him, but then he just cleaned the room again. When asked why he did it again, Luke explained: 'Yeah, I cleaned it so that he could see me cleaning it ... I can understand how he could be. It was like six months that his son was here. He'd be a little frustrated, and so I cleaned it again.' When asked to talk about his job, Luke related stories that told the researchers that his 'official' duties were only one part of his real job. Another, central, part of his job was to make the patients and their families feel comfortable, to cheer them up when they were down, to encourage them and divert them from their pain, to give them a willing ear if they felt like talking. Luke aimed to do something different from mere custodial work.[1]

Relational caring is not a 'principled' approach to caring, an approach in which caring is steered and evaluated by principles coming from outside the practice itself as sources of action – principles such as equality, trust, reciprocity, traceability, joint ownership and role clarity. However valuable these principles may be, the source of action in relational caring is the idea of a specific good that emerges from within the relational network in which caregivers and care receivers find themselves and interact with each other (cf Habran and Battard, 2019). Two intertwined concepts are therefore essential: relationality and

Figure 10.1: Relational caring, defined by relationality and finality

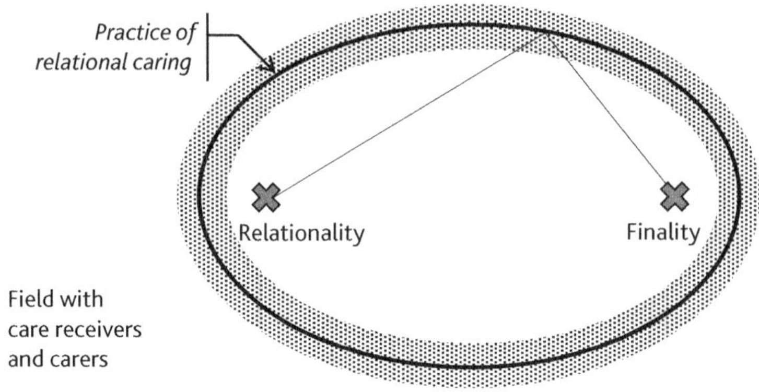

Note: Relational caring is defined by relationality and finality, not as principles but more as two point of reference, like the two focal points of an ellips. In mathematics, an ellipse is a plane curve surrounding two focal points in such a way that for all points on the curve, the sum of the two distances to the focal points is a constant. The consequence is that the farther away one is from one of the two focal points, the closer one is to the other. The closer the two foci are to each other, the more the ellipse is like a circle. The analogy suggests that an action can be everywhere on the plane but the closest it is to the ellipse (signified by the shaded areas), the more it is an instance of relational caring. Where on the ellipse an action of a relationally caring professional is situated may depend, on among other things, on the urgency of the issue, assessed on the basis of discipline-specific knowledge.

Taking the analogy of the ellipse a step further, the characteristics of a particular profession can be related to the 'distance' between the two points of reference. This distance is small in a profession like that of the outreach chaplains in the 2001 study, where the professional is present in the lifeworld of the residents and finality is more determined by relationality, and large in a profession like that of a highly specialised heart surgeon, where the patient comes to the hospital and relationality is, in most cases, more dominated by finality.

finality, not as principles but more as two points of reference, like the two focal points of an ellipse (Figure 10.1). The concrete form relational caring may take depends on the concrete context, on the care receivers and carers involved, and on the nature and urgency of the issue at hand.

Relationality is about who participates, how they are positioned and how they position themselves and each other, what happens in the interaction between them, and what this means to them. In a weak sense of relationality, caring relationships are conceived of as merely conditional or instrumental to good care, and not as themselves a good and an integral part of good care. It is an essential aspect of relationality in a 'strong' sense that what happens, emerges and is discovered in relationships between caregivers, care receivers and the persons around them has real consequences for what is done and to what end, and not only *how* it is done. Relationality also has consequences for how the context, the situation and the persons within the situation are perceived. And vice versa: relationality is always situated.

Finality is about the ultimate end of the practice, also from a historical perspective, and about what the participants actually aim at in what they do, as distinct from what they set as their goal. Finality must not be understood as a fixed *telos*, fixed by nature or by God, or as the operational goals set by partakers in the practice or by the organisation that sustains the practice. An essential aspect of finality in a strong sense is that the specific aim of the practice cannot be determined without considering the concrete relationships between caregivers, care receivers, the persons around them and their lifeworld, life course, concerns and so forth. A good relationship is a good in itself.

These two points of reference and our conception of them make our idea of relational caring a radical notion. This radicalism makes it unique and means it has comprehensive and far-reaching consequences, as we will elucidate and argue in this chapter.

First point of reference: relationality

When a professional in healthcare or social work knows immediately what to do in a particular situation and context, the best thing is probably to act straight away. Especially when the urgency is high and the issue is not contested, and an evidence-based protocol is available. But situations in which a care professional immediately knows what to do occur much less frequently than a lot of professionals, their managers and most people tend to think. Issues are usually not that simple. Often, it is worthwhile to think twice. And in cases in which professionals do not know immediately and indubitably what to do, they are best advised to start to work relationally rather than self-referentially (in the sense of starting from and sticking to their professional frames of reference, however proven and sensible these may be).[2] In this chapter, we will present a view on the relationality of care that is much more radical than that as it exists within theories about the care relationship, the therapeutic alliance or the working alliance (Rogers, 1957; Bordin, 1979; Kozar and Day, 2012). Similarly, we take the importance and relevance of relationality more seriously than theories about patient-centred care (Balint, 1969; Stewart, 2001), person-centred care (Kitwood, 1997; Mitchell and Agnelli, 2015; Tieu and Matthews, 2024) and relationship-centred or relationship-based care (Tresolini and Pew-Fetze Task Force, 1994; Malloch et al, 2000; Wyer, Alves Silva et al, 2014) do. We think it is important to appreciate and foster the caring relationship and its contribution to good care. But we have found that a focus on the relationship is too narrow (Baart, 2018c: 74–6). In fact, our inquiries into practices of good care are gradually radicalising our relational thinking about care. This radicalisation is necessary in order to perceive and think about good care, about why care receivers benefit from it and how it can be promoted. Our search in this chapter is therefore for a concept of care, help and support as a practice of 'relational caring' – using 'caring', a gerund, instead of 'care', a noun, to designate the dynamic and emergent character of care as a practice. We will start by looking more closely at a story from a chaplain in outreach pastoral care that shows relational caring in detail (paragraphs are numbered to assist in later discussion).[3]

CASE FRAGMENT 10.2

Elif and her tonsils

13-year-old Elif has had a sore throat and a bad breath for some time now. I talk to the playground manager about this and we both think her tonsils are the problem. [1]

I ask Elif whether she has been to the doctor and she answers that the doctor removed something from her and that someone was supposed to call back but that her mother is always forgetting. She is in a lot of pain and is being bullied at school. I suggest she should just make the call herself. She does this on the playground in my presence. The assistant says it is important that she make an appointment with the doctor and that she can come that afternoon if she wants. [2]

She wants to, but her mother is not at home. She calls her at a relative's house and asks if she can go to the doctor with me. She gets permission to do this. [3]

As we ride the bike, with her on the back seat, I rehearse together with her what she will say to the doctor, what she will ask. I think of the kinds of things the doctor might reply, and the responses she will have to give. Even though it is scary for her, she speaks to the doctor herself. (...) [4]

She is given a referral to the ENT (ear, nose and throat) doctor and Elif asks if I will go with her again: 'My mother doesn't speak Dutch, she is no use to me.' I say I would do that if her parents think it is a good idea too, or that I could come along with her mother. [5]

The first time I go with her. The doctor confirms that it would be best to operate on her tonsils, but that they need permission from the parents. So we go back to this doctor again, with her mother. [6]

She is operated a few weeks later and is brought and taken home by her parents. I go to visit her when she is back home. She is very happy that she won't be in pain anymore, but especially that children at school can no longer say they don't want to sit next to her because she stinks. [7]

What do we see here? It is a minor story, but told in great detail. It is a story about removing tonsils and about teaching a 13-year-old girl some basic skills. And about rejection and isolation, pain, fear and inability, and an absent mother.[4] But what interests us is another, third, meaningful layer in this story. It is striking that the underlying problems of isolation, pain and the absent mother are hardly addressed in anything the chaplain says. They *are* addressed in what the chaplain *does*, but in a very specific way.

The first thing to note is that the chaplain is apparently in a position to notice that the girl has bad breath. And she does not only notice it, but also talks about it with Elif and does something about it. This three-tiered approach, noticing–thematising–reworking, ultimately leads to the girl being socially included again. The girl's loneliness is noticed and alleviated through a temporary relationship with the chaplain.

How does this relationship develop? The chaplain asks the girl to call the doctor herself. She makes the action of calling the doctor look small and safe: 'just call' and 'in my presence' [2]. The doctor wants to see the girl, with her mother. However, the girl's illiterate mother of Turkish descent is not only omissive [2], but also absent [3]. The girl trusts the chaplain enough to ask her to take up her mother's role, and to come with her immediately. The chaplain temporarily takes the mother's position, in terms of both availability and task. And this happens with the mother's approval. It is worthwhile to look for a moment at how the chaplain tells this part of the story: 'She (...) asks if she can go to the doctor with me. She gets permission to do this' [3]. It reminds us of the way mothers allow their children to go play with one of their friends. It could be said that the chaplain is presented as a kind of peer, which is particularly remarkable because the girl's peers have rejected her because of her bad breath. This is the second position the chaplain takes. She takes a third position, very briefly: that of an imaginary physician, rehearsing together with Elif what she is going to say and ask [4].

The doctor refers the girl to a specialist and the girl asks the chaplain to go with her. It is interesting to note that the chaplain is asked to go in the position of her mother, as can be inferred from the girl's explanation that her real mother is of no use to her [5]. Again, the chaplain responds with a double message: yes, I will do that for you but I'm not going to exclude your mother. Given how isolated the girl is, further exclusion must be avoided. This can be interpreted as the chaplain correcting the girl. The chaplain will come along with the mother, not the other way around. The parental position remains intact. Through this inclusion of the mother, the mother is included (through her daughter) in the network of current relationships.

After the girl's first visit to the ENT doctor together with the chaplain, the role of the mother begins to grow again [6–7]. The chaplain leaves the position of mother and returns it to the girl's mother. The last visit takes place at the girl's home, and it confirms what the whole story was about: being included again. The chaplain positioned herself alongside the girl, the very place no one else wanted to be because of the odour. She hands back that particular spot to the girl's classmates: the odour has disappeared together with the pain. Elif can be included again [7].

This case fragment is one of many fragments that were presented to the researcher by this chaplain in outreach pastoral care. As the researcher analysed all these fragments and tried to figure out what this kind of work is about, an image began to emerge of relational caring and what it yields. This professional's work is generally characterised by apparently insignificant everydayness. But its meaning lies beyond itself. She is intent on establishing a relationship with the persons she works with and for, whether or not this will be successful or fully developed. As soon as a relationship has been established, the chaplain allows her actions to be steered by what emerges as a good within that relationship. Whenever possible, she establishes and manages a relationship with the other person while herself occupying a social position near to them, a position that has often been abandoned and is in any case not occupied by anyone else. By doing this, the other is seen and their concerns, their burning issues, are recognised and acknowledged. Whenever possible, the chaplain eventually hands back this position she is occupying temporarily to people who are close to the other. The benefit of this relational work is: the other is able to live their life again without being burdened too much by shame, neglect, violence, lovelessness, suffocating identity models and other such things. The chaplain connects with the other person in what is broken, in the evil, in the suffering that they undergo, and she seeks to foster a way of living with brokenness, evil and suffering that offers the perspective of a freer, safer and more appropriate life.

Over the years, as researchers we have become convinced, and we have been confirmed in this conviction, that this relationality is essential not only to outreach pastoral care but to all professional work with and for people, especially, but not exclusively, in healthcare and social work.

Four dimensions of relational caring

In the case we discussed in the last section, we have seen how important the relationship between the professional and the other is: as a good-in-itself and as a steering and organising mechanism. In addition, the relationship is the place where connecting-with and attuning-your-practice-to takes place. The importance of the relationship in good care is being acknowledged in practice and in theory. However, in practice the relationship between the caregiver and the care receiver is often utilised as an instrument or strategy, as something useful from a policy implementation view. It is understood as what precedes good care and is associated with treating the other well on a personal level, communicating well, inviting the other to participate in decision making, promoting equality and reciprocity, and so on. The relationship between the professional and the care receiver is sometimes treated as a service relationship, designed to retain people in need of care as customers. There is also a substantial amount of literature about therapeutic relationships or relationships as a working alliance. Much research has been done on the effectiveness of relationships (especially in mandated social work, Menger, 2018). But we have a different conception of relationships in relational caring.

Table 10.1: Four dimensions of relational caring

Dimension of relational caring	*Modes of relational caring*
Provisional dimension: Care, help and support as a provision that cannot be delivered outside relationships.	A. Caring *from* the relationship: Relationship as a steering mechanism for care, help and support. B. Caring *as* relationship: Relationship as a good-in-itself.
Contextual dimension: The care receiver as a contextual and relational being.	Caring *in* relationships: Relationships as the network and the life context of the care receiver.
Political-ethical dimension: The caregiver as a political, embedded and relational professional.	Caring *by* relationships: Relationships as the embedding of the caregiver.
Existential dimension: Humans as relational beings.	Caring *inherently aimed at* relationships: Relationships as the destiny of each human being. The ultimate end of care is that the care receiver, with their vulnerability and interdependence, is as good a member of society as possible and thereby stands in their own, more or less satisfactory relationship with the world, with others, with themselves and with the fragility of existence itself.

On the basis of our empirical research, we think that the relationship is not just an instrument and should not be conceived of as separate from the caring itself. We also think that it is necessary to look beyond the relationship between the person in need of care and the caregiver as individuals. Both the care receiver and the caregiver live in networks of relationships, not only in the context of the care involved, but also in their lifeworld. Care receivers are often cared for by a team of carers, including both professionals of different professions and informal carers. And caregivers often deal with groups, families, wards, neighbourhoods, populations and so forth.

As we conceptualise care, help and support as a practice of relational caring and probe concrete care practices, we have come to distinguish five modes of relational caring that can be subsumed under four dimensions of relational caring (Table 10.1).

1. The first dimension of relational caring pertains to the caring relationship between the person in need of care and the caregiver. In relational caring, this relationship is both a good-in-itself and a steering mechanism of care. We know, of course, that relationships are not always good and beneficial. Relationships can be violent. A lot of physical and mental violence occurs in the context of both private, professional and institutional relationships. This should be borne in mind, but it should not stop us from conceiving of the relationship as the place or the space where care must be realised.

The relationship structures the way the professional perceives, weighs up, cares, evaluates, acts and refrains from acting. The relationship is both a potential instrumental good and a potential intrinsic good. In other words, its relevance to relational caring is primarily intrinsic and structuring, and not (only) instrumental and strategic. All this does not mean that such a relationship is necessarily conflict free, time consuming and reciprocal, or involves frequent contact and in-depth conversations. But it does mean that the caregiver addresses not only the other's condition, what is happening or has been done to them, but also what these things mean to the other.

2. The second dimension is the fact that care receivers are contextual and relational beings. Care receivers live their lives in a relational network, and care, help and support should not cut them off from it. Care receivers have a history, a social position, an identity, obligations and loyalties towards others, and they have honour. Care can be good care only if it is well attuned to care receivers-in-relationships and the lives they live.
3. The third dimension is that care professionals are also contextual and relational beings. As professionals they are embedded in a care organisation (a hospital, for example) that itself is embedded in an institution (healthcare, or hospital care in case of a hospital). More often than not, they work in a team. Care is given in ordered relationships in which rights, tasks, liabilities, conditions, regulations, restrictions and so forth apply, while others are asking for care too and where selection criteria apply. Care is given in the context of the wider society and it also contributes to society. Care professionals continuously navigate all these background relationships and are therefore also political professionals.
4. The fourth and last dimension is the existential fact that human beings are relational beings, both ontologically (that is, with regard to how humans exist) and teleologically (that is, with regard to their destiny). The ultimate end of good care is that care receivers, with their vulnerabilities and interdependencies, are as good members of this society as possible, and thereby stand in their own, more or less satisfactory relationship with the world, with others, with themselves and with the fragility of existence itself.

Strong and weak relationality

The distinction between the relational and clinical-technical aspects of care is often referred to in terms of warm–cold, soft–hard or red–blue. We think this is not a fruitful way to conceptualise relational caring. We would instead like to introduce the distinction between strong and weak relationality.[5] This is meant as a descriptive, not an evaluative distinction. However, it is a descriptive distinction that stands at the service of an evaluative conclusion: from a presence-theoretical perspective, strong relationality is conducive to good care. The distinction between weak and strong relationality is primarily an epistemological and not an ontological one, in the sense that it is not fixed for all time. The decisive distinction between weak and strong relationality is that, when professionals work on the basis of strong relationality, what appears to be important in the relationship involved determines the caring itself, and not just how it is implemented or dressed up. In other words, the good emerging in the relationship determines the 'what', 'how' and 'by whom' of the care needed. The transition from weak to strong relationality cannot be made gradually by simply moving along the scale. If the integral practice is strongly relational, it also contains weakly relational aspects and it may be a matter of gradualism to move from these weakly relational aspects to strongly relational variants thereof. However, if the integral practice itself is weakly relational, the transition to a strongly relational practice is a matter of a qualitative leap or turnaround. This means that if you observe, weigh and act in terms of relationships, the transition to relational caring is a matter of conversion at some point. If you look, think and act in terms of relational caring, then there is no need for a qualitative leap to shift your attention to relationships at a certain point. Put simply and starkly, it boils down to the fact that the good to be pursued is sought and determined from the perspective of the relationship and is not self-referentially selected or prescribed by the discipline, the applicable policy, the institution and so on, whether or not these are dressed up in a relational manner. In order to be able to recognise strong relationality in healthcare and social work practices, the most important criterion and the tipping point on the scale of weak to strong relationality is that the good pursued is developed in an inquiry that is informed by both relational and discipline-specific reasoning that starts and ends with the person, group of persons or community in need of care.

Functions of strong relationality in relational caring

To further characterise strong as opposed to weak relationality, we will now discuss the function of relationality, its contribution to good care. After analysing many case fragments from many domains of care, help and support, we found different functions, different categories of what relational caring can do. We conceptualise these around that with which relational caring is concerned: particular relationships, and we do this in terms of space and time. The more strong relationality is practised, the more the function of relationality is realised. We distinguish six functions of relationality in relational caring. Later on in this section, we will add three more (for an overview, see Table 10.2).

1. Relational caring is intent on relationships that function as an open stage where the other person can show, present and articulate themselves and

let themselves be known. The relationship offers the scope, the stage, the invitation and the safety to appear. In the relationship, an answer can be found to questions such as: who is the other? What is their life about? What could be good here? This is often also an answer to questions that the care receiver poses themselves: who am I? What is my life about? This showing oneself is a very delicate process. When the care receiver cannot show themselves properly and freely, it remains unclear what kind of care, help and support is adequate and appropriate for this person in this moment, situation and context. The result could be that a woman in her 80s is compelled to face an unnecessary and unwanted mastectomy (Case fragment 10.3). But the caregiver must also show themselves. In this sense, the relationship becomes a source of knowledge for the professional as well as for the care receiver.

2. Relational caring is intent on relationships that not only convey information, knowledge, interventions, help, support, trust, feedback and so forth. By entering into a relationship, the professional becomes able to better understand who the other person is, how justice can be done to them at that moment and in that specific situation and context, and where boundaries are to be expected. The relationship becomes a space for epistemic fine-tuning, a framework for what the professional can do, should do and is allowed to do. Information about the care receiver is always relational. It is a story in which the narrator – a relative, a caregiver, a colleague, a volunteer – is also personally involved, and this in three ways. First, it is the narrator's story, told from their perspective. Two persons who view the same painting will nevertheless tell different stories about it. Second, the narrator was present – often doing something – in the context in which the things happened which they are recounting about the other. The other's behaviour may be a response to the narrator's prior actions. And last, the story narrates how the other shows themselves, and they show themselves in a way that is made possible in part by the relationship between them and the narrator who was present (Case fragment 10.4). It is important therefore to collect different stories and acknowledge them as stories that all say something that matters about the other.
3. Relational caring is intent on relationships that are also a place of beneficence and recognition. In these relationships, the other is safe, is seen and heard, confirmed in their existence, acknowledged as a person with dignity and honoured in their position. The other is recognised with love, respect and social esteem and protected against neglect, lawlessness and humiliation (Honneth, 1995; van Heijst, 2008).
4. Relational caring is intent on relationships as places where the care receiver becomes a human being and a subject again, and is not just a number or an object to be processed. Relational caring makes a relationship a safe place to express yourself, to face up to yourself, show your strength,

reinvent yourself. And it is also a safe place to articulate your needs or allow yourself to be cared for.

The next two functions are more about the caregiver.

5. Relational caring is intent on relationships that are worthwhile in themselves, because they express who the other is to the professional and who the professional can be to the other. At least for this moment and at least with this professional, the other person is seen and heard, is counted, is socially included and is 'elected', and the meaningfulness of their life is acknowledged. In relational caring, the relationship is the place of expressionate acts, acts in which two goods are non-instrumentally realised: the preciousness of the other and the professional's 'dedicated connectedness' with the other (van Heijst, 2011: 119–23). The relationally caring professional does practical and useful things in such a way that they simultaneously express that the other is worthwhile, dear and a respected member of the human family.
6. Relational caring is intent on relationships that are a source of legitimation for the caregiver. Why should the professional be allowed to undress the other, cut them, give them advice, constrain them, punish them, pressure them into doing things? Although this is usually based on formal and legal provisions, legitimacy is best built up and strengthened within the caring relationship itself. In relational caring, the relationship is a site of legitimation, approval, fruitful fighting and commitment to a common concern, especially in difficult situations and contexts. It is also the place where the other person, if necessary, is relationally bounded and even relationally punished. What it means to relationally bound or punish has to be discovered in the concrete situation and relationship.

CASE FRAGMENT 10.3

Mastectomy

A researcher in a hospital one night encounters a woman who cannot sleep. She is in her 80s and has breast cancer. She is awaiting a mastectomy the next day. The researcher talks to her and discovers that she does not want the mastectomy. She thinks this mastectomy will not benefit her. The cancer is not acutely life threatening and, due to her advanced age, the cancer is not growing very fast. Removing her breast will not substantially prolong her life, whereas recovery will take considerable time. When the researcher asks her whether she has discussed this with the doctor, she answers that she didn't feel free to discuss it with him. The researcher advises her to do so after all and, after saying goodbye, informs the nurses about the patient's wish to talk to the doctor. Later, he learns the operation was cancelled.[6]

CASE FRAGMENT 10.4

Different stories about Anne

Anne lives in a nursing home and has been diagnosed with dementia. Her son regularly takes her on outings in his car. He says she really likes it. In fact, he thinks that the nursing home should involve his mother in more activities. The professionals, however, are concerned about the toll the outings take on his mother. They see that whenever Anne returns, she is so tired that they have to let her rest in bed. Taking her to bed is a hassle, as Anne always protests fiercely. The caregivers and her son have often spoken with each other about their different perspectives. These are also discussed in the research meeting in which the researchers discuss the preliminary findings of their following of Anne with the caregivers and Anne's son. In the safety of this meeting, which is moderated by the researchers, they can speak freely about their concerns and their perceptions and gain greater understanding of each other. They can express mutual recognition of the other person's story and come closer to each other. The occupational therapist then proposes that the next time Anne should be allowed to rest in an adapted wheelchair. This means she doesn't need to change clothes and it is easier for her, and the caregivers, to return to the table.[7]

In short, the relationships which relational caring envisages do much more than convey information and interventions, but they are essential to caregivers, and they are places of comfort and consolation that are beneficial to care receivers.

Connecting with and attuning your practice to the person or persons in need of care

In Case fragment 10.2, we have seen the three-tiered approach of noticing, thematising and reworking that is made possible by the professional's relational caring. This relational caring itself can be conceptualised as a three-tiered approach, with the first and second layers consisting of a radical connecting with and attuning your practice to the lifeworld, including the life course and its turning points, the longings and concerns of the people cared with and for. It is important to note that this is very different from the common idea of diagnosis, in which the patient or client is isolated from their environment and relational network, invited to enter the world of the care setting and treated as an individual with their own individual disease or problem. In relational caring, the person in need of care is perceived in their own environment and their relational network. Before turning to the second layer of attuning or fine-tuning, we have to specify what 'connecting with the other's lifeworld as the starting point or first layer of relational caring' means (see also 'Attunement to lifeworld and life course' in Chapter 4).

What do we mean by 'lifeworld'? In general terms, a person's lifeworld is their self-evident understanding of reality, enshrined in contexts of meaning and images of the world, society and the self, connected with a time perspective. However, it is characteristic of relational caring that it attempts to connect with categorical lifeworlds: lifeworlds of certain social groups or categories of people, especially of those who experience themselves as socially redundant. There are not just neighbourhood residents, teenage mothers, caravan dwellers or hospital patients, there are different categories of neighbourhood residents, teenage mothers, caravan dwellers or hospital patients. Our intention is not to pigeonhole people, to treat them as exemplars of certain well-defined categories, but to reflect the fact that people are not completely unique individuals. Distinguishing empirically grounded categories contributes to understanding the reasonableness of certain phenomena. Considering people as competent actors for as long as possible, connecting with their general and categorical lifeworld, requires reconstructing the inner rationality and logic behind patterns, types, survival strategies and cultures. This is a first specification of our understanding of connecting with the lifeworld.

A second specification is that the lifeworld can be considered as something dynamic, and this is why we wish to introduce the concept of life course. Connecting with the lifeworld also entails connecting with the life course, that is, the course of a life with its phases of socialisation, developmental trajectories, career, status transitions and turning points. Turning points are moments in a career or a trajectory (Riemann and Schütze, 1991) that can become points of engagement during which a trajectory is bent into another, possibly better direction.

A third and last specification is about what we have come to call 'concerns'. It is common to think that when people ask for care, help and support, it is the professional who has to do work. But people who ask for care, help and support have to do work themselves too – and sometimes the workload is substantial. There is the work they are urged to do by the professional because of their supposed self-reliance. But there is also work they have to do to help the professional do their own work, for example presenting their needs in terms the professional can or is allowed to process. Or standing up for themselves, their child, their neighbourhood while avoiding being perceived as a troublesome patient, parent or neighbour. In addition to the problem or question that caused them to ask for care, help or support, people in need of care have other issues they struggle with. For example: someone comes to the doctor with a broken arm, but the real problem is: how can I continue to do my work? Someone seeks addiction care to treat their addiction, but the issue they are struggling with is: how do I make sure nobody finds out? We call these issues concerns. In general, concerns have four aspects in common: they indicate a certain struggle, they are personal in nature, they impose themselves with urgency and they often require substantial effort from the patient or client. A study of emergency care found that concerns centred on five issues: anxiety, expectations, the care itself, endurance and recognition (Olthuis et al, 2014). The concerns of care receivers can be taken away and alleviated, but also created and aggravated by caregivers and their responses to what they perceive the care receiver's concerns to be. The caregiver must come close to the care receiver, think relationally and try to find out what is bothering them, must look relationally at signs of possible concerns, fears, longings and so on. If an adequate, fitting response is to be given, it will be necessary to perceive the care receiver's real concerns.

In relational caring, the aim of connecting with someone's lifeworld and life course, turning points, concerns, is to understand the other's life, not to identify with their position. More specifically, its primary aim is to achieve a reconstructive–rational understanding, from a reflective internal perspective, not solely an emotional understanding, nor an explanatory–rational understanding from an external perspective. Connecting with and attuning your practice to someone's lifeworld and life course is not about being nice, attentive and sympathetic. Nor is it about explaining the care receiver's mood, behaviour or reaction patterns from a psychological or sociological perspective. It starts with reconstructing and understanding the rationality and logic of the other person's lifeworld, what is at stake for them and what are their most urgent concerns. Whenever the caregiver connects with these concerns, this clarifies to them how to thematise what is at stake so that something can be done about it. Perhaps the responses cannot include helping the other escape from prison, but they may include helping him to be a good father to his children while he is in prison. Connecting-with-and-attuning-your-practice-to is not the same as: 'Your wish is our command'. Connecting-with means: drawing near to the other and remaining near to them, finding out what is at stake for them and how this can be thematised so that this 'theme' can become one of the professional's own concerns. The professional recognises and acknowledges the relevance and importance of the theme to the other. But the professional does not necessarily confirm the care receiver's articulation of the theme, nor the precise realisation or solution that they desire.

Attuning-your-practice-to is a step within connecting-with, a step that can be compared to fine-tuning. The professional who engages in this fine-tuning shows themselves, saying something like: 'I do not think that what you ask is wise; this is what I can do and these are my boundaries.' It is an ongoing, mutual and iterative process. And it is a process fraught with tensions, conflicts and struggles. We will now look at another case fragment (Case fragment 10.5).

CASE FRAGMENT 10.5

Breast augmentation

A woman with a psychiatric background and a history of being mistreated and abused by successive partners desperately wants a breast augmentation.

> She is convinced that by having her breasts enlarged she will be able to bind men to her and thus meet her own need for sex, new clothes and occasional outings. The care professional counters that enlarging her breasts is not necessary and is not a good idea anyway. The woman starts to put all her energy into persuading the professional instead of thinking for herself about whether it was a good idea or not. Knowing her, the professional decides not to help her in the way she wants.[8]

It is clear what this woman's concern is in her own mind: she wants to persuade the professional to help her fulfil her wish for a breast augmentation. In relational caring, the professional will inquire what lies behind the patient's wish for sex, new clothes and outings. It can be a sincere, very human desire for friendship and intimacy to which the professional can respond adequately. By inquiring, the professional shows themselves in order to give a relational answer.

Response, mismatch and relational programming

Our concise discussion of Case fragment 10.5 has now brought us to the third tier of relational caring as a three-tiered approach: the layer of the care professional's response to the other person's concerns. Does the professional perceive the care receiver's concerns? Does he or she identify these concerns as having become one of their own concerns as a professional? How do they respond to them? And what impact do these responses have on the concerns of the other? The study of emergency care mentioned earlier has shown that the impact of the response to the patient's concerns can be placed on a spectrum, from alleviating and even remedying the concerns to prolonging, complicating and worsening them (Olthuis et al, 2014b). The question is whether the response is adequate to the concerns. If it is not, the care provided is not good care.

Relational caring requires connecting with and attuning your practice to the other and their lifeworld, life course, concerns and so forth. Connecting-with and attuning-your-practice-to are prerequisites for good care and are the criteria for whether the care provided is relevant and appropriate. There are also many other promoters of good care: methods, routines, manuals, protocols, guidelines, provisions, facilities, laws and so forth. When care, help or support is given in accordance with these other promoters but is not experienced and valued as good and beneficial by the care receiver, we call this a 'mismatch'. Mismatches occur when the care, help or support offered is good by some external standard but is not well attuned to the care receiver themselves and their life, longings and concerns (Baart, 2002; Baart and Steketee, 2003; Baart 2013; Goossensen et al, 2014).

In relational caring, the other's 'theme' is reworked in a specific, relational way. We call this 'relational programming': out of all the possible things that can be done, professionals choose the one thing that fits the way the other has shown themselves in the relationship. The concept of 'relationship-based programming' was introduced by Jason Bocarro and Peter Witt in a paper about designing pedagogical and recreational programmes for children in addition to what schools do. They argue for programmes that focus not on activities but on entering into and maintaining relationships (2003). Relational programming as we understand it is aimed at honouring, acknowledging and confirming the other as a full, knowledgeable member of the human family.

Three additional functions of relationality in relational caring

Relational caring helps to draw reasonable and acceptable boundaries in care, help and support. Otherwise, care, help and support are likely to exceed all boundaries and will not be sustainable. We have elaborated three perspectives, each of which considers a problem in care, help and support: difficult clients, overtreatment and professional perpetuation of need (Baart, 2013). We will number them from where we left off when we discussed the functions of relationality earlier.

7. Relational caring is intent on relationships as places where power and the abuse of power, as well as the violence that is sometimes unfortunately unavoidable in professional care, help and support, can be bridled. When they work with difficult clients, clients who show aggressive, transgressive and sometimes violent behaviour, professionals are sometimes swayed by the desire to punish and constrain the client, to separate themselves and distance themselves from their client. Working relationally, which is in fact often the only effective way to do this work, helps to avoid and postpone that moment. And when it does become necessary to punish the other, the relationship is the place where the professional regrets the punishment together with the other, endures it and, wherever possible, makes it fruitful. Even if the professional in question is the person who has imposed the punishment.
8. Relational caring is intent on relationships as places to restrain the – sometimes understandable – inclination of caregivers and care receivers alike to continue treatments and interventions far beyond what is meaningful and responsible. By becoming close to the care receiver, by being reflexive and by deliberating with them, the professional can find out what will contribute to a good life for this person in this situation and context, and what anxiety underlies their request for care, help or support. Reflecting on treatments and interventions and taking decisions about them within the relationship between the professional and the other helps to curb overtreatment. The availability of moral and existential

capital is necessary to think about the meaningfulness of further treatment or intervention. It is the relationship that makes it possible to introduce moral and existential capital and even to build and share it.[9]

9. Relational caring is intent on relationships as places where the professional perpetuation of need can be countered. We distinguish three forms or layers of the perpetuation of need: *methodical*, due to the professional methods, guidelines and protocols; *systemic*, due to the requirements of the system; and *cultural*, due to certain characteristics of our culture.

The *professional–methodical* perpetuation of need is a result of neglect or of failing to properly attune your practice to the other. Professional neglect is the result of not doing anything or not bringing the care that has been started to an end relationally. Doing nothing may be legitimised by functional differentiation or by certain rules that professionals impose upon themselves, such as respect for the client's autonomy or the requirement that the client should be motivated. Not completing care that has been started may occur wherever the situation is too complex, the professionals are too specialised or the chain of care providers is too long. The focus on competences instead of professional virtues such as courage and dedication in education and training of professionals does not help either. Another cause of methodical perpetuation of need is the occurrence of mismatches: the care provided is good care by the standards of professional methods, guidelines or protocols, but is not well attuned to the care receiver, and must therefore be provided again and again but remains unsatisfactory.

The *bureaucratic–systemic* perpetuation of need occurs when professionals are not able or allowed to use or enlarge their discretionary and systemic space or safeguard it against the system's unhelpful rules, organisation, finances, control, registration and quality criteria (cf Achterhuis, 1979). It also occurs when they are unable to resist the tendency to identify the person with their behaviour, so that when certain behaviours by the care receiver have to be punished, they are unable to stay near to the person concerned.

The *cultural–ideological* perpetuation of need is a result of the fact that our culture cherishes the idea that human and social life can be engineered, and of the specific way in which we deal with emotions in care, help and support. The ideology of the manufacturability of human and social life expresses itself in the confidence that suffering can be taken away, defects can be eliminated and problems can be solved. Organic and soft powers, carefulness and the awareness of tragedy are neglected. Faith in strict, proven and evidence-based interventions undoes the effect of the caring relationship, the mutual trust between the professional and the other person and their joint effort. Trust in treatment plans, in rationally planned, defined and solution-oriented interventions precludes relational, professionally loving and sensible 'muddling through'. Muddling through means: understanding what the practice is about (its finality), taking small steps and looking where each step gets you, looking at what is possible, deliberating, taking a next step, persevering but staying sensitive and constantly attuned to the field. It is an incremental way of doing, in which goals and means, values and methods, observations and judgements overlap and merge (see also Chapter 11).

The cultural perpetuation of need is also a result of the specific way in which we deal with emotionality in care, help and support. Emotions are often considered to be uncriticisable and therefore remain largely unprocessed and they are often not subjected to conscious, critical reflection. Professionals are supposed to neutralise or even suppress their emotions and not allow them to influence their practice. Bureaucratic, methodical and professional rules prevent professionals' emotions from influencing professional judgements and the way they treat people. In fact, however, emotions are more informative than this suggests (cf Nussbaum, 2001). They are a source of knowledge that can be made fruitful for good care if they are processed, that is, subjected to critical reflection and critically considered in moral deliberation.

In summary, the relationships which relational caring envisages are also the place where caregivers can bridle difficult, transgressive care receivers, restrain overtreatment by introducing moral and existential capital and counter the professional perpetuation of need in its methodical, systemic and cultural guises (see Table 10.2 for an overview of all nine functions).

Table 10.2: Functions of strong relationality in relational caring

Relationality as the place ...
... where care receivers show, present and articulate themselves
... where caregivers attune their practice to care receivers and set goals
... where care receivers experience benevolence and recognition
... where care receivers become human beings and subjects again
... where caregivers express what the other person means to them
... where legitimation for the care by the professional can be found
... where the power of professionals is bridled
... where the continuation of meaningless treatment and intervention is restrained
... where the professional–methodical, bureaucratic–systemic and cultural–ideological perpetuation of need and neediness is countered
... *but also where chafing, conflict, struggle and violence occur!*

Second point of reference: finality

At the start of this chapter we introduced the idea that relational caring has two points of reference: relationality and finality. So far, we have been discussing relationality, and especially strong relationality, although we did mention finality, the understanding of which is essential to muddling through. Finality is the other reference point of relational caring. It is what the practice is ultimately about, conceptualised in terms of its end, its *telos*. This is not the same as a fixed *telos*, fixed by God or by nature, or as what people or organisations set as their particular operational goals. In order to realise the finality of a practice, discipline-specific knowledge as well as relational knowledge are essential.

By introducing the concept of finality, we are connecting with philosophical thought about acting in terms of ends. According to Aristotle, every action has its own end, its own goal, its own purport (Aristotle, 2013). That end is not necessarily identical to the acting person's objectives. If we continue that line of thinking, finality is something a particular type of action, a particular practice, a particular type of work, a particular organisation or a particular institution have. Unlike classical teleological thinkers such as Aristotle, we do not understand finality in the sense of a metaphysically determined, ontologically anchored or God-ordained goal. We do not think of finality as a predetermined and external end, derived for instance from 'human nature'. But nor do we see finality as a goal that can be freely chosen, or that a particular organisation or society can simply agree upon on the basis of rational debate. The finality, end or purport of a particular kind of action, practice, type of work, organisation or institution can be discovered, over time, only within the action or practice or institution itself (MacIntyre, 2007). This can be done by asking: what is at stake in this action? What does it seek to aid? What is the good it is aimed at? From what evil does it seek to distance itself? This is not to say that only those who act, only the practitioners, the professionals, can answer the finality question. Everyone involved in and affected by the act, every participant in the practice, and ultimately every citizen, can have a say in it. So, we do not use the word finality metaphysically, but heuristically: it allows us to discover what this particular practice is ultimately about, not in theory but in practice, and to articulate in words what we have discovered. Articulating the finality of a practice is a discursive achievement.

Practices are intrinsically connected with institutions. Institutions are a particular historical community's structures of *living together*, which have their own specific ends that also limit the structures in question. These structures cannot be reduced to interpersonal relationships, but are nevertheless linked to them (Ricœur, 1992). Institutions support practices by formulating and distributing rights, duties and responsibilities (MacIntyre, 2007). Some of the social institutions, for example healthcare, social welfare and education, are also organisations or systems of organisations: healthcare organisations, social welfare organisations or educational institutions.[10] While practitioners focus on the internal goods of their practice, organisations are engaged in acquiring and distributing external goods: money, power and status. Without support from the institution and the organisation, a practice will not survive for long – as evidenced by the highest general administrativecourt's failure to protect individual citizens in the childcare benefits scandal in the Netherlands (van Domselaar, 2021).

However, in late modernity organisations themselves are also coming under pressure, because organisations have begun to accommodate various distinct institutions that are not self-evidently compatible. If, for example, a healthcare organisation also becomes a for-profit production business, the institution of healthcare with its own internal goods will come under pressure from a variety of rule-based and self-enforcing systems of registration, control and quality assurance. These systems' own legitimate ends are transparency, efficiency and cost control, but these do not automatically lead to good care for sick and precarious people. If these systems gain the upper hand, the institutional character of the hospital will be abrogated, and doctors and nurses will become 'bundles of desired functions' (Dubet, 2002), increasingly at risk of loss of motivation and burnout. The high complexity of society obscures institutional goals. As a consequence of systemic pressure, these institutional goals are not only obscured but are even exposed to the threat of being totally expunged (Vosman, 2008; van Heijst, 2011). This expresses the importance of institutions for society. Institutions underpin society. If they are depoliticised, they will be blown off course. It is necessary therefore to raise the finality question and try to answer it again and again.

In Case fragment 10.1, the custodian Luke is asked to explain why he cleaned the room again after the father of the patient in that room snapped at him. He replies by articulating what he sees as his duty as a custodian in a hospital. His work is not just to clean, but to clean and reassure patients and the people around them. If the task of reassuring requires him to clean a room twice, even though this is superfluous from the perspective of his cleaning duties, he will clean the room twice. Without saying all this in so many words, Luke is giving an account of his work – cleaning in a hospital – in terms of its finality. The finality of this work is related to the finality of the hospital, that is, the finality of the institution of hospital care. And the finality of the institution of hospital care is related to the finality of the social institution of healthcare, which in turn is related to the finality of society.

The question is what this relatedness entails. One answer is to conceptualise this relatedness as a kind of deduction or translation. In that case, the finality of a custodian's work, a nurse's work or a physician's work in a hospital is derived from or is a translation of the finality of the institution of hospital care. This means the custodian's work, or the nurse's work, or the physician's work does not have its own finality in the sense that practice theory expects any practice to have. Moreover, the finality of, say, a physician's work in a hospital may be more similar to that of a nurse's work in a hospital than to the finality of a physician's work in, say, a general practice. This is counterintuitive: there is a lot of literature about 'the goals of medicine' (Cassell, 1991; The Goals of Medicine, 1996; Kaldjian, 2014).

Following Ricœur, we conceive of the relatedness between different levels of finality as 'the nesting [*enchâssement*] of finalities, one inside the other' (Ricœur, 1992: 178). In this case, the finality of Luke's work as a custodian is nested in the finality of the institution of hospital care, which is nested in the institution of healthcare, which is nested in the finality of society. This is, of course, rather schematic. It must be realised that an organisation can be situated at the intersection of different social institutions. A nursing home, for example, belongs to the social institution of healthcare, but also to that of residential care and of social welfare. One way to solve this problem is to speak about the overarching social institution of care, including healthcare, residential care and social welfare. Another way to deal with this problem is to realise that the concept of institution applies to different levels, from less complex social forms such as conventions, rules, social norms, roles and rituals, to more complex and more complete social entities, such as societies or cultures (Miller, S., 2019). Healthcare, hospital care and intensive care can all be conceptualised as institutions in the sense of a particular historical community's structures of living together, with their own specific ends (Ricœur, 1992). We prefer this second option: nursing homes belong to the institution of nursing home care.

Raising the finality question

We have argued that it is permanently necessary in late modernity for teams or groups of practitioners to raise the finality question and try to answer it: what is our practice, essentially, ultimately about? Why do we do what we evidently do? What is it that motivates us most deeply in our work, keeps us going, drives us, gives us satisfaction? What is our ultimate contribution as professionals to society? What is the ultimate purpose of our practice? Teams or groups of practitioners can discover what their practice is ultimately about precisely by articulating an answer, explaining it to each other, elaborating it, reflecting on it, confronting it with concrete cases, trying out alternative articulations and so on. We do not assume that finality can ever be given once and for all, and that all we need to do is articulate it to have an answer that is then valid forever. Instead, we assume that reality resists arbitrary articulations. This is why it is essential to confront articulations with concrete cases: what does this articulation clarify? What further questions does it raise? In what ways could alternative articulations be more adequate or helpful to this case? This procedure can help to see whether a particular articulation indeed clarifies something and is helpful. Every answer to the finality question is therefore always provisional. At this moment, for these people here, and for what they have to do now, this articulation of the finality of the practice is sufficiently directional and satisfactory, and sufficiently challenging. But raising the finality question and articulating an answer is something that has to be done again and again.

Although finding an answer starts with considering one's own practice, articulating the answer starts with the finality of the institution in which that practice is being practised. There is a choice here regarding the level of institution that one decides to consider: it could be the institution of healthcare, for instance, of hospital care or of intensive care. It depends on the reason why or occasion upon which the finality question is raised. We recommend that the practitioners involved should take some distance from the actual work. Raising the finality question so as to articulate an answer helps practitioners to keep their priorities straight, to know whether they are doing their job well, to make room for muddling through and practical wisdom, to install a basic frame of reference for perceiving, interpreting, acting and evaluating within a given practice or type of work, and to keep at arm's length goals that have been imposed from outside.

At the same time, raising the finality question is difficult in late modernity, for a number of reasons. First, the idea that a particular kind of action or practice has its own, inalienable end was abandoned in modernity and remains suspicious in late modernity. Second, the classical category of ends has been corrupted in ethical considerations and has come to mean self-determined goals or objectives. And last, ends have been replaced in ethical considerations by foreseeable consequences. Articulating an answer to the finality question is often difficult for professionals, especially when the organisation for which they work has declared something to be its purpose: 'Our hospital is about …'. Or when politicians promote neoliberal values such as autonomy, self-reliance and participation as goals for professions in the domains of healthcare and social welfare.

How does discerning and articulating the finality of one's practice work? In the process of articulating an answer to the finality question, an essential role is reserved for what practitioners have discovered in their practice. It is not enough to exchange views, opinions and experiences. Instead, it is necessary to look for what advanced, reflective, deliberative and practically wise practitioners have discovered with respect to what that practice is ultimately aimed at. This cannot be done by a practitioner on his or her own. It must be done together, in a process of reflection and deliberation. Articulating the finality is a highly contextual, relational and discursive process. It requires supervision, for example to ensure that the participants do not settle for a particular answer too quickly. There are other sources for this process besides that which the practitioners have discovered in their practice themselves (1): that which their predecessors (especially the virtuosos among them) have discovered, and which may be available through manuals and the canon of the profession (2); that which those who are being acted upon, the patients, clients, residents, pupils – and those around them – have discovered, and which may be available directly through relational caring and indirectly through research (3); and that which colleagues have discovered in other places, and which may be available through research (4). The political character of institutions should also be taken into account: citizens and politicians have a say too about what a practice is about (5). Discerning and articulating the finality should therefore be done discursively, with historical awareness, nourished by a political care ethics and informed by an analysis of where the institution functions badly or falls below its bottom threshold. The finality question must be answered on the spot, so to speak, but the answer has a meaning that extends beyond that moment and location. It is possible to say something in general about the finality of various institutions. From the perspective of the care receiver, a hospital is about 'experiencing solicitude', care for older persons about 'being able to live as a human being among human beings', social work about 'living an honourable life', youth work about 'being able to flourish'. To give an example from a field outside healthcare and social work: Nel Noddings has described the 'primary aim' of education as 'the maintenance and enhancement of caring', not 'trained intelligence' (Noddings, 1984: 172).

When is it time to conclude the process? Raising the finality question so as to articulate an answer never leads to a definitive, once-for-all answer. In this sense, it never ends. But practitioners raise the finality question because they want to get their priorities straight, because they want to know whether they are doing their work well, because they want to make room for practical wisdom, because they want to know how to look at their work, how to perceive, interpret, perform and evaluate it. That is why, at some point, the discerning of the finality must be concluded – at least for the time being – by articulating a provisional answer to the finality question, an answer based on what practitioners have discovered and what they have agreed on, using various sources. This answer is an (always provisional, always adjustable) articulation of the finality of the practice or type of work in question. If practitioners invest in this articulation, then the finality articulated also becomes their goal. Then other objectives – in the sense of: self-imposed goals, such as receiving appreciation, earning money, gaining status, growing in responsibility – become subordinate to this finality. And this lasts until the finality articulated no longer suffices, until new situations or issues arise or colleagues leave and others take their place. Then it may be necessary to raise the finality question again.

Relational caring, defined by relationality and finality

We have argued that relational caring has two points of reference: relationality and finality. Relationality in the sense of taking relationships and working relationally seriously, and finality in the sense of taking what caring is ultimately about seriously. If we think about relational caring using the analogy of an ellipse around two points of reference, we can imagine every concrete instance of relational caring as being informed or determined by relationality and finality in an inverse relationship.[11] Depending on the context and situation, on the care receivers and caregivers involved, and on the urgency of the issue at hand, relationality can become more salient and finality less salient, or the other way around. This can be illustrated by Case fragment 10.6.

CASE FRAGMENT 10.6

A potato chip

On his day off, a young hospital doctor is walking through a shopping centre with a friend. They pass a snack bar. A family just in front of the restaurant are enjoying their chips: a mother, a father, and their daughter of about 16. The moment the doctor and his friend pass, the girl begins to choke on a potato chip that went down the wrong way and she begins to suffocate. Without any hesitation, the doctor stands behind the girl, places his clasped hands on her stomach just below the diaphragm and thrusts them into her stomach with a jerk. The chip is dislodged from her throat and the girl starts breathing again. At this point the father turns around. You can see him thinking, 'What is that man doing to my daughter ...?' The doctor's companion pulls him into the crowd and hauls him away. The young doctor protests, 'I can explain!', but she answers decidedly, 'His daughter will do that! I don't want you to get hit! Did you see how angry the man was getting!'[12]

In Case fragment 10.6, the doctor very quickly reduces the complexity of the situation to just one issue: a potato chip in the trachea – a non-contested issue. He knows what to do, and he acts. That is what doctors are extremely good at: reducing situations to the problem, knowing what to do, and acting. In this case, his acting is informed by one of the goals of medicine: prevention of death. In his acting, the doctor is not interested in establishing a professional relationship, neither with the girl nor with her father. But the care in Case fragment 10.6 is not entirely without relationality. The doctor's act may be seen as a response to the girl's appeal for help, an appeal to which he is sensitive. There is someone who is sensitive to the need of another person and who is willing to respond, given the institutionalised identities of physician and citizen. Someone is in need, and the other person notices this need. This is at least the beginning of a professional relationship. One can imagine a case in which things are the other way around, a case in which relationality is more salient than finality. Case fragment 10.3 is one such case, with the doctor being informed of what the researcher discovered.

Two relational issues

Relational autonomy

Autonomy is an important value in healthcare and social work, and respect for autonomy is an important principle, one that often overrules other principles. But autonomy is a political-ethical concept which is often evoked to ward off a specific menace. It has a long history and has acquired, and continues to acquire, many contextually conditioned aspects and meanings. Many of these aspects and meanings still resonate even today. Whenever someone evokes autonomy in some context or discussion, meanings from other contexts and discussions influence the way it is understood, the value that is attached to it and the consequences of evoking it. This is due to the fact that autonomy is a catchword of modernity, one which exemplifies the modern turn to the subject and subjectivity. Another catchword of modernity is authenticity, to which autonomy is closely related, as the respective histories of these terms show (Timmerman, 2010; 2011).

Autonomy plays a role in the contexts of morality, of politics and power and of identity, in which humans are conceived as moral beings, citizens and unique, historical beings, respectively. In the context of *morality*, autonomy plays a pivotal role in the foundation of a modern conception of morality. The premodern conception of morality as obedience has been replaced by the conception of morality as autonomy (Kant, 1998; Schneewind, 1998; Larmore, 2008). In the context of *politics and power*, two different debates are ongoing that both use the concept of autonomy. One is the debate about the demarcation of mutual rights and duties between citizens and the state (Kant, 1992; Mill, 2012). Autonomy is evoked to counter state paternalism. The other debate is that about control over one's body, mind and life in relation to different kinds of professional interventions (Dworkin, 1988; Mackenzie and Stoljar, 2000; Beauchamp and Childress, 2009). It originated in the discussions after World War II that led to the Nuremberg Code (in 1947) and the World Medical Association's Declaration of Helsinki (in 1964). In combination with authenticity, and often in the guise of 'personal autonomy', autonomy is evoked to delimit the power and unjustified paternalism of professionals. What is often overlooked is that respecting and promoting personal autonomy always occurs in a relationship, and that the person of the professional, and their autonomy and authenticity, are also involved (Timmerman, 2010; 2011). In the context of *identity*, autonomy and authenticity are seen as central to the formation of modern identity (Taylor, 1989; 1991). Autonomy and authenticity are mustered in the battle against alienation and self-alienation.

In all these debates, the question of autonomy and respect for autonomy raises the following issue: does it matter – and if so, how – that it is me (or us)? But this question, and thus also autonomy, are considered in the abstract situation of a healthy, confident and self-sufficient adult, usually a male. In the case of persons who are sick, mentally disabled, traumatised, dependent, dying and/or living in precarious situations, countering professional paternalism is similarly discussed in terms of respect for autonomy, usually on the basis of concepts such as 'derived consent' and 'proxy consent' (Tibbles, 1985). We do not argue that autonomy as a political-ethical concept has no role to play at all in thinking about persons who do not meet the ideal of the fully autonomous person. In the context of recuperation and recovery, in which human beings are conceived of as embodied beings embedded in relational networks who are therefore vulnerable and liable to precarisation, autonomy and authenticity are about managing to keep afloat and regaining the existential core of one's existence. They are evoked to ward off the risk of getting lost. But this requires a concept of relational autonomy and respect for autonomy that starts by recognising that humans are embodied and relational beings and are therefore vulnerable.

Our plea is to think about autonomy not from the abstraction of a healthy, confident and self-sufficient individual, but from the concrete situation of vulnerable persons who are dependent on care. And when it comes to persons with multiple profound mental and physical disabilities and who show behaviour that is difficult to understand, autonomy is a highly problematic and demanding concept. The usual idea of autonomy, which rests on (a) a person's choice, wish or longing and on (b) a meta level on which that choice, wish or longing is managed,[13] fails. Nevertheless, in current care for these persons, at least in the Netherlands, autonomy, and respect for and the promotion of autonomy, are highly valued as ideals and quality measures. When we analysed the literature, Dutch policy documents, and the everyday language of professionals in one particular organisation, we found a multifaceted, layered concept of what we call 'hermeneutic relational autonomy' (Baart, 2024). We have heuristically distinguished five levels in this concept.

On the first level, autonomy is mainly seen in the light of choosing and deciding, and of being allowed to express one's will, desire or need with regard to the what and how of the care provided. In this context, autonomy means self-determination – the right everyone has to make their own choices – and self-regulation – the use a person makes of that right. Not respecting autonomy, understood in this sense, is unjustified paternalism.

On the second level, autonomy is viewed mainly in the light of participation, of being involved and being able and allowed to influence the organisation and the course of the care that is provided to you. Professionals should leave clients to do what they can do themselves. In this context, autonomy is self-direction – the influence that clients have over the trajectory of care as it is realised – and self-control – the control that clients have over themselves and their attempts to establish mastery over the care. Not respecting autonomy, understood in this sense, is interference.

On the third level, autonomy is seen mainly in the light of being able to live your own life while depending on others. In this context, autonomy is self-reliance – the ability to deal with your own problems – and independence – occupying your own place among other people. Professionals should allow clients to live their own lives as much as possible. Not respecting autonomy, understood in this sense, is perpetuation of neediness, by the professionals or by the client themselves.

On the fourth level, autonomy is viewed mainly in the light of being yourself in the best possible way and being left free to become who you are. In this understanding, autonomy is explicitly related to authenticity. In this context, autonomy is self-development – developing your own talents and possibilities – and self-realisation – realising yourself with all your potentialities, in a sustainable way. Not respecting autonomy, understood in this sense, means containing or even writing off, cancelling the client by others or by the client themselves.

On the fifth level, autonomy is mainly seen in the light of being accepted in society as who you are, in your otherness, also when it disturbs others. In this understanding, autonomy is self-confidence – the public acceptability of one's identity – and self-affirmation – daring to do what one is able to do. Not respecting autonomy, in this sense, results in alienation, stereotyping and stigmatisation.

Respecting and promoting autonomy is a relational process of coming near to the client, connecting-with and attuning-your-practice-to them, and taking responsibility for enabling the unfolding and development of the client's person. It is a process in which these five levels are addressed. If the client's process of becoming themselves is regarded over a longer period of time, there may be instances where their autonomy was overruled on one level, but promoted and respected on another level, whether simultaneously or not. To the extent that the concept of autonomy can be applied to real people, people are autonomous *because of*, not despite, their social embedding in their relational network. Relationality is a condition for the development of autonomy in this broad sense of the word. The actual promotion of the client's relational autonomy requires relational caring on the part of the professional, including a continuous, everyday hermeneutics. The caregiver themselves is included in this hermeneutics, as an instrument and as a horizon of understanding. This hermeneutics can discover the care receiver's inner perspective or experienced meaning and articulate its moral meaning: given that their situation means this to the care receiver, what can we do at this moment? It is in this way that it matters that the care receiver is *this particular person*.

Relational bounding

Most caregivers have experienced moments of which they say afterwards, 'Something went wrong there. That should have gone differently. I'm not proud of that.' A common way of speaking about this is to broadly and formally recognise that there is a boundary that the professional should not cross. Examples are physically attacking the other, taking something away from the other by force or humiliating the other. And it is also common to condemn behaviour that crosses these boundaries – the caregiver themselves is often the first to do so. If the subsequent deliberation is conducted with colleagues, it is often about how what went wrong can be prevented in the future. But this approach is no help to the caregiver in question. It does not acknowledge that some residents, clients, patients and pupils can be very disruptive, recalcitrant, demanding and even violent. And this means that nothing is learned that might contribute to good care.

We have looked at what happens in those moments with a view to learning about good care, and without the illusion that it is possible to prevent things going wrong again in the future, and this led us to develop the notion of 'relational bounding'.[14] We concluded that professionals in healthcare and social work have to learn from boundary transgressions in professional relationships with patients, clients, pupils and residents, and should not foreclose this learning process by starting the deliberation with a moral condemnation. After all, relational caring that aims to make a difference requires the professional to come near to the other person. And coming near requires discovering, approaching, exploring and often challenging boundaries, by both sides. Crossing boundaries is sometimes inevitable in relational caring. If this is navigated well, it can turn out to have sown the seeds of good relational caring.

A boundary is always about a good that has to be protected. If you back away from every boundary, if you never even approach a boundary, you never learn what is at stake there. When you encounter the other person's boundaries, that person's reaction may be to strictly police it: the matter at hand cannot be discussed further. In this case, the professional has two options. The first is to accept the boundary and indicate that they have no intention of crossing it. This means something has been learned, and the confrontation was necessary to arrive at this insight. But there are situations in which a professional may have good reasons not to accept the boundary set by the other. The professional may challenge the boundary, because the other is of concern to the professional, and for the other person's good. That requires the professional to come forward, to show themselves personally, in the hope that the other will trust them enough to show themselves too. There may be a struggle, but there will also be joint learning. The professional can also experience a boundary and negotiations will then have to take place: what does each side need from the other, where may they not go, where should boundaries be moved?

Boundaries are usually imagined as lines, but they can also be regarded in terms of zones. A boundary zone is a transition zone from one sphere of life to another: a different morality, a different purpose, a place of pride and honour, a place of pain and shame and so on. Unlike a line, you can enter and explore a zone. That does not mean you have crossed a boundary yet, but you can feel the resistance gradually increasing. You sense where the resistance is, where the other sphere of life begins and what that sphere of life means for the other person. Depending on this, you can decide to move into the other sphere of life, and sometimes also to move the boundary altogether or invite the other to move the boundary. This can be done, for example, by escalating something a little bit, in a gentle, predictable and managed way. If you think in terms of border zones, you may also notice interference between your own border zone and that of the other. It can be revealing to think in this way about the disruptive, recalcitrant, demanding and violent behaviour of some residents, clients, pupils and patients and the response that professionals give to these behaviours.

Working in boundary zones in this way, on and across boundaries, is an important resource for learning to understand what is at stake for the other, what you can do and cannot do and who you can be to the other. Connecting-with and attuning-your-practice-to are therefore certainly not always harmonious, but they are necessary to be able to practise good relational caring. For this to happen, the professional needs space to be allowed to learn situationally, to better understand the care receiver. Inevitably, this goes hand in hand with strife and conflict. And tragedy must be accepted: caregiver and care receiver may not find each other. Or they do find each other, but it does not help, or helps only for a little while.

Crossing boundaries can become part of relational bounding if the professional learns what is at stake and, therefore, what good care can be in this instance. And it becomes part of relational bounding by including the active re-establishment of the relationship in the process. Learning from boundary transgressions can be done both within the situation and afterwards. Learning *within the situation* is about recognising, acknowledging, appreciating that the other person is showing themselves and then showing yourself too. Learning *afterwards* is preferably done together with colleagues. These colleagues should not place themselves in an outsider's position, the position of an observer who objectifies and moralises, the distant position, but come near and ask themselves: what would I have done if I had been that colleague, if I had been in their position? The most important thing is to actively re-establish, restore, recover the relationship with the care receiver. Such episodes can deepen the relationship. And it can be formative for the other person. Often it is necessary to apologise, and sometimes to help the other person to deal with the apology. This is also an instance of introducing social and moral capital.[15] And if it is possible to re-establish the relationship, this is liberating for both sides, for that moment. But this process must be carefully navigated, otherwise it may hurt the relationship and the other even further, sowing the seeds of violence.

Conclusion

We have argued that relational caring has two points of reference: relationality and finality. Relationality in the sense of taking relationships and working relationally seriously, and finality in the sense of taking what caring is ultimately about seriously. We have discussed the distinction between weak and strong relationality and argued for strong relationality. We take relationships seriously, not as mere conveyors of care, help and support, but as steering and organising mechanisms, as goods-in-themselves, as the care receiver's networks and context of life, as the embedding of the caregiver, and as each human being's destiny. And the question of what caring is ultimately about is given its due weight by conceptualising it in terms of its ultimate end, including that of social institutions that support caring practices, and acknowledging the political character of institutions. Raising the finality question and articulating an answer in a way that starts with the finality of the institution that supports that practice is a contextual, relational and discursive process by a team or group of practitioners. Taking relational caring seriously requires a radical implementation of relationality in all of our thinking about good care, help and support. Respecting and promoting autonomy is to be viewed as a relational process, as are constraining care receivers, setting boundaries to them, punishing their behaviour or ending the caring relationship with them. In these radical relational processes, practical wisdom is indispensable. We will return to practical wisdom in the next chapter.

11

Practically wise professionals

Motto
When you have to act, act in a practically wise way – and don't be afraid to make a leap.

CASE FRAGMENT 11.1

'I'm not sure I would do it again'

Marie-Anne is one of the mentally disabled residents of De Boeier, an assisted living facility in a residential area in Zwolle. At one point she was diagnosed with breast cancer. Breast-conserving surgery was needed, but Marie-Anne didn't want it. Marja Rumpf is the coordinating supervisor. Three years later, she recounts the following story:

'When we told Marie-Anne that she had breast cancer, she was of course terribly sad: "What's going to happen next? Am I going to die now?" Nobody knew the answer. It turned out that breast-conserving surgery was necessary. Marie-Anne immediately panicked. Six people from the home had died shortly after each other, all in hospital. Marie-Anne called off the operation a few times.

'On the day it was finally supposed to happen, my colleague and I woke her up as gently as possible. But the battle started immediately: she didn't want to go. Her trusted caregiver couldn't get her to move either. Marie-Anne weighs 100 kilos and we couldn't get her out of her chair despite all our pushing and pulling. We called off the whole thing ourselves. A few moments later, Marie-Anne had dressed and was ready to go to work. I got so angry that I called her names. I lost my patience with her ... She broke down, clung to me all the way and cried that she was terrified of the operation. I told her I was afraid too: for her life. That was a turning point: she was no longer alone with her fear. Now she dared to go to the hospital, but only with me.

'Once we got there, Marie-Anne had to be put in a hospital bed immediately, wearing a surgical gown and an oxygen cap. That was a bridge too far: she ran away. When we found her outside, my colleague coaxed her into going to the doctor to tell him herself that she didn't want the surgery. The doctor asked my colleagues in for a consultation. If it was necessary and he had permission, he could drug Marie-Anne by force. I stayed behind with Marie-Anne. I thought

> force would be disastrous for her. I had to come up with something. The consultation went on and on. I started to play with the blue gown and the oxygen cap. Marie-Anne didn't want to try it herself, but thought it was funny when I showed her what I was doing. On a whim, I took off my sweater and put on the blue gown. Marie-Anne was as surprised as I was. We had to laugh at it together. She also took off her clothes and if we did everything together, she was willing to go further. She put on a gown too and we crammed into the narrow bed together. There we were when the doctor came back.
>
> 'From then on, everyone participated in the realisation that it could work this way. I felt very unhappy during the many hours we had to wait: I was half-naked in bed alongside a client, with two male colleagues at the foot of the bed. And this while Marie-Anne could change her mind at any moment. She kept asking if I was really going to go through with it. In the operating room we were both given an oxygen mask. Marie-Anne fell asleep very peacefully and I was finally able to get out of the bed.
>
> 'The operation was successful, Marie-Anne is doing well. When she talks about that day now, she always starts by saying, "They grabbed me and I didn't want to come". I think it's very unfortunate that it has stayed with her like that. She herself is especially proud that she succeeded, she will tell everyone who wants to hear it. But she only does that when I'm there too: it's not her story, it's our story.'[1]

This chapter deals with the professionalism of relationally caring professionals. Usually, professionalism is discussed in terms of knowledge, skills, attitude, ethos and accountability. All these five interdependent dimensions are relevant for relationally caring professionals. Our emphasis on relational caring as the heart of all good professional care, help and support in healthcare and social work is not a plea for deprofessionalisation, for 'just following your heart', for setting aside discipline-specific knowledge, skills and so on. But these things must all be understood in a way that is adequate to relational caring. The care receiver, that which is at stake for them and that which is relationally possible and desirable between the care receiver and their caregivers determine how knowledge, skills, attitude, ethos and accountability must be understood, which and whose knowledge and skills count, and how they can contribute to the good of the other. Each of these dimensions must be conceptualised as a multipolar field of tension – tension that must not be eliminated but maintained and adequately handled.[2] As regards knowledge, professionals must have the will and the ability to understand, acquire and exert both explicit, discipline-specific and relational knowledge and tacit knowing, to inquire continuously and to imagine future courses. As to skills, professionals must have the will and the ability to act in a practical way, to give scope to the other in their otherness, to what is at stake for them and to what can be done in the relationship with the other. As regards attitude, professionals must have the will and the ability to regulate themselves, to navigate their feelings and see them as sources of knowledge, to be accessible and touchable and to engage in reflection and deliberation. As to ethos, professionals must have the will and the ability to navigate morality, to practise virtues, to be sensitive and ready to respond to emerging goods and to raise and answer the question of the finality of their practice. As regards accountability, professionals must have the will and the ability to render an account of the quality of their care, to cultivate quality awareness, to inquire into the quality of care and to present their work contextually and in a combination of complementary ways – not only as facts and figures but also in the form of images and stories.

It has always been the case that professionals must be able to act, despite uncertainty whether their actions will produce the desired outcomes. In late modernity, however, this ability has come under increased pressure as a result of several interconnected developments. Complexity has increased enormously in most institutional contexts in healthcare and social work, especially in hospitals (Vosman et al, 2016). The desire to have widely available, sound knowledge and adequate techniques, together with the need – inspired by the free market economy – to present evidence of productivity to investors, has increased investment in finding out, defining and documenting what professionals need to do. This investment has grown even more because confidence in professionals has decreased in society because of a cultural resistance to paternalism and patronage, as well as revelations of malpractice by individual professionals and the inability of professional organisations to prevent it. However, imposing rules and regulations in response to malpractice further erodes public confidence in professionals and leads to the undermining of professional pride, and increased absenteeism and burnout among professionals themselves.

A classical concept such as practical wisdom can help resist the pressure that is being put on professionals, precisely because of its long history of interpretations and reinterpretations in different times and different contexts. In particular, practical wisdom can help navigate complexity.

Phronetic professionalism

In modernity, especially in the twentieth century, professionalism came to refer not just to the classical professions of doctor, lawyer and clergyman, but to a whole range of professionals in the fields of healthcare and social work. Professionalism acquired the following meanings: (a) knowing the theory, techniques, rules and guidelines of one's profession, (b) being capable of using and applying them, and (c) being able and willing to render public account of one's actions. Each of the three classical professions had specialised knowledge of and skills for a particular existential domain of life.

Someone who felt under threat in this domain could turn to the relevant profession for relief. Someone whose physical health was compromised turned to a doctor, someone whose societal freedom was under threat to a lawyer and someone whose spiritual welfare was in peril to a religious minister. It was characteristic of these professionals that they acted under a great deal of uncertainty as to whether their actions would have the desired effect. They could function because of a high level of societal confidence in their expertise, altruism and willingness to serve the community. They were allowed to supervise themselves through self-regulation. This was no longer regarded as sufficient in the twentieth century. More and more, professions began to lay claim to the idea of professionalism, which had hitherto been reserved for the classical professions. A technical-instrumental concept of professionalism was developed and began to be applied to all kinds of professionals in healthcare and social work. This concept requires professionals to base their acting on scientific knowledge ('evidence-based'), to apply rational methods and techniques to their work and to strip physical, mental or social problems of their moral and political implications in order to find technical solutions. The societal investment in these professionals is matched by the societal control exerted over them.

In the 1990s, a new concept of professionalism was developed, particularly by Harry Kunneman and Douwe van Houten of the University of Humanistic Studies in the Netherlands, and by Geert van der Laan and Andries Baart. This concept acknowledged that every professional practice is a moral enterprise with different moral layers. It was called 'normative professionalism' (Jacobs et al, 2008; van Ewijk and Kunneman, 2013), but we prefer to call it 'normative-reflective professionalism' to emphasise that reflexivity is an indispensable aspect of it (Baart, 1996; 2001: 827–43; Baart and Steketee, 2003). 'Normative' refers to the professional practice as a moral endeavour with different moral layers. One of these layers is the professional's ethos: their character and virtues, such as moral discernment and courage. Another layer consists of the good of the participants in which the professional is involved. Other layers are the end, goods and norms of the profession and of the professional community, and the common good and the norms of society. 'Reflective' refers to the continuous, personal and self-critical reflexivity that accompanies the practising of the profession (Schön, 1983; 1987). It involves the professional's intellectual and institutional freedom to form their own situational judgements, interpretations and actions, applying general knowledge to particular cases, and to justify these. Various sources of knowledge are utilised in this reflexivity, including the professional's emotions once they have been analysed. Ideally, all this happens in the context of a learning community of practitioners involved in moral deliberation.

The concept of normative-reflective professionalism was a great improvement on the traditional, technical-instrumental view of professionalism. We do not wish to deny its merits, but feel it is necessary to go a step further, because it is problematic, especially the reflexivity part. We feel that the way in which reflection is often elaborated and shaped is too formal, procedural, discursive and incorporeal. Greater importance often appears to be assigned to right procedure ('rule-driven reflection') than to a good outcome. Alternative sources of knowledge – emotions, tacit knowing, bodily knowledge, intuitions, patient and family knowledge – are scarcely considered. Reflection alone, especially when it is confined to its discursive aspects, offers insufficient resistance to systemic pressure. The professional's character and virtues, such as courage, seem to be more decisive to resist pressure than reflexion. And more importantly, reflecting does not automatically lead to acting. There is a gap between formally, discursively, incorporeally reflecting and actually acting. Reflection can be distinctly unhelpful, especially when things happen in a flow or under time pressure. Lastly, reflection is a luxury professionals cannot afford when they are placed before a situation where they have to act. In response to these difficulties, we have further developed the concept of normative-reflective professionalism, which has resulted in the concept of phronetic or practically wise professionalism. This view of professionalism retains social-technical knowledge, normativity and reflexivity as important aspects, but positions them in a larger framework.

Muddling through

Before we turn to practical wisdom, we will first address another problem that besets a lot of thinking about professionalism. Professionalism is often regarded as a warrant for good care. The idea is that enhancing professionalism will lead to better care. The assumption is often that professionalism is the systematic and planned application of evidence-based explicit knowledge. But there is another, darker side to professionalism: professionals can also professionally perpetuate suffering. We distinguish three forms or layers of professional perpetuation of suffering: methodical, bureaucratic and cultural (see Chapter 10). On the methodical level, we see 'mismatches': care that is good according to some method or rule, but that is not attuned to the concrete person in need, and professional neglect by not completing care or doing nothing, often due to the imposition of rules that justify doing nothing. On the bureaucratic or systemic level, we see professionals who are not given the scope to provide what they deem to be good care, and persons in need of complex care who are being passed around from one care organisation to the next. On the cultural level, we see the troublesome consequences of a problematic faith in progress and social engineering and of a specific perception of emotions as distracting the professional from what they have to do. What we call a problematic faith in social engineering is evident in the belief that suffering, defects and problems can always be solved, that solutions can be advanced by what professionals do and that what professionals do must be guided by rational, 'evidence-based' treatment plans. The problem behind the professional perpetuation of suffering is the division between theory and practice, between planning and implementation and between good and bad, a division that does not exist as neatly in practice as it does in some theories.

In fact, the problem is that professionals and professional organisations are finding it difficult to acknowledge the roughness, the improvisation and the nasty side of their practice. The mechanism of 'self-consolation' is an expression of this: when faced with the inefficacy of their plans and efforts, professionals seek comfort in the beauty, rhetoric and internal reasonableness of their plans and efforts, instead of in their loyal and dedicated being with the other (Baart, 2001: 717–19).

In 1959, the political macroeconomist Charles Lindblom came up with the 'science of muddling through' (Lindblom, 1959; 1979). While studying welfare policies throughout the industrialised world, Lindblom realised that most of the literature proposed an approach to policy making that could actually function only for simple problems. A different approach was needed for complex problems, one which he called the 'successive limited comparisons' or 'incremental' method. This approach is able to deal with situations 'where means and ends are sometimes impossible to separate, where aspirations or objectives undergo constant development, and where drastic simplification of the complexity of the real world is urgent if problems are to be solved in the time that can be given to them' (Lindblom, 1959: 88). According to Lindblom, this method is the system behind what is known as 'muddling through'. Muddling through is not the same thing as messing around. It requires a good sense of the direction in which you are heading and relevant knowledge of the field in which you are working. It consists of taking successive small steps, and then seeing where you stand, what can be seen from there and what next step could be taken (cf Mechanic, 1997). Instead of straightforwardly implementing your plans, muddling through requires reflection and deliberation, continuous adjustment of the plan, a determination to carry on, including in difficult situations, and courage to act (Baart, 2013: 84–7).

In our view, muddling through is a moral enterprise, and moral choices, moral deliberation and moral learning processes are indispensable to it. It is performed in the perspective of the 'broken good': the good of the other cannot be appropriated by the other themselves, cannot be completed, is mixed up with bad things, lies beyond what the professional can perceive, is turned into a bad (*malum*) or is unimaginable (Baart, 2004b). In our care-ethical, presence-theoretical perspective, we use the expression 'lovingly and sensibly muddling through'. 'Lovingly' refers to the professional's will and ability to relate to the other in their otherness for the other's good. 'Sensibly' refers to practical wisdom, one of the virtues that must be practised for relational caring as muddling through.

Practical wisdom in late modernity

The concept of practical wisdom originates from Aristotle. In his *Nicomachean Ethics*, he introduces the concept of *phronèsis* as a kind of knowledge that forms part of the threefold division into *technè*, *phronèsis* and *epistèmè*: professional skill, practical wisdom and scientific knowledge (Aristotle, 2013). Professional competence or technical skill is a processing kind of knowledge and expertise, and is about things, about making them and about their efficacy. Practical wisdom is a practical kind of knowledge and expertise, and is about the lives of others and one's own life and how these can be good lives. Scientific, universal knowledge is a theoretical kind of knowledge and expertise, and is about truth and unchanging laws. Practical wisdom connects skilled capability and thorough knowledge with the good life, so to speak. To Aristotle, this practical wisdom is a character virtue, a disposition that has to be pursued and that helps a human being to act morally excellently.

Following the example of Aristotle, ancient Greek philosophy regards *phronèsis* as the ability to recognise and respect the purport of acting towards an end (*telos*) (Vosman, 2008). *Phronèsis* has to do not only with finding suitable means for a given end, but also with recognising the end of the type of acting involved. This latter point is not about setting goals, but about recognising the moral good that is pursued in that kind of acting. The Roman concept of *prudentia*, which was further developed in the Middle Ages, is about observing and estimating – with all one's capabilities and in all directions – what is morally relevant in the context of acting amid uncertainties. This also includes the perception of freedom and anxiety both in the other and in yourself, without, for example, allowing your own anxiety to become the determining factor. And it includes looking back at what was done wrongly and what went wrong, all with a view to establishing what needs to be done.

Paul Ricœur has combined the characteristics of *phronèsis* and *prudentia* mentioned earlier to propose a conception of practical wisdom as 'wisdom thought within practices' (Vosman, 2008: 30). According to Vosman, Ricœur maintains three bipolar tensions that are characteristic of the complexity in many care practices in late modernity (Vosman, 2008: 31–2). In each tension, one pole receives more support from society than the other. First, there is the tension, already mentioned, between finding suitable means to an end, on the one hand, and recognising what the end is, on the other. Second, there is that between making and repairing things and situations, on the one hand, and morally excellent acting in relationships and within a community, on the other. Third, Vosman discusses the tension between having to act, on the one hand, and being opaque to oneself, on the other, a tension that exists for both the person who must act and the person who must undergo the action. For example, a clinician must always act decisively, but the purpose of their acting – why do I do this and why do I do it in this way? – is often not so clear. It lies hidden in the concrete good that is pursued and in the concrete evil that is averted for this concrete patient here-and-now, in their relationship with these concrete caregivers.

Like Ricœur and Vosman, we consider practical wisdom in the context of practices and institutions. Professionals are not the performers of individual acts. Their acting is determined by the larger whole of the professional practice of which they are practitioners. A professional practice is the coherent whole of what practitioners do individually and collectively, of what they say separately and collectively and of the things and techniques that they use for this. This historically and socially developed whole of 'doings and sayings' (Schatzki, 1996) has its own meaning, its own internal goods and its own inherent ends (MacIntyre, 2007). For example, the ends of Western medical practice are traditionally: (a) to ward off death, (b) to help cure illnesses and ailments and (c) to combat pain and distress. In each specific case, these ends will relate to each other differently. These ends, and the associated standards of excellence, can be determined only by practising that practice. Only practitioners will experience what actually matters, what is good in that practice (Ricœur, 1992; MacIntyre, 2007).

Practices are intrinsically connected with institutions. Institutions are a particular historical community's structures of *living together*, which have their own specific ends that also limit the structures in question. These structures cannot be reduced to interpersonal relationships, but are nevertheless linked to them (Ricœur, 1992: 194). Institutions support practices by formulating and distributing rights, duties and responsibilities (MacIntyre, 2007). An institution, such as healthcare, social welfare or education, is given concrete shape in various organisations: healthcare organisations, social welfare organisations or educational institutions. While practitioners focus on the internal goods of their practice, organisations are engaged in acquiring and distributing external goods: money, power and status. Without support from the institution and the organisation, a practice cannot survive long. However, organisations can also have a corrupting effect. To resist these corrupting powers, practitioners need virtues such as justice, courage and truthfulness (MacIntyre, 2007). Institutions and organisations themselves are also under pressure in late modernity because organisations have started to accommodate several distinct institutions that sit together uneasily. If a healthcare organisation also becomes a for-profit production business, the healthcare institution, which has its own ends, will come under pressure from all kinds of regulatory systems of bureaucracy, registration and quality assurance. These systems' own legitimate ends are transparency, efficiency and cost control, and these have their merits, but they do not automatically lead to good care for sick people. Hospitals thus become systems that destroy the institutional character of the hospital. And doctors and nurses are turned into 'bundles of desired functions' (cf Dubet, 2002; discussed in Vosman, 2008: 38–43). This means that practical wisdom becomes both more relevant and less obvious at the same time. Vosman has therefore argued that 'systemic space' is needed in addition to free-range or discretionary space: space within the system in which various practitioners within the institution (for example, doctors, nurses and managers in a hospital) can jointly consider the tenor, substance and purport of the care practices involved. By giving scope to moral deliberation, the exploring of emotions and the elucidation of goals and ends, organisations and communities of practitioners can contribute to learning or, rather, to cultivating practical wisdom (Baart, 2008; Schwartz and Sharpe, 2010; Kinsella and Pitman, 2012).

Practical wisdom in general practice: a study

There is a lot of literature about practical wisdom in medicine. Practical wisdom helps doctors to resist forces that undermine their profession, including a medical ethics that no longer speaks of ends but only of principles, consequences and procedures (Kaldjian, 2014). Practical wisdom helps doctors to incorporate different types of knowledge and different domains that are relevant for decision making into their own acting. These domains concern medical science, patient preferences, the doctor's own moral perspective and society's expectations. Practical wisdom helps doctors to recognise the goals of their medical practice in that mix-up of powers, to translate them into the concrete situation and to respect them in their own acting. Practical wisdom requires estimating the nature, severity and prognosis of the patient's situation. Not only the moment itself matters, but also the entire process that precedes it (Goudsmit, 2005). Practical wisdom is what gives doctors a gut feeling that something is wrong, a feeling that serves as a guide for diagnostics or, if acting quickly is required, as a mental shortcut (Stolper et al, 2011). Practical wisdom helps doctors to make transitions between the various discourses with which they are dealing, in particular between professional discourse with colleagues and everyday discourse with patients and their relatives (Goudsmit, 2005). Finally, practical wisdom helps doctors to act, to take the leap from perceiving, reflecting and deliberating to acting.

End-of-life care by general practitioners

In 2015–16, we carried out a study of end-of-life care by general practitioners (GPs) in the Netherlands (Timmerman and Baart, 2016a). It was inspired by our amazement at the way one specific GP was treated, and how his acting in a specific case was judged. The GP in question gave a long-time patient whose condition had deteriorated sharply a high dose of morphine, after which the patient died, to the relief of the patient's spouse. Before the GP had the opportunity to explain and justify his actions, he was subjected to a public debate that pointed the finger at him, and he was accused of improper conduct by the National Health Inspectorate. He then committed suicide. We were surprised at how ill-informed society was about what GPs in general perceive and how they reflect, assess, weigh, act and evaluate at the bedsides of their sick and dying patients, even though there is a great deal of quantitative and qualitative research. Our intuition was that, first, it would be worthwhile and relevant to remedy this lack of understanding, and second, heuristic use of the concept of practical wisdom would be helpful in doing this. Instead of assuming that GPs use principle-driven reasoning, we decided to undertake an empirical and practice-driven reconstruction of GPs' perceiving and *in actu* judging.

The empirical material consisted of the extensive and comprehensive description of six cases, one from each of the six participating GPs, and fragmentary information about approximately 80 additional cases. We reconstructed the end-of-life care process in such a way as to retain rather than reduce and unduly simplify its complex, dynamic and emergent character. To freely and truthfully reconstruct the whole process, we had to develop our own vocabulary, grammar and syntax. To preserve the emergent dynamics of the process, we introduced the idea that the current situation and process is continuously interpreted through images and stories, references to lived reality and an imagined synthesis ('what will the final situation be?'). We interpreted our reconstruction of the end-of-life care process by GPs as a practising of practical wisdom, conceived as 'knowing how to act in a concrete situation (and acting accordingly)'. We saw that GPs act not only discipline-specifically – related to the fact that they are medical doctors – but also relationship-specifically – related to the fact that the patient and the GP stand in a relationship with each other, with both persons living and working – and dying – in relationships with others (Table 11.1).

Reconstructing a complex process

Practical wisdom means acting context-, patient- and situation-specifically. What is at stake here, morally speaking, is always particular and unstable and it cannot necessarily be deduced from external standards. There were no instances in the material of GPs simplifying anything unnecessarily or prematurely. They moved with the dynamics of the process and responded to what presented itself as a possible good. Practical wisdom means being aware of the objective framework of your work and introducing substantial ideas about good living and dying into the deliberations with patients and their loved ones. Practical wisdom requires moral perception, not only of the patient's physical condition and complaints but also of their primary, derived and secondary suffering and that of their relatives, of the patient's and their relatives' capacities and of what is at stake for them. GPs also perceive themselves, including their own emotions. Finally, they also extrapolate their perceptions towards the future ('moral imagination', Johnson, 1993): what if it continues like this? And how do I evaluate that in terms of good or bad? GPs must act in situations where knowledge and guidelines fall short and uncertainty cannot be eliminated. It is not clear how they should proceed, no logical deductions can be made, rules and insights are not decisive or are even contradictory, and deliberating does not result in any outcome – or there is no time to deliberate. There is no escape from the necessity of acting: no matter how difficult and uncertain the situation is, something has to be done and what is done must be good. We also saw GPs do their utmost to anticipate unexpected developments. They endeavoured to prevent forced-action situations, but without intervening prematurely and/or too drastically (avoiding irreversible trajectories). Unexpected developments nevertheless occurred (such as a sudden deterioration) and we saw the GPs respond to these, interrupting the course of their acting or changing their policy (for example, by increasing pain relief, but only to such an extent that consultation remained possible). Finally, we also saw situations in which the GPs feared that things would not end well, even though the best possible knowledge had been used, the procedures had been followed and skilful action had been taken. Practical wisdom then means to have the courage to change course, to give up the strict interpretation of the rules and then look for the unknown. This way of doing, refraining, going another way, and so forth by GPs is an instance of muddling through.

As we have mentioned, practical wisdom requires that GPs estimate the nature, severity and prognosis of the patient's situation. The GP can make this assessment only in the practising itself. The moment itself matters. At the same time, the entire process also matters. After all, their own observing and acting is part of the image that the GP is trying to form. The GPs in our cases constantly made estimates. In their stories about these cases, they remained very close to the moment, but without losing sight of the entire process – both everything that had already happened and the end they were pursuing. It is precisely this process-dependent and self-referring nature of the estimating that GPs do – and of their perceiving, considering, assessing and acting – that prompted us as researchers to reconstruct a complex image of that entire process.

Attentiveness, metaphorical positioning and taking a leap

We wish to emphasise three elements from the complex process of GPs' care for the sick and dying patient: attentiveness, metaphorical positioning and the necessity of taking a leap. In the cases we analysed, we saw GPs looking very narrowly and precisely at the patient and, at the same time, looking very broadly at the people around the patient. We saw that GPs always kept the patient in the focus of their attention and, at the same time, made constant adjustments to the other persons and things in their focus and in their 'scopus' (the full width of their attentiveness), and/or to the persons and things that had to be brought from the wider context into their scopus or even their focus.

We saw that GPs acted fully as medical doctors, but in the course of the process we also saw them 'metaphorically positioning' themselves. Within the informal network around the patient, the GP occupies a position that often has the characteristics of an informal neighbour, a brother or sister, a friend or close neighbour, even though the GP does not actually become any of these things. Taking this position means deepening the relationship with the patient and allowing the patient to show themselves more openly and more completely, with their desires, fears and concerns. Taking this dynamic and case-specific metaphorical position creates the conditions for being able to identify what is at stake and what is a potential good, and thus also for good care by GPs.

Often the GPs had to take a leap, not without reflexivity, not without considering everything that they had perceived, assessed, weighed and done, and not in the sense of acting randomly, but still they had to take a leap and just hope for the best. For example, one of the doctors told us that he had bought a flower for a terminally ill female patient who had just turned 40. Even though afterwards he had a lot to say about his reasons for doing this, ultimately he had to acknowledge that he simply 'found himself buying a flower'.

Practically wise professionals, communities and organisations

Any understanding of practical wisdom that seeks to be helpful to our thinking about professionals in complex organisations in late modern society must do justice to the complexity, dynamics and emergence in the everyday lives of patients, clients, pupils, residents and their relatives, and in professional practices and organisations (see also Bontemps-Hommen et al, 2019). Complex processes must be conceived in a complex way,

Table 11.1: Practical wisdom requires and contributes to making scope for ...

Scope for ...	Understood here as ...
Moral intuitions	Admitting and articulating that something is not right, that you wanted, meant, pursued and so forth something different (moral intuition as a contrast experience), and practising the virtues that go with it, such as courage, honesty, boldness and integrity.
Moral imagination	Close your eyes and imagine: what will this lead to if we do nothing? What will become of the patient or client if the policy remains unchanged? Who will suffer harm from this and what harm specifically, and who will benefit?
Interruptions	Stop acting, take time out, interrupt and suspend routines, procedures, step-by-step plans: create breathing space.
Raising and answering the finality question	Consider the question together with others: what is this really about? What is the ultimate end we should strive for? And what goal are we actually pursuing?
Deliberation	The joint reflection should take place on the basis of ... • a preferred option for the weakest: who comes first here? • hermeneutics: what does it mean? What value do we attach to it? • sound knowledge: why is this happening? How can we understand and possibly explain this? • mature experiences: what experience do I have with this? What was wise and what was unwise? • available alternative skills: what is possible? What am I/are we capable of? • moral imagination (in the positive sense): what good is conceivable here? • virtues: what can I do and what virtues must I practise (because I am treading on dangerous ground)?
Daring to take a leap	Practising the virtues necessary for this (for example, dedication, loyalty, *acribie* and tenacity) while continuing to perceive how one's actions turn out.

and simplifications must be avoided. We have shown that the concept of practical wisdom – as we conceive it – enables us to say much more about the process, from perceiving and assessing to acting and evaluating, and to say it much more precisely.

In our research into care practices, we assume that practically wise professionals have good reasons to act as they do, even when they sometimes deviate from the existing laws and regulations and the applicable guidelines and protocols. Practical wisdom is not at odds with rules, guidelines and protocols, but it contrasts with anxiously following these, on the basis of knowledge of the ultimate end of the practice. For the professional who knows what their profession is ultimately about – even though this can be determined only on a situational and relational level, and in conversation with the patient, client or resident and their relatives – rules, guidelines and protocols are signposts that indicate how to act and that are based on informative experiences of practically wise colleagues in similar situations. Practical wisdom helps to determine in what relevant respects the situation in which professionals, their colleagues, their patient, client, pupil or resident and the latter's relatives find themselves corresponds to and differs from the situations on which the rules and guidelines are based. Practical wisdom also helps to determine how and to what extent those instructions must be followed or may be disregarded. And finally, practical wisdom helps to take a leap.

For Aristotle, practical wisdom was primarily a virtue on the level of individual actors, but we think it is helpful to realise that practical wisdom manifests itself also on the level of practices, institutions and society as a whole. We have already mentioned Ricœur's conceptualisation of practical wisdom as 'wisdom thought within practices'. Marij Bontemps-Hommen conducted four qualitative studies into practices of medical specialists in a general hospital. In one of these studies, she analysed the self-reported lessons that medical specialists learned from 100 multidisciplinary case discussions (Bontemps-Hommen et al 2020). Based on a literature review and her empirical studies, she has proposed a definition of the practical wisdom of medical practices: 'the capability which emerges in joint actions, that incorporate the logic of good care and are aimed at discerning and focusing on each particular patient's good, that is also in accordance with the telos of the practice, in a dynamic process, using the most appropriate means, while dealing with complexity and with operational and systemic pressures' (Bontemps-Hommen, 2020: 165). In his study of practical wisdom in governance, Henk den Uijl has distinguished between the individual level, the level of practices and the level of institutional arrangements. He has concluded that practical wisdom in governance on the individual level is about 'judgment, interpretation and […] understand[ing] the moral and political aspects of decision-making'. On the level of practices, it is about 'common sense: a sense for what matters to people in the plural', and on the level of institutions it is about 'promoting and sustaining association and participation of involved people in ordinary and administrative questions' (den Uijl, 2022: 395).

Borrowing den Uijl's idea of distinguishing different levels of manifestations of practical wisdom, we have summarised our discussion of practically wise professionals, communities and organisations in Table 11.2. We have added the level of society at which practical wisdom manifests itself as the scope for professional autonomy and civic participation.

Conclusion

Although the individual professional is not the sole actor or the only initiator of actions, and practices, institutions, organisations and society

Table 11.2: Manifestations of practical wisdom

Level	Bearers	Manifestations of practical wisdom
Actors	Individuals	Virtues, tacit knowing, judgement, responsively adequate actions, moral intuitions, moral imagination, breaking rules, taking a leap
Practices	Communities, teams, learning communities	Routines, rules, joint actions, raising and answering the finality question with others, joint reflection, deliberation, scope for interruptions
Institutions	Organisations, executive and supervisory boards	Facilitation of discretionary and systemic space for professionals, scope for interruptions, scope for participation of professionals and clients or patients in decision making
Society	Society as a whole	Scope for professional autonomy and civic participation

must also be considered, it is still true that there is no practical wisdom without practically wise professionals and therefore no good care, help and support either. If we want professionals in healthcare and social work to perceive openly and inquire carefully, to relationally connect with and attune their practice to clients, patients, residents and pupils and the latter's relatives, to care in a contextually and situationally adequate way, to be loyally dedicated to clients and not to abandon them, to be able to muddle through, and to be willing and able to continue learning and inquiring, we need to give scope, facilitate and promote practical wisdom. Let us summarise for their benefit what can be expected from practically wise professionals. Such professionals:

a. know what their professional practice is and what its aim is, and seek this end in concrete situations;
b. accept that they must act, even if goals are conflicting, rules contradict each other and the outcome of their acting is uncertain;
c. understand that complexity, dynamics and emergence belong to their professional practice and should not be unduly simplified or suppressed;
d. look wider and further, use multiple sources of knowledge, including their own experience, intuitions and emotions, and employ moral imagination;
e. bring their entire personality to their practice, know their working style and are able to identify the metaphorical positions they occupy;
f. conceive rules and guidelines as indications of how to act, based on the instructive experience of practically wise colleagues in similar situations;
g. are willing, courageous and able to 'lovingly and sensibly muddle through', in the perspective of the 'broken good';
h. practise virtues such as courage, discernment, truthfulness, loyalty, justice, tenacity and so forth, in all their relationships;

i. respond to the question of accountability by telling the whole story from the inside;
j. learn, individually and jointly, from what has not gone well and what was not done well in the past.

It will help, of course, if not only individual professionals exercise practical wisdom, but also teams of professionals and the organisation itself.

INTERLUDE

A note on technology

Our conception of relational caring stresses the importance of social relationships, physical nearness, bodily contact, embodied knowledge and emotions as sources of knowledge. We are often asked how we look at the use of technology in healthcare and social work. Having laid out the groundwork of relational caring in Chapters 9 to 11 – carefully perceiving, attuning one's practice to the other and practical wisdom – it may be time to turn to that question.

Technology is a big issue in healthcare and social work, as it is in society in general, and it is only getting bigger. Currently, in the 2020s, machine-learning information technology systems, (general purpose) artificial intelligence and big data are accelerating the growth in the ubiquity, opportunities and challenges of technology in society. But we also realise that technology is as old as mankind. For example, language, clothing and writing can also be considered as technologies. However it may be, the use of technology in our understanding of relational caring actually deserves its own chapter in this book, but we do not currently have the scope to write such a chapter. We therefore confine ourselves to a few fundamental comments on this issue.

We think that technology can assist and relieve caregivers, both professionals and informal caregivers, and contribute to the self-esteem, freedom of movement and autonomy of care receivers. In fact, it does already assist and relieve caregivers and it does already contribute to care receivers' self-esteem, freedom of movement and autonomy. For example, care robots give physically disabled persons back their independence in everyday life in relation to other people.

But we also see how technology is promoted in an attempt to solve societal problems, which are first depoliticised. Nowadays, the appeal to technology is often an attempt to avoid real (political) thinking and acting, for example in the climate crisis, the energy crisis and the agricultural crisis. And also in the care crisis, for example in the care for older persons in the Netherlands, where the government promotes the idea 'Self if possible, at home if possible, digital if possible'; and has decreed that the overall number of staff in nursing homes should not increase, because personnel must be available for other sectors. Which sectors are not specified.

We believe that good care can be improved by technology, but bad care cannot be compensated by it. We realise that patients, clients, residents, pupils and so forth are also connected to non-human actors, embedded in a web of human and non-human actors, but we hesitate to call those connections relationships. We are wary of attempts to trick people into interacting with artificial intelligence as if with a human being. However successful it may be to make progress in imitating human relationships, the question is whether we want to view human relationships based on how well machines can imitate them.

As we explain in this book, we tend to think about healthcare and social work from a substantial, moral concept of good care. The core of good care is freely perceiving and imagining, properly attuning one's practice to the person in need of care and practising practical wisdom. Technology has to be incorporated in these three moments, of perception, of practice and of evaluation. And all these three components involve corporeality. Where the use of technology in healthcare and social work ignores people's physicality, for example when the embodied knowledge of the doctor or the social worker is overruled, technology becomes problematic. But where technology supplements the physical limitations of caregivers and care receivers in their daily lives, technology can contribute to good care and to living a good life. As it already does.

12

Cultivating quality awareness

With Jan den Bakker

Motto
But is this good care, and can you give an account of it and account for it properly?

CASE FRAGMENT 12.1

The case of Pia

A case description about a young adult with intellectual disability is thematically analysed for a workshop about quality of care. The conclusions are discussed in the workshop. The detailed case description is about Pia, a young adult, heavily-built woman. The description is supplied by the organisation that is currently caring for Pia. She has the emotional level of a toddler and autism. Pia has little faith in her own abilities and needs guidance all day long to initiate any action. She gets anxious very easily, and expresses this by screaming, biting and pulling her own and other people's hair. She often suffers from constipation. According to the case description, Pia needs safety, security and warmth, and predictability, clarity and structure. This requires regular coordination and fine-tuning by the team. Carers must properly recognise and correctly interpret the signals Pia gives out. Until recently, Pia lived in a home with children and young people, but her development stagnated there. Now she is living in a home for adults. The team is primarily working to create a stable environment to live in and conduct her daily activities, an environment that will give her a feeling of safety. These are the elements provided by the summary of her case description. An experienced researcher gives a thematic analysis, from which the participants in the workshop conclude that the sources of knowledge upon which the description is based are very malady-oriented, and that the reported handling of these sources is highly implementation-oriented. There is little about relational sources of knowledge and relational care for the client. The case description says something about the person of the client, but from an outsider perspective. It says little about the client herself, as a relational and vulnerable person, who is also paying a

> price for being admitted to the facility. The participants of the workshop gather from the description that the organisation is concerned about the environment that it can offer the client. But it says nothing, for example, about the organisation's view on good care. The participants conclude that a more substantive idea of quality, using more perspectives, could be helpful to get a more diverse, richer picture of the care for Pia.[1]

Good care requires relational caring. However, relational caring becomes difficult if professionals are evaluated, judged and rewarded by quality systems that are not equipped to perceive, recognise and acknowledge it. This has led us, together with colleague Jan den Bakker, to develop a way of thinking about quality that is able to do justice to relational caring, as well as a model to guide inquiry into and critically determine the quality of care received. Our way of thinking includes not only a perspective 'from nowhere' but also perspectives from within; not only 'facts and figures' (abstracted reality) but also phenomenology (lived reality), narrativity (signified reality), participation (shared reality) and deliberation (evaluated reality). This thinking and the resulting Care-Ethical Model of Quality Enquiry (CEMQUE model) are based on more than ten years of research, study and deliberation about quality with care professionals and their organisations (Baart, 2004d; 2008; 2014b; 2018c; Baart and Grypdonck, 2008; den Bakker, 2018).[2]

Assessing quality of care

The usual method for determining whether care receivers have received good care is to ask them or their relatives afterwards whether they are satisfied. They are asked to systematically share their experiences with different aspects of the care provided, for example by completing a survey. But the answers that care receivers give to these kinds of questions are often ambiguous. Care receivers are likely to express satisfaction even with results that others would judge to be unsatisfactory or even bad, simply because they deem a good relationship with the caregiver or the organisation to be more important. Also, care receivers may articulate dissatisfaction because they did not get what they wanted. Determining the meaning of expressed satisfaction or dissatisfaction therefore requires careful examination of the case, and interpretation of and deliberation about them. Although satisfaction, dissatisfaction and discomfort expressed by care receivers should be taken seriously, the outcomes of patient satisfaction surveys are not a good measure of good care. Care receivers, or their relatives, certainly have a voice in determining the quality of care and should be allowed to express themselves. But we think the way to do this is to perceive them carefully, connect with and attune your practice to them and deliberate with them during the entire caring process itself.

In many quality systems, care professionals are generally evaluated and judged according to whether they adhere to the prescribed system and have followed rules, guidelines, protocols and procedures. These systems and rules originate in the wish to improve care, to share helpful knowledge, to make good practice transferable and to prevent harm. However, over time they have begun to dominate, pushing the question 'but is what is being done here and now good care?' into the background. This shift in emphasis has led to much improvement in the quality of care since the 1990s, but also to an increase in the administrative burden for professionals, which in turn is causing loss of motivation, burnout, moral fatigue and other similar problems for many of them. In addition, incidents with casualties continue to occur, and so does not-so-good care. This has of course been noted in many forums and in many studies, reports, newspaper articles and documentaries, but the question remains of what went wrong and how this can be dealt with.

Our point is that good care is not simply a matter of following rules, however helpful these may be in general, nor is care that is provided in strict compliance with the rules necessarily good care. Many quality systems are unable to perceive mismatches: care that is given according to external rules but is not attuned to the care receiver. This is where practical wisdom is important, because practical wisdom is required for care to be both guided by rules and well attuned to the care receiver, to find out what good care may be for them.

In this chapter we will present and elucidate a way of thinking about quality that can:

- do justice to relational caring;
- give voice to care receivers and their relational networks according to their concerns;
- perceive mismatches without disregarding rules, guidelines, protocols and so forth;
- appreciate the practical wisdom of care professionals in view of the uniqueness of each and every case.

We will also present the CEMQUE model, a model that can guide inquiry into the quality of care received and critically determine this quality.

Stagnation in quality thinking

There is much excellent literature about quality, quality assurance, accountability for quality, strategies for improving quality and quality systems, also and especially in healthcare and social work (de Jonge et al, 2011). To mention just a few, there have been discussions of the significance of measuring patient satisfaction (Tzeng and Yin, 2008), alternatives to the traditional ISO-oriented approach (Harteloh, 2003), the contribution of publishing performance data to the improvement of quality of care (Fun et al, 2008; Metcalfe et al, 2018), the impact of quality systems on the daily practice of mental healthcare (van Geffen, 2019), regulatory pressure (Banerjee and Armstrong, 2015; van de Bovenkamp et al, 2020) and administrative burdens on professionals (Banerjee et al, 2015; de Veer et al, 2017; Woolhandler and Himmelstein, 2014), the performance paradox (van Thiel and Leeuw, 2002), the performativity of accounting in care (Drost et al, 2017) and indeed of accountability itself as a 'matter of care' (Jerak-Zuiderent, 2013; Ubels, 2015). However, when it comes to the practical implementation of quality thinking, including of its theoretical foundation, we see a lot of thinking that has reached a dead end, despite scholarly criticism.[3] We believe four factors have contributed to this stagnation. First, as soon as designers of quality systems start to think about quality in healthcare and social work, interest in substantive thinking seems to subside. What care really is – a moral practice through and through that is guided by the situation – and the purpose that social interventions actually serve – to organise the political-ethical order of society – no longer receive attention. The important normative aspects of healthcare and social work are constantly concealed and moral issues are addressed as existential and psychological issues, if at all.

Second, quality thinking and the systems that we build to guarantee quality irrevocably seem to end up with a heavily skewed set of checks and balances. According to Thomas Schmidt (2017), our fixation on quality means that we are becoming entangled in all sorts of paradoxes (cf van Thiel and Leeuw, 2002) and that we initiate mechanisms we can no longer stop (Shojania, 2019). Quality policy is about striking an acceptable balance between what is good and what is not good, and these two things occur simultaneously. There is practically nothing in care that is entirely good and not, at the same time, or when seen from a different perspective, not good.

Third, several logics and discourses are dominant in healthcare and social work that are not easily compatible with the 'logic of care' (Mol, 2008), in which relationality plays a key part. Quality policy is often derived from the field of the production of goods, where it serves the market, ensures that supply matches demand and binds customers to the product. This 'logic of production' is not appropriate for care. Nor is medical thinking, which is also very dominant and is not easily compatible with the logic of care. Not only is there a difference in intentionality (cure versus care) but also in the underlying science, epistemology, conceptualisation, research methodology and normativity (cf Mol, 2008). In this chapter we want to 'think care from caring' (Vosman, 2014) and not from healing, solving problems, manufacturing or service provision.

The fourth factor refers to common ideas about organisation and management that often prove to be inconducive to solving the problems that have just been mentioned. We need to consider the institutional embeddedness of the care that is offered: the style of management, the processes of policy formulation and, for example, all the routines, scripts, roles, conventions and expectations that prevent thematising what is taken for granted and thereby inhibit innovation. This often falls outside the usual quality frameworks. Also, moral deliberations easily conform to what seems self-evident.

Thinking about quality should start with thinking about care. Care is not a set of separate care actions, but a practice, an interplay of sayings, doings, undergoings and artefacts, that is intersected by other practices and involves many different aspects and levels (see Chapter 6). All these things need to be factored in if we are to think fruitfully about quality. As the care ethicist and political theorist Joan Tronto pointed out, good care is integrated care (Tronto, 1993). Attention to quality is not an isolated issue, but is interwoven with all kinds of learning and reflection processes (McPherson et al, 2001). Moreover, care is a complex practice in which care receivers and caregivers must deliberate to find out what good care is. Quality cannot be determined on the basis of general criteria, but must be discovered locally per person and situation, and together with the person involved. Finally, care is a moral practice. Determining quality is impossible without considering moral issues, asking moral questions and making moral judgements, without disregarding the ambiguities of human life (Vosman, 2018).

Cultivating quality awareness

Mainstream quality systems are hardly able to perceive and appreciate relational caring because they are oriented to 'objective' norms and values. Most care practitioners, however, will acknowledge that care is 'good' primarily in a particular context, in a specific situation and at a determined moment in the tangible life of a particular person. These two approaches of looking at the quality of care correspond to the two modes of 'doing accountability' that Sonja Jerak-Zuiderent distinguishes: 'from nowhere and for everyone' and 'from somewhere and for someone' (2013; 2015). Our approach is more related to the second mode. It is based on three pillars: (a) the relationality or situatedness of care and, thus, of assessing quality; (b) the practical wisdom of professional caregivers; and (c) the cultivated, self-regulating awareness of quality. The first two are discussed in Chapters 10 and 11, respectively. This chapter discusses the third pillar.

Professional caregivers have been taught to follow rules and guidelines, and have learned that they will expose themselves to criticism if they deviate from these. This fetters them in their perceiving, acting, reflecting and evaluating. By contrast, assessing the quality of relational caring can be done only (a) on the spot, (b) within the relationships between caregivers and care receivers and (c) as a temporary thing. Care is a moral practice, and therefore assessing its quality is also a moral practice. This is a radically different approach from that offered in mainstream approaches.

What about public accountability? Measuring and presenting numbers is just one way of examining quality and accounting for good care. Usually this is done by producing a broad variety of quantitative performance data used to compare care organisations. Numbers can be very informative but 'have to be seen in relation to the ambiguities of the work and investments they entail' (Jerak-Zuiderent and Bal, 2011: 240). Other ways of examining and giving account are the narrative or hermeneutic approach and the phenomenological approach (Charon, 2006; Burhans, 2008; Baart and Willeme, 2010; Vosselman, 2014). In this chapter, we will focus on a fourth method: a developed and cultivated, reflective and self-reflective quality awareness that is nourished by and expressed in perceiving, understanding, responding and giving account properly (Baart, 2014b). The other methods of quality examination mentioned earlier can be used within this context by bringing them into communication with each other, so that they can inform and fuel the ongoing inquiry into good care both horizontally and vertically (cf Jerak-Zuiderent's (2013) concept of 'generative accountability').

It is not enough to use external tools in order to properly examine the quality of relational caring; the caregivers must become an instrument themselves, continuously and carefully inquiring into and within the concrete situation. This applies not only to the individual professional, but also to teams of professionals and to the organisation as a whole. We propose that the cultivation of critical, vigilant quality awareness should be made the core of quality policy.[4] Permanent quality awareness maintains the connection between learning to perceive, understand, evaluate and act. It looks at the entire process, including the person who does the counting and who gives the account, and thus keeps the different ways of looking at quality together. Giving an account takes place at three levels: the internal level within the organisation, including the care receiver, the internal level with third parties, and the external level outside the organisation itself. First of all, caregivers must render account of the care provided to the care receiver, on a continuous basis during the care that is given or proposed, and this receives an immediate response. Relational caring, examining quality and giving account both horizontally and vertically are all intertwined (den Bakker, 2018).

Regardless of what learning and reflection practices are chosen, sooner or later we will need a substantive idea of what constitutes good care, or at least questions that can help them approximate such an idea. In the next section, we will present a detailed model of good care that both nourishes quality awareness and makes it concrete.

The Care-Ethical Model of Quality Enquiry (CEMQUE)

Drawing on the conceptual foundations of relational caring, practical wisdom and cultivating quality awareness, this section presents and operationalises a detailed and innovative model. It was developed on the basis of the acknowledgement that the quality of care that is relationally arranged, attuned and navigated can be determined only locally and not on the basis of a definition or theory of quality. We developed our model based on (a) a strong philosophical and theoretical underpinning of what care actually is and (b) our experience in empirical and theoretical research. We validated and fine-tuned it in (c) training of professionals and teams of professionals and (d) discussions with professionals and organisations in healthcare and social work during an ongoing quality workshop held from 2012 to 2018. Our model is first and foremost a heuristic model that is intended to help professionals and organisations to describe, assess and improve care, to give an account of good care, assess existing quality frameworks and formulate quality policies. We have found it particularly helpful for evaluating complaints and incident reports.

Before we present our model, we must first explain two decisions we made. The first is that we decided to take the perspectives rather than relationships as the constitutive dimensions of the model. More precisely, we took as dimensions of our model the four frames of reference rooted in the perspectives of the care receiver, the caregiver, the organisation and society, respectively. One pragmatic reason for this is that taking frames of reference rooted in these perspectives as dimensions of the model is more attuned to how care receivers, professionals and organisations currently tend to think. A more fundamental reason is that connecting with and attuning your practice to the care receiver and their lifeworld, life course, concerns and so forth are essential in our conception of relational caring. To connect with and attuning your practice to the other requires trying to enter into the perspective of the care receiver, this particular care receiver, in all their relationships with other people. We want this perspective to be central to our model. Although we rejected relationships as dimensions of our model, the different aspects of the model have been elaborated in terms of social relationships and are themselves related and correlated to each other. The people involved in the practice must themselves discover in their deliberation about good care how these relationships function in concrete cases, in what combinations and what weight must be assigned to them; the model can be used to do this.

The second decision we must explain is that we have made our idea of the ultimate goal of good care, its *telos*, a focal point in the model. To continue the previous discussion: good care must make a difference in the lives of care receivers. Care ethics has traditionally seen care as a response to the 'moral injunction' 'not to turn away from someone in need' (Gilligan and Attanucci, 1988: 73) and has situated the 'purpose of caring' in 'the care-receivers' experience of being supported and not left on their own' (van Heijst, 2011: 3). The good cannot be realised without the tragic, which is woven through everyday life in a complex structure. Even if nothing can be done to heal or solve a problem, if life stagnates or collapses, it is always still possible to stay with the other. The ultimate goal of good care is to help the care receiver find their own, more or less satisfactory, relationship to the fragility, perilousness and transience of human existence: accepting, fighting, cursing, repairing, celebrating, undergoing or evading it (or a combination of these things).

The COVID-19 pandemic has shown that 'helping the care receiver to find their own relationship to the fragility of existence' is indeed a much more adequate articulation of the purpose of good care than 'adding quality to the patient's or client's life'. When a person is dying, lonely and in agony, good care has nothing to do with adding quality of life. 'Quality of life' implies that this is something objective that (a) can be accomplished, (b) can be determined to be good from the outside and (c) is indubitably good. We question all three statements: (a) it is possible to provoke or promote good in someone else's life, but what is good must ultimately be found or discovered by the person themselves; (b) determining that something is good in someone's life is an evaluative act that the person themselves performs in that particular situation; and (c) the good is always and inevitably a 'broken good', mixed up with things that are not so good or even evil. Good care is care that helps the care receiver realise their good. But the care receiver's good itself lies beyond the caregiver's and the care system's scope and responsibility (as is indicated in Figure 12.1). Healthcare and social work can be helpful, but should not pretend, as Ivan Illich argued, that they are able to remove the necessity of coming 'to terms with pain, impairment, and death' (Illich, 1975: 90), or of living what the psychiatrist Arthur Kleinman has called – borrowing an expression from William James – 'endurance and acceptance of genuine reality' (Kleinman, 2006: 9). What care can contribute, however, is that it can alleviate the care receiver's concerns, although it can also aggravate them. We will return to the issue of concerns later.

The CEMQUE consists of four normative dimensions (Figure 12.1):

- humanity, from the care receiver's perspective;
- solicitude, from the professional caregiver's perspective;
- habitability, from the perspective of the care organisation; and
- justice and decency, from the perspective of society.

The fourth dimension of the model is about the embedding of care in society with its care paradigms, which determine the societal, legal, scholarly and financial frameworks of care.

In the following sections, we will elaborate on each of the four dimensions of the model. For each of them, we will start with a 'brief philosophy' of

Figure 12.1: The Care-Ethical Model of Quality Enquiry

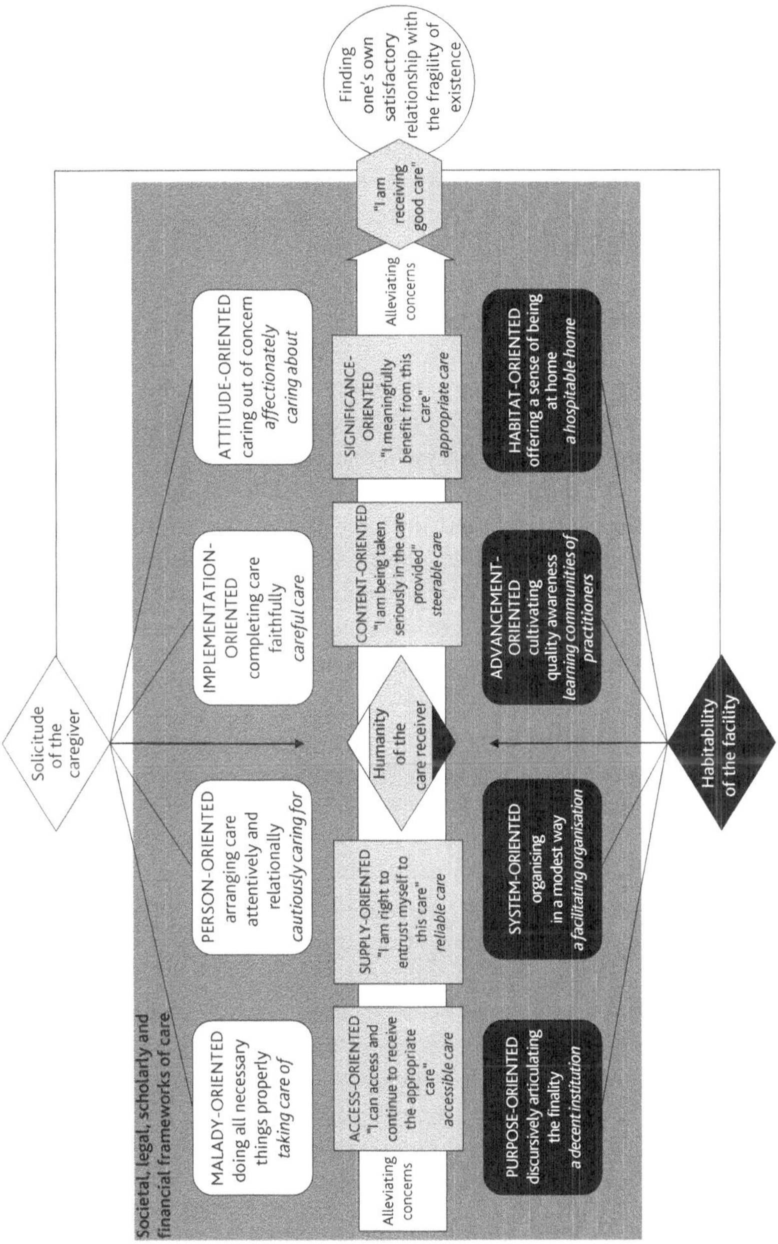

Source: Adapted from Timmerman, Baart and den Bakker, 2021: 196, which was retrieved, in translated form, from Baart 2018c: 150; graphics by Erik van Gameren

the keyword or overall criteria for quality at that level: humanity, solicitude, habitability and justice. These small philosophies not only draw on the literature about the concept involved but also outline our own conceptual space. The four keywords represent sets of questions that drive the inquiry and at the same time keep it multidimensional and broad; they are not principles that must be applied and balanced against one another. For each of the dimensions, the quality criteria have been clustered according to a qualitative procedure that seeks both maximum internal homogeneity and maximum external heterogeneity. As it turns out, this procedure clustering at each level resulted in four clusters, each under a heading that is not completely independent of theoretical thinking.

The dimension of the care receiver

Care receivers are central to any attempt to assess the quality of care (Hewitt-Taylor, 2015; Amelung et al, 2017; Carey, 2017; de Chesnay and Anderson, 2019). They are implicated everywhere in our model, but they are explicitly present in this first dimension. It is represented in Figure 12.1 by the middle row, with the wide arrow and the grey boxes that we regard as buttons. The idea is that each of these buttons 'activates' numerous questions and worksheets that inquire into that particular aspect of good care. Because care is complex, 'pushing' each button also activates other buttons.

The ultimate goal of good care is to help the care receiver find their own satisfactory relationship to the fragility of existence. What care can contribute is that it can alleviate the care receiver's concerns. This is what the wide arrow at the centre indicates. As has been seen earlier, people who ask for care, help and support may expect the professional to do the work, but they must do work too – and the workload can be considerable. In addition to the issue that prompted them to ask for care, help or support, they often have other issues that they struggle with. We call these issues 'concerns'. In general, concerns have four aspects in common: they indicate a certain problem, they are personal in nature, they impose themselves with urgency and they require an effort from the patient or client. Care receivers' concerns can be taken away and alleviated, but also created and aggravated by caregivers and their responses to what they perceive the care receiver's concerns to be (Olthuis et al, 2014b). The caregiver must come close to the care receiver and seek a relationship with them in order to properly perceive their real concerns and provide an adequate, fitting response.

> The overall quality criterion at the level of the care receiver is not quality of life or autonomy, but what we call their 'humanity'. In using this term, we are entering a complex field of meanings, definitions and usages from different disciplines. Because we are interested in

> those aspects of humanity that can be affected by care, we regard four elaborations of the concept as relevant. First, humanity is due to every person, it does not have to be earned and cannot expire. Anyone who tramples on somebody else's humanity destroys something that we collectively find precious. Humanity is often a counterfactual concept. Second, human existence takes place in extensive networks of interdependencies and reciprocities, including 'relational autonomy', a conception of autonomy that is more social than personal, more diachronic than momentaneous, more a matter of degree than of whether or not a person has the rational capacity to make decisions regarding their own life (see Chapter 10). Every person is part of the human family; humanity means fellow humanity, and that means citizenship. Third, humanity is also connected to general and deep-seated human desires, including the desire for recognition. These desires must be fulfilled in one way or another if people are to be 'human'. Fulfilment will require customisation. Humanity in health care means not adding to suffering and finding the right balance between general supply and unique focus. Humanity as an umbrella concept also introduces the idea of personal identity. Fourth, people are vulnerable because humanity is connected to what is precious and no one wants to lose. Vulnerability is inherent in humanity. There are many types of vulnerability. It is possible to distinguish between intrinsic and extrinsic vulnerability, and between potential and current vulnerability, but in many cases these distinctions turn out to be unhelpful. People can also become more vulnerable through receiving care. The bottom line here is: do not increase or prolong suffering, do not expropriate the other person's life, and do not refuse access to health and/or social care.

The quality criteria for the level of the care receiver can be clustered into four categories, according to whether they are oriented to the access to, the supply, the content or the significance of the care offered or provided. If the access-oriented criteria – the first category – have been met, the care receiver could say: 'I can access and continue to receive the appropriate care.' Good care is structurally, relationally and culturally accessible, findable and attainable. If the supply-oriented criteria – the second category – have been met, the care receiver could say: 'I am right to entrust myself to this care.' Good care is transparent, sound and reliable. Three issues are relevant: what does care do for me? What does care ask from me? How does care protect me, especially my privacy? If the content-oriented quality criteria – the third category – have been met, the care receiver could say: 'I am being taken seriously in the care provided.' Good care is respectful, shared and steerable. This steerability is related to recognition: relational recognition of the care receiver's unicity, discursive recognition of their knowledge and political recognition of their position. If the significance-oriented quality criteria – the fourth category – have been met, the care receiver could say: 'I benefit from this care.' Good care is appropriate – that is, helpful, tolerable, acceptable and a good fit with the care receiver's life – and beneficial – it helps to find the receiver's own satisfactory relationship to the fragility of human existence. Does this care focus on allowing them to live their life in whatever modality they can call theirs?

The dimension of the caregiver

The second dimension of the model is about the frame of reference rooted in the perspective of the professional caregiver; it is represented in Figure 12.1 by the top row, with the white boxes.

> The overarching quality criterion for the caregiver is their 'solicitude', not their expertise, competence or ability to intervene, repair or cure. Solicitude is a relational concept: becoming involved with another person who is in need. It is also a reciprocal concept: it is involvement with another person's suffering that has affected the caregiver. Solicitude includes a bandwidth of motivation: from worrying at a distance (worrying about) to feeling called on to act (caring about). This raises an interesting dialectic: the practising of solicitude is itself also a vehicle for developing ideas about how solicitude can best be practised. Solicitude is not just an emotion, but also a will that must become practical and be sustained. It is also an evaluative term – something or somebody else is in miserable circumstances – and it entails an element of moral imagination – not doing anything will lead to more misery. Solicitude is set against the background of social precarity.

The quality criteria for the level of the caregiver can also be clustered into four categories according to whether they are oriented to the malady or the person of the care receiver, to the implementation of care or the caregiver's attitude. The malady-oriented criteria gauge whether all necessary things are done properly, fairly, safely, competently, in a timely fashion, transparently and so on (cf Moulin, 2002; Donabedian, 2003; Hughes, 2008). They ask whether what is happening in a specific situation is good care, given the available discipline-specific knowledge regarding the person's malady, defect, trauma, need or injury and the available remedies. Given the situation, the malady and the available remedies, what goals are being pursued professionally and practically? Good care means taking care of the care receiver in an adequate manner. The thing that these criteria assess is professional competence.

The person-oriented criteria are about organising care attentively and relationally (Baart, 2004a; Klaver, 2016). They ask whether what is happening in a specific situation is good care, given the available knowledge about the suffering person's lifeworld, life course, longing and concerns and, in that context, about the concrete meaning of this malady for this person. Are we adequately connecting with and attuning our practice to their lifeworld, life course, concerns and so on? Given their lifeworld, life course, longing and concerns and the significance of the malady, what goals are the professionals pursuing for this person in an attentive and practical manner? Good care means caring for the care receiver cautiously. The things that these criteria assess are attentiveness and dedication (cf Schaufeli, 2014).

The implementation-oriented criteria pertain to faithfully adjusting and completing care. They ask questions about starting, giving and implementing care, about keeping on course, adjusting and completing care. Are the professionals taking responsibility, even if those who should in fact do not? Good care means faithfully completing care. The thing that these criteria assess is responsibility.

The attitude-oriented criteria are about caring from engagement. They raise the question of what form engagement should take with regard to how the client is being treated and which emotions are shared. Is this being done in such a way that both the care receiver and the caring professional benefit from it? Are professional carers emotionally involved in an appropriate, controlled and managed fashion? Are they making sure they are not themselves becoming burned out? Self-care is part of good care. The thing these criteria assess is engagement, being involved with the other person 'with distance' but not 'at a distance' (Stoopendaal, 2008).

The dimension of the care facility

The third dimension is connected with perspective of the care facility – represented in Figure 12.1 by the bottom row, with the black buttons.

> The overall quality criterion for care facilities is 'habitability', not hospitality or safeguarding. Habitability is a relational concept. It refers to an organisation as a materialisation or bearer of an institution, that offers those who take refuge there and those who must be there because of their work a space to live, work and maintain an identity. It is also a political concept: what room are we prepared to make for our guests, who are also strangers and often in some sense rivals, enemies or intruders? Is what makes the facility habitable for one guest perhaps excluding another? First of all, entering care entails crossing a border, going from 'outside' to an 'inside' that has its own objectives, regulations and logic. Emphasising habitability when thinking about the organisation of care foregrounds the precariousness for the care receiver of entering another space and putting themselves under a different regime. Habitability includes the notion of bringing people

> into a safe place and preserving or sheltering them there. Sometimes the opposite of habitability is to uproot people.
>
> Secondly, people who receive care in a habitable resort are almost always guests. They live in someone else's world. This place of temporary shelter can easily become a 'total institution'. Erving Goffman describes the terrible 'mortification' of residents who have become embedded in a system of adaptation, of gaining privileges and dodging responsibilities (Goffman, 1970). If care offers too much comfort and too little challenge, it can happen that care receivers give up, become dependent and ultimately lose themselves. The guest's status as a 'stranger' in the institution is lost sight of and they are thereby alienated from their inner world and lifeworld. Habitability is only habitability if it can control the totalising danger of caring. Thirdly, habitability corrects hospitality, disconnecting it from the feeling of 'being at home' that can also be accompanied by the exclusion of other people. We regard hospitality as the organisation of the open reception of both care receivers and caregivers. Finally, habitability is also a keyword for a societal order in which potential caregivers and potential care receivers are always already engaged with each other.

The quality criteria for the level of the care facility can also be clustered into four categories according to whether they are oriented to purpose, system, advancement or habitat. Corresponding to these four categories are four organisational facilitators of good care: the institution, the organisation as facilitator, learning communities of practitioners and the organisation as a 'home'. The normativity derives from the finality of the institution, an institution that must be at least 'decent'. Articulating the finality of the institution and maintaining this articulation is a discursive achievement, the result of a deliberation of all involved in the institution. This deliberation is fed directly, by learning communities of practitioners, and indirectly, through learning communities, by the organisation as facilitator and as a 'home'. Unlike similar approaches to caring organisations such as those proposed by Moore and Beadle (2006), we consistently conceptualise our approach as relational. We view care organisations as a collection of practices that need to be connected. The concept of a 'decent institution' is central here. Organisations have an ultimate end and must contribute to a decent society. We conceptualise good care as solicitude. The four facilitators of habitability are dynamic practices that are connected. Habitability is the embedding of solicitude, and solicitude makes demands on habitability.

The purpose-oriented quality criteria are oriented to a decent institution of which the finality is articulated and informs the finality of practices within that institution. A care organisation must be able to find the right balance between the finality or *telos* of the institution (what are health and social care ultimately about?), the political-public rules of implementation (governance) and its own actual possibilities and limitations. This means compromising, but doing so 'decently' (Margalit, 1996). Discerning and articulating the organisation's end (its *raison d'être*, core business, internal goods, scope, inner destiny, main tenet), even if temporarily, is a difficult process in which three dominant practices – those of the professional, the management and the board – need to be involved. A supporting environment should be sought to do this.

The system-oriented quality criteria are oriented to a facilitating organisation that organises its processes in a modest way and provides a habitable home for its employees. Does the organisation give space to its professionals' knowledge and understanding, does it permit them to discover what good care is and to learn to take responsibility and manage themselves properly? This requires a modest kind of organisation and management: simple structures, trust in craftsmanship, adopting only rules that are supportive, managers who function as 'heat shields', protecting professionals from unhelpful initiatives from higher up the chain.

The advancement-oriented quality criteria are oriented to creating learning communities that cultivate a shared quality awareness. This also implies vertical facilitation through consultation, feedback, deliberation, support, normative reflectivity and joint experiments.

The habitat-oriented quality criteria are oriented to offering people a hospitable environment that offers a sense of being at home. Habitability implies compassion at the institutional level for both clients and staff. This translates into a particular organisational culture and practical, physical and organisational conditions and provisions.

The dimension of society with its societal, legal, scholarly and financial frameworks of care

The fourth dimension of the model is about the frame of reference connected to society with its care paradigms, and is represented in Figure 12.1 by the grey plane, the background to the three rows that represent the other dimensions. We call this the 'copper plate': copper is an excellent conductor. What counts as good care is to a large extent determined, made possible and limited by powerful forces in the background that influence relational caring but can hardly be seen or manipulated by care receivers, caregivers and care organisations. The political ideal of self-reliance and participation, the paradigm shift in the way people with intellectual disabilities are perceived, from patient to citizen, and the system of financing health and social care are examples of these hidden forces. Ordinary quality systems have little influence over these forces because they are themselves embedded in these frameworks. A political-ethical orientation of thinking about quality is much needed.

> This dimension involves continuous and systematic thinking about whether the care provided contributes to 'the good life with and for others in just institutions' (Ricœur, 1992) 'in a decent society' (Margalit, 1996) – and in a sustainable world. 'The good life' also implies the ability to live in a satisfactory relationship to one's own fragility. 'With and for others' entails a double recognition: I must acknowledge myself (*soi-même*), but also the others (*autrui*) who are just like me. 'In just institutions' expresses the idea that the good life takes place in an orderly society in which institutions make living together possible, but also delimit it. Justice also includes recognition. A decent society is a society in which people are not humiliated by its institutions.

For now, we will confine ourselves to four categories of systemic frameworks of care. Societal and cultural conventions and hypes determine who and what are deemed to be worthy recipients of care and who are supposedly fit to take care of themselves. The legal definition of rights and obligations, tasks and accountabilities determines who can claim care and who must provide it. Scholarly and scientific paradigms determine what and whose knowledge counts and is worthy of being applied, and how much room is given to alternative modes of knowing and moral considerations. The system of financing healthcare and social work determines what care is available and attainable, for whom and under what conditions.

Conclusion

The CEMQUE is helpful and revealing because it perceives, organises, makes explicit, questions, evaluates, promotes and gives an account of good care in healthcare and social work. Its strengths are its three pillars (relational caring, practical wisdom and cultivating quality awareness), its comprehensiveness and coherence (the four dimensions), the centrality of concerns in relation to the fragility of existence, and the inclusion of the political and care-ethical dimension. The CEMQUE model can help professionals in their deliberations to see a larger margin of manoeuvre than they are likely to think they have. It draws attention to aspects that may be temporarily suppressed, but that deserve much more explicit attention, even in times of crisis, if the care provided is to be good care.

13

The continuing formation of relationally caring professionals

Motto

Becoming able to understand what the impact, meaning and relevance is of living in a certain situation or with a certain condition, requires going through a process of formation.

CASE FRAGMENT 13.1

A nurse in exposure

A South African nursing scholar who is familiar with caring presence in nursing practised exposure by spending a month at the frail care department of a centre for adults with intellectual disabilities. The purpose of this period of exposure was to experience the interaction between nurses and caregivers and residents, and to have reflective conversations with the nurses and caregivers regarding their experience of providing care. She kept a reflective journal and had several reflective conversations with a mentor, an expert in presence. Looking back in order to learn from that experience, she writes: 'I experienced the exposure as a process of slowly awakening, and slowly deepening insights. I learned about myself, my way of thinking about presence, and about the caregivers and the residents. It was a continuous process of delving deeper and deeper into myself, and into what "presence" means. I had the feeling I was moving from "making your acquaintance" to "getting to know you" through deep conversations. I was learning through exposing my thoughts, engaging, making contact, and connecting to the real world. I began to ask questions on a different level; not only looking for information, but specifically looking for "meaning". [...] Constantly, I had to learn to notice and silence my own inner voice, slow my pace, really listen, truly respect boundaries, and let go of my own agenda, regardless of the fact that I thought I had the best of intentions.'[1]

Although it is difficult to imagine care that is non-relational, it is not so easy to actually do relational caring – that is, care that consistently results from and is structured by relational thinking, inquiring and steering. Relational caring can be found in actual care practices in healthcare and social work.

There are professionals in these domains who are practising presence and relational caring (see Chapter 3). But many professionals find it difficult, think it requires a lot more time than they actually have, do not see how it can be combined with what they consider to be their profession, or regard it as something for virtuosos. This chapter deals with the question how relational caring and the practising of presence can be learned. It also looks at what is needed to design and organise educational curricula so as to foster relationally caring professionals, and to provide for their continuing education (Baart, 2014a; Timmerman and Baart, 2022). We are attempting to mediate between empirically grounded theory and practice in care practices and education, care in healthcare and social work, strong relationality, a political take on care ethics and critical-reflexive *Bildung*.

Our proposal is based on the learning and transition processes our colleagues and we have studied, initiated, implemented and evaluated (see Chapter 7). Learning to practise presence and relational caring requires learning processes that differ from those required for learning to apply theories or follow methods. Engaging in 'exposure', being trained to practise open and attentive perception, learning from exemplary practitioners, changing your perspective, practising case-based learning, reading novels, watching documentaries and films together and participating in learning communities first and foremost affect your attitude, understanding, inquisitiveness and other qualities, and only secondarily your knowledge and skills. There is an existential aspect to this: you have to understand certain things about life and the fragility of human existence. It requires a degree of self-confidence and the ability to receive feedback. Usually, it requires unlearning many reflexes, habits and routines: labelling, knowing in advance what is up, jumping to solutions, shying away from what is unknown or too complex and, interestingly, the persistent tendency to add rather than subtract components when attempting to solve a problem (Adams et al, 2021). One important thing it fosters is solicitude, a genuine commitment to people in need of care and support. It is a process of formation, not just qualification.

We draw heavily on discussions about the reflective practitioner (Argyris and Schön, 1974; Schön, 1983; 1987), normative professionalisation (Jacobs et al, 2008; van Ewijk and Kunneman, 2013), *Bildung* (Klafki, 2007) and practical wisdom (see Chapter 11). Our proposal must be situated in the context of comprehensive transitions in care and care organisations (Loorbach and Rotmans, 2010) in late modernity (Vosman and Niemeijer, 2017) in the domains of both healthcare and social work. If the education of relationally caring professionals is to contribute to these transitions, it needs to involve in-depth learning, and professionalisation as a counter-programme, that is, an alternative professional way of giving care (Daaleman et al, 2011). Our proposal is ultimately aimed at fostering mature, competent, reflexive and practically wise professional caregivers who are able to relationally connect with and attune their practice to care receivers, and to adequately handle existential, moral and political-institutional tensions in relational caring within complex organisations in late modern societies.

A formation process

Learning to work as a relationally caring professional is not only a process of vocational qualification (acquiring technical, communicative and attitudinal competences) or professional socialisation (becoming a valued member of the community of professionals). It is also and above all else a formation process: a process of professional subjectification (Biesta, 2020), of transformative learning (Laros et al, 2017), of *Bildung*, and especially of critical-reflexive *Bildung*, aimed at a 'values-driven transformation of both individual learners and society' (Sjöström et al, 2017). Whereas qualification is about teaching the professional the knowledge, skills, dispositions and competences of the profession, formation is about forming the professional to become a mature, sensitive, inquisitive, responsible person, who is familiar with and able to understand and handle existential, moral and political issues in their professional position in society. Because giving and receiving care are political activities that are constitutive of the *polis*, such positions are also political positions (Vosman, 2020). Ultimately, the formation of the relationally caring professional is not only about the professional's sustainable development, transformation or self-transformation, but also about that of the professional practice, of care organisations and of society as a whole.

As professionals, trainees need to master the necessary knowledge, skills, dispositions and competences. However, a process of formation is needed to prevent students from developing an instrumentalist attitude to the resources of their profession (Reichenbach, 2014). Because the professional's self is their most important 'instrument' in relational caring, practising being *a* self, that is, the subject of their own acting, who is open to the appeal that other persons make on them and is free to respond to that appeal, is the core of their formation. This core is what Gert Biesta has called 'subjectification' (Biesta, 2020). Moreover, relational caring is not just a method, a set of methods or a system of principles, but an approach, that is, a comprehensive way of perceiving, reflecting, evaluating, being courageous, doing and refraining, using artefacts and knowing, within the framework of a substantial idea of good care. Whereas a method is an effective procedure in which a particular, pre-given goal can be achieved with a degree of certainty by undertaking certain steps in a specific order, an approach is conjectural: the practitioner must do everything possible to achieve the emerging goal, but can never be sure in advance that they will succeed. Therefore, the formation of the relationally caring professional is not only about learning methods but also about becoming familiar with and appropriating the metatheoretical background theories of relational caring and becoming able to criticise these from within (see Chapter 14). Because of the nature of such an approach, learning to practise relational caring requires a formation process, and without continuing to engage in such a process, care professionals are likely to cease practising relational caring. Because relational caring is an approach which essentially involves the professional as a person, the qualities that the formation process aims to instil are personal qualities and not simply 'competences' that the person must acquire.

Rather than proposing an elaborate model of professional formation, this chapter presents a map of five domains of formation: those of the relational caring approach, of perception, of knowledge, of interpretation and of practical wisdom, including their associated theoretical stances and preferences, and together with formational goals for each of these domains (Figure 13.1). It is essential to understand that this map does not represent the acting of the professional or the practising of relational caring, nor is it a model of how to organise the formation process. It is not a trajectory of formational goals, nor a unidirectional process of causes and consequences. It is a map of the domains of the main formational goals that need to be included in the formation of relationally caring professionals who practise presence. The map is not simply a list; the domains have been arranged in a deliberate manner, from left to right and with vertical interplay. Both the five domains and the way they have been arranged are special and unusual.

In the centre of the map there is a horizontal arrow pointing to the right, which expresses the empirical truth that every formation process is embedded in an ongoing practice. There is always a way of doing and learning, both before and after the formation process, which is institutionalised in protocols, methods and artefacts as well as in taken-for-granted habits of caring, reflecting and collaborating. This embedment of the formation process ensures the continuity of care, but it is also a source of resistance, repelling attempts to change how care is given and organised. We consider the formational process – regularly leaving the practice, reflecting on it, deliberating with colleagues and so on before entering it again – as a recurring 'detour' of the ongoing practice. This detour encompasses not only learning but also unlearning and relearning. To the left of the arrow there is the domain of the relational caring approach, the all-encompassing 'philosophy' of relational caring which informs all the other domains. By calling it an approach, we distance it from the false idea that care is a method, that following specific steps in a specific order will necessarily result in specific outcomes. To the right of the arrow there is the domain of practical wisedom, which is needed to act in situations of uncertain outcomes, conflicting guidelines and contradictory goals.

Another feature that is central to the arrangement of the map is the vertical interplay between perception and knowledge. The domain of perception is about how the professional perceives the situation, the relationships in the situation, the resident, patient or client with their vulnerabilities, needs and concerns, the professional's own position including power relations,

Figure 13.1: The five core domains of the formation of relationally caring professionals

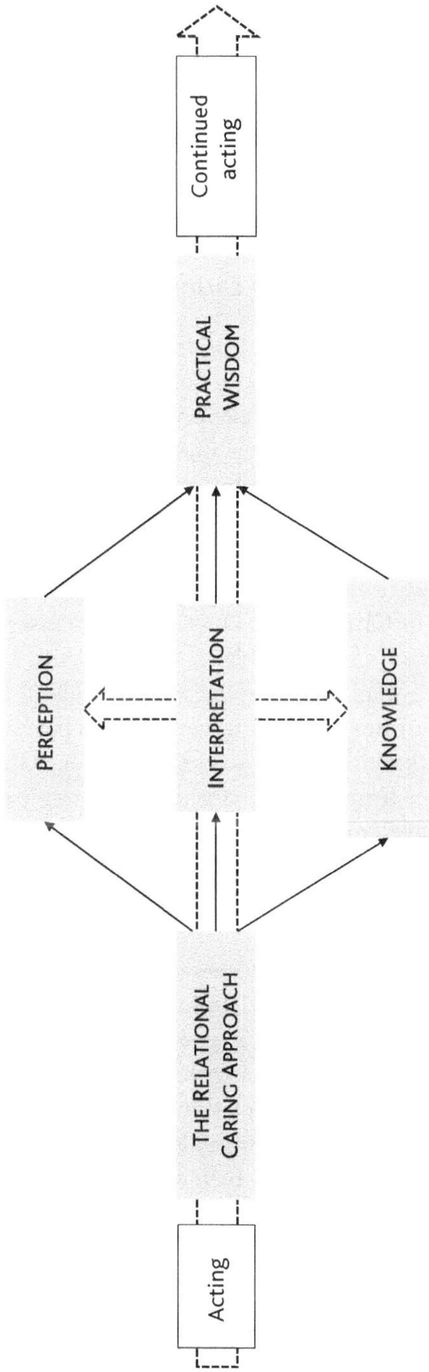

Source: Adapted from Timmerman and Baart, 2022: 589

the care organisation and society. The domain of knowledge in this vertical interplay is about the knowledge and know-how the professional can access and is supposed to use, including patient or client and family knowledge. It is an interplay, because all perception is theory laden and what is perceived determines what knowledge is activated. At the intersection of these two movements there is the domain of interpretation, the process of determining the meaning, relevance and significance of what is at stake and of what the professional can and cannot do.

The domain of the relational caring approach

The formation of relationally caring professionals involves familiarisation with how care ethics and presence theory conceptualise and theorise healthcare and social work: as a practice of relational caring. The formational goals in the domain of the relational caring approach help professionals to become able and willing to: (a) raise the finality question, (b) relationally connect with and attune their practice to the care receiver or care receivers, (c) tolerate the tragic aspects of life, (d) comply with emergence, and understand the importance of these things (Figure 13.2). The first two goals concern issues that are discussed in Chapter 10. This section discusses the last two goals.

Care does not always solve problems, cure patients, help clients, improve a person's lot. Life is frail and complex and, although it can be manipulated, it is impossible to ensure that an intervention will have a desirable outcome. Professionals must have the ability to perceive, understand, endure and relate to – rather than flee from – hopelessness and the tragic failure of care. They must know and have come to terms with the notion that, even if nothing further can be done, they can still stay and be with the other (see Chapter 9). Relational caring is more like lovingly and sensibly 'muddling through' – meandering, continuously learning and adjusting, always with the *telos* of care in mind – rather than straightforwardly fixing problems according to a predetermined plan (see Chapter 10). In the context of 'broken goods', that is, results that are not in all aspects 'good' even though they are successful, relational caring needs to be done with dedication. Tolerance of the tragic is an indispensable goal in the formation of relationally caring professionals.

Care is the intersection between multiple practices and is as such highly complex, unstable and emergent. Relevant variables may be unpredictable, non-reducible and untraceable. Professionals have to be trained to be open and receptive to this complex, dynamic, multivocal, unstable and emergent character of care, and must avoid becoming social technocrats in a communicative guise.

The formation process aims to give professionals a basic attitude of thinking about healthcare and social work from the perspective of relational caring, the ability to recurrently and jointly raise and answer the question of what the practice is about, and an awareness of and an ability to handle complexity, dynamics and emergence. It will foster their tolerance of the tragic.

The domain of perception

According to Joan Tronto, the first phase of care is 'noting the existence of a need and making an assessment that this need should be met' (Tronto, 1993: 106). The need must first of all be perceived, and this requires an open, receptive and inquisitive way of perceiving (see Chapter 9). The professional identifies this perception of need in interaction with their knowledge and this leads to an interpretation that is meaningful and sensible (Sayer, 2011). The formational goals in this domain are related to the development of a competent (a) attentiveness, (b) moral sensitivity and (c) phenomenological sensibility (Figure 13.2).

Perception of someone's need requires attentiveness, which is both instrumental and beneficial in itself (see Chapter 9). An attentive professional takes the other person seriously. Relationally caring professionals are interested in what is at stake in the life of the care receiver, in their concerns at that moment. The focus, scopus and wider context of the caregiver's attentiveness determine the answer to the questions: who and what is relational caring aimed at and what do caregivers consider to be their task and responsibility? This involves a process of inclusion and exclusion that is continuously adjusted, narrowed down and expanded during the caring process. This attentiveness implies more than being concentrated and alert, it has to do with being interested in the care receiver. Watching films, especially documentary films, can be a particularly revealing and painful experience in this respect. Relevant themes present themselves to someone's interested attentiveness. This interplay between foreground and background, centre and periphery, focus and margin is what determines the caregiver's agenda and playing field. It is not a stable thing, because the perspective constantly shifts from the centre to the periphery, and themes develop and gain or lose importance. Being attentive is an act of giving, it constitutes a relationship, and it is the beginning of social inclusion and recognition. It is something that has to be learned and constantly refined.

Judging that a person's perceived need should be met is a moral act that requires sensitivity to the appeal of the other. This sensitivity is what prevents the professional from simply turning away from the other in need. It requires developing the willingness and capability to (i) marvel at and be open to unexpected meanings; (ii) be receptive to appeals and change between proximal and distal consciousness, between focal and subsidiary attentiveness; (iii) take the 'perspective from within' on indigence (Housset, 2003).

Care is about concrete needs, experienced from the first person's point of view. Perception therefore requires a phenomenological perspective, one that is aimed at how things manifest themselves to the care receiver; how they present themselves in experiences and thus come to have meaning. Methodologically, this means learning to (i) practise bracketing, bridling or managing one's own preconceived meanings and expectations (LeVasseur, 2003); (ii) become aware of and critique modern 'social imaginaries' (Taylor, 2007); and finally, (iii) reconstruct the quintessence of the phenomenon in the care receiver's receptivity (Benner, 1994; Vosman, 2018). Regular 'exposures' are very helpful in this respect.

The formation process is aimed at giving professionals the ability to perceive the care receiver and themselves as freely, openly and carefully as they can, and at teaching them attentiveness, moral sensitivity and phenomenological sensibility.

The domain of knowledge

Professionals lean heavily on all kinds of professional, discipline-specific knowledge. There are different sources and modes of knowledge in the complex reality of relational caring in healthcare and social work, and a power struggle is ongoing about which and whose knowledge is paramount when deciding what should or should not be done. The formational goals in this domain contribute to professionals' ability to: (a) acknowledge different sources and modes of knowledge and (b) criticise power and power discourses (Figure 13.2).

The professional's professional knowledge usually takes priority over other parties' knowledge, especially that of the care receiver and their relatives. The formation of the relationally caring professional should be aimed at teaching them to make room for (i) the informal insights of the care receiver and their family members, for example about what will work in the life of the care receiver; (ii) their semiotic interpretations based on familiarity, for example their understanding of the meaning of the care receiver's behaviour, posture and facial expressions against the background of their shared life and history; and (iii) their moral preferences and boundaries, for example about what they regard as morally appropriate with regard to continuation of the treatment. Making room for these three types of knowledge curbs the professional's 'epistemic paternalism', diminishes 'epistemic injustice' and promotes a more just distribution of 'epistemic authority' (Fricker, 2007; Brister, 2012). Being aware of cultural differences is conducive to promoting 'cognitive justice' (de Sousa Santos, 2018).

Our political take on care ethics makes us aware of the power of knowledge, and of the institutions and societal structures in which people are being cared for (Barnes, 2012). We distinguish between a local, first-level discourse of power, which is situated in concrete care practices, and a more general, second-level discourse of power, which is situated in politics and governs such things as the distribution of care and caring responsibilities that are generally taken for granted, as well as the privilege of not having to care. The latter discourse 'encompasses' the former and is influential as the embedding politics of caring. In every concrete care practice, there are already deeply rooted powers at play that discipline the way the individual participants act. These powers come in the form of compulsory procedures, rules and routines, but also of people in certain positions with whom the professional has to interact. The distribution of care and caring responsibilities reproduces a differentiated society in which certain categories of people deserve care and others do not, and in which certain categories of people are predominantly the carers while others claim to be free of the responsibilities of caring. This distribution of care and of caring responsibilities is internally linked to the distribution of power, precarity and recognition.

The formation process in this domain aims to give professionals the ability to access and introduce different sources and modes of knowledge, critical awareness concerning the discourses of power on different levels, and a certain resilience (Benard, 2004).

The domain of interpretation

At the intersection of perception and knowledge, interpretation looks for 'understanding' and seeks to expand the 'horizon of understanding' (a term of Hans-Georg Gadamer). Here, again, it is important to realise that care is a moral practice; it is not a morally neutral phenomenon that requires ethical principles only when it is confronted with 'ethical dilemmas'. The formational goals in this domain contribute to the development of the professional's ability to: (a) practise hermeneutical benevolence, (b) recognise and work with emotions as moral intuitions and with 'ethos' as a source of ethics and (c) use moral deliberation (Figure 13.2).

Professionals need to be able to handle everyone impartially, including persons who are different from the people with whom they are familiar. They need a certain degree of benevolence when interpreting the other. Hermeneutical benevolence has at least three aspects. The first is an interested attentiveness that does not expropriate the other's concrete specificity and uniqueness by categorising and 'othering' them. The second is the assumption that there is interesting, rich meaning in the other, in their life and in what is at stake for them, a meaning that the professional is not immediately able to understand, and that will always escape them to a certain degree even though they must attempt to understand it. Full understanding is impossible, and caution and reticence are always necessary. The third aspect of hermeneutical benevolence is the idea that this particular meaning and significance that exist for the other have moral relevance to the professional. It assigns a position to the professional: to be the other person's advocate, helper, friend or guest. The professional's

Figure 13.2: The goals of the formation of relationally caring professionals

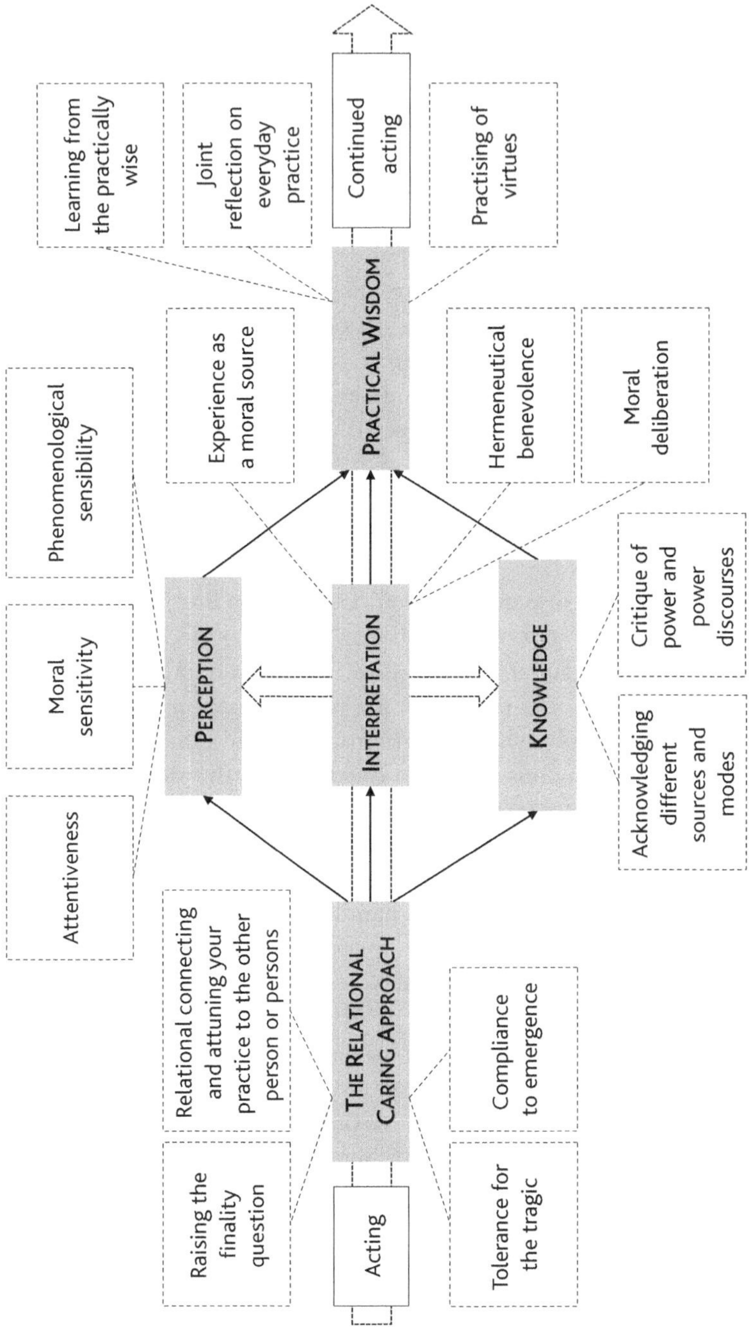

Source: Adapted from Timmerman and Baart, 2022: 590

role is 'inscribable': the care receiver can decide 'who' the carer is to them, mostly metaphorically.

According to cognitive theories, emotions inform moral intuitions: they tell us what is good and just, what values are to be promoted and what is praiseworthy. They also tell us what is abhorrent and wrong, what values are harmed and what is regrettable (Nussbaum, 2001; 2004; 2013; Roeser, 2011). They encourage us to say 'no', not to go any further, to stop. They tell us that something is wrong and unjust, that someone is undeservingly being made a victim, and they tell us what should be done or refrained from. Interpreting emotions as moral intuitions does not require asserting that they are infallible (van Tongeren, 1999). Of course, moral intuitions can be misguided and be rooted in controversial sentiments and unjust evaluations (Baart, 2013). But at the same time, they can also be a critical moral memory that breaks through the bureaucratic regime of rules, procedures and institutionalised cruelty and neglect. We do not know a priori what they are, and that is why they should be morally explored and criticised (Dancy, 2017).

That which is good is that which empirically shows itself to be good. Empirical analysis is therefore indispensable in moral deliberation. Based on the distinction between three types of feelings – sentiments, emotions and affects – it is possible to distinguish between three types of moral deliberation (Baart, 2013). The first is the ideological critique of sentiments, of society's feelings about categories of people, be they migrants or babies, and of 'social imaginaries' (Sevenhuijsen, 2004; Engster, 2007). The second is the critical hermeneutics of moral experiences (van Tongeren, 1994; 1999), and the third is the critical investigation of defensible moral particularism (Dancy, 2017).

The formation process in this domain aims to give professionals a critical awareness of the inherently moral aspects of relational caring, hermeneutical benevolence, the ability to explore and manage emotions as criticisable moral intuitions and ethos as a criticisable source of ethics, and the capability to use different types of moral deliberation.

The domain of practical wisdom

In some cases, acting is preceded by making a judgement and taking a decision or a series of decisions in which perception, knowledge and interpretation come together, leading to an intention to act in a specific way. More often, acting in a broad sense is done in the course of perceiving, reflecting, consulting, knowing, considering, interpreting, assessing, weighing, acting in a narrow sense and evaluating. Especially if a professional has to act in a case of conflicting goals, contradictory rules and uncertain outcomes, practical wisdom is a more helpful concept than judgement or decision alone (see Chapter 11). This is even more strongly the case in late modernity, where health and social care is provided in a society and in organisations characterised by complexity, ambiguity and systemic pressure (Vosman and Niemeijer, 2017). The formational goals in the domain of practical wisdom are to (a) learn from practically wise persons when and how to act in a practically wise way, (b) engage in joint reflection on everyday practice to acquire practical wisdom and (c) to train virtues such as parrhesia, dedication and tenacity (Figure 13.2).

Professionals have all kinds of formal, explicit and codified knowledge, including knowledge of proven interventions learned from books, at school or from databases. Advanced professionals also have their experience, their embodied know-how (Sennett, 2008), their tacit knowing (Polanyi, 1958; 1966). Tacit knowing is the result of what they have gone through in life, what they have perceived from what experienced colleagues have shown, what they have learned from what went well and what did not. Using explicit knowledge is always embedded in tacit knowing. However, acting requires practical wisdom: the ability to discern what might be morally good and to make morally sound decisions. This discernment does not take place exclusively on the basis of explicit, intellectually motivated reasons, but also of the professional's own mature, moral experiences and the wisdom to use those experiences in complex and non-standard situations. Someone can learn how to act in a practically wise manner by studying the way experienced, advanced, practically wise colleagues act.

There is some discussion in the literature about whether practical wisdom can only be learned implicitly and individually through practising itself or can also be acquired through intentional learning processes in groups (Kinsella and Pitman, 2012). Recent research has shown that physicians in hospitals can acquire and develop practical wisdom in their practices through regular, learning-oriented case discussions (Bontemps-Hommen, 2020; Bontemps-Hommen et al, 2020).

Three specific virtues are required to support practical wisdom in difficult situations where the temptation is to end the caring process despite the care receiver's evidently continuing need. The first is the courage to speak the truth in the face of danger, to say what one has to say regardless of the consequences for oneself. This is called 'parrhesia' (Foucault, 2001; 2011). The second virtue is 'dedication', a complete and wholehearted loyalty to taking care of the other, whatever it requires (Grøthe et al, 2015). The third virtue that is needed is 'tenacity', the strength not to give up, not to choose the easiest path or to select only the promising patients or clients, but to stay with and persistently search for the good of the care receiver, however difficult, nasty or unthankful they may be (Kuokkanen and Leino-Kilpi, 2001).

The formation process in this domain is aimed at giving professionals a critical awareness of the relevance that virtues in general and practical wisdom in particular have for acting. Practical wisdom will have to be fostered by learning from practically wise colleagues and engaging in joint reflection on everyday practice focused on practical wisdom. Virtues such as parrhesia, dedication and tenacity will have to be nurtured.

In Figure 13.2, the formational goals in the five core domains of the formation of relationally caring professionals are shown schematically.

Formational resources

Having so far discussed the 'what' of learning to work with and for people, we will now turn to the 'how'. At the very least, the formation process requires exposure, inquiry, deep learning and participation in learning communities. It must be embedded in ongoing practice. Case-based learning and quality deliberation cultivate quality awareness and contribute to the formation process. Art can also be helpful. It is essential that care organisations facilitate permanent learning by providing time, resources and skilled facilitators and fostering a culture in which professionals can show themselves and speak about their fears, doubts and mistakes.

Exposure

Exposure as we understand it, is a supervised mode of exposing oneself to life in a particular situation, context or practice, through a thorough, methodical and intentional immersion in the situation, context or practice in question and the lifeworld of the people involved in it (cf Case fragment 13.1). The aim is to promote and facilitate a change of perspective by confronting yourself with the perspective of the people you encounter, rather than regarding everything exclusively from the perspective of your own frames of reference. By becoming aware of your responses to what is strange to yourself, and reflecting on these, it is possible to gain insight into the situation, context or practice involved, and into yourself too. In the practice of relational caring as we understand it, exposure is not only a precursor to or a way of entering into this practice, but it is the relationally caring professional's permanent, professional and basic attitude (see Chapter 9 and the literature references there).

Inquiry

Inquiry is a continuous learning process in practice that is driven by an attentive, wondering, critical and self-reflexive attitude. It is embedded in what John Dewey has called a 'community of inquiry' (Dewey, 1938). Inquiry as we espouse it combines elements of inquiry-based learning, fostering inquisitiveness, heuristic inquiry, acquiring understanding of the lived life of others, appreciative inquiry, looking for what went well and can be helpful for the future, therapeutic inquiry, finding one's freedom and open-mindedness, and moral inquiry that fosters compassion by cultivating moral imagination, especially through art and literature. It is focused on practical wisdom. Recurrent exposures fuel this inquiry (see Chapter 9 and the literature references there).

Deep learning

We understand deep learning as in-depth and long-lasting learning that affects the person and their motives and intentions, their understandings and feelings. It is a kind of learning that uses real-life problem solving in designed and supervised experiences that foster critical thinking, collaboration, character building, creativity and citizenship. In deep learning, teachers and learners engage in learning partnerships (Fullan et al, 2017). Working with and reflecting on your own experiences in life, for example by writing a diary, can be particularly fruitful to achieve deep learning. Training to become an 'experience expert' is a very advanced variant of this (Weerman and Abma, 2018).

Learning communities

Learning communities are communities of practitioners that are aimed at learning. Etienne Wenger has defined communities of practitioners as 'groups of people who share a concern, a set of problems or a passion about a topic, and who deepen their knowledge and expertise in this area by interacting on an ongoing basis' (Wenger et al, 2002). A crucial feature of any community of practitioners is that there are a shared domain of interest and joint activities that are related to the work that make it a community, and that there is a shared practice. The community of practitioners may have been formed explicitly to learn, or it may be an incidental outcome of interactions between the members. As a learning community, communities of practitioners must have learning as their aim, a kind of learning that is itself aimed at good work. Learning communities of the type that we envisage are committed to free and open inquiry into people's own everyday practising of relational caring (van Elst and Baart, 2012; van Elst, 2015).

Case-based learning

Case-based learning (CBL) is a powerful way of learning: it involves professionals learning about their profession by carefully scrutinising specific cases from their work together with a group of colleagues and mentored by a trained tutor. One of the professionals contributes a case and the group creates a joint image of what happened by interrogating the contributor. This image must include the contributor's logic and motives and the reconstruction of the client's own reasons and perspective. This will ultimately lead to the question: now that we have investigated all this, what might be good actions to take? An essential feature of CBL as we advocate it is that sufficient time is taken to find out together what actually happened, including the interpretations that played a role in the case, and that a precise description is compiled before the ethical question is addressed. A session can easily take two to three hours, and sometimes turns into moral deliberation (Srinivasan et al, 2007; Baart, 2010; Thistlethwaite et al, 2012).

Quality deliberation, cultivating quality awareness

Assessing relational caring needs to be done on the spot, within the relationships between caregivers and care receivers and in the moment the care is given. The professional needs more than just external tools; they must become an instrument themselves, continuously and carefully inquiring in and into the concrete situation. This applies not only to the individual professional but also to teams of professionals and the organisation as a whole. The cultivation of critical, vigilant quality awareness is the core of a quality policy that does justice to relational caring. Cultivating quality awareness contributes to the formation process, while quality awareness itself is also an outcome of such a process. Permanent quality awareness maintains the connection between learning to perceive, learning to understand, appreciate and act. It looks at the entire process, including the person who counts and renders account, and thus keeps the different ways of looking at quality and the different ways of learning together. A powerful way to cultivate quality awareness is to engage in a sort of 'quality deliberation', a joint inquiry into care from four perspectives: the care receiver's, the caregiver's, that of the organisation and that of society (see Chapter 12).

Art

Art, as one of the classical sources of *Bildung* (in the classical idea of this concept, cf von Bonsdorff, 2012), can help to cultivate free, open and broad perception and moral imagination. And to acquire a basic understanding of what it means to be lonely, excluded, vengeful or humiliated, for example. A distinction can be made between perceiving art, perceiving with art, perceiving by art and perceiving as art. *Perceiving art* means participating in the experience of perceiving works of art, opening yourself up to what the artist perceived and experienced, being enriched by the artist's knowledge and ideas. *Perceiving with art* means being criticised and corrected in the way you perceive and process the world through perceiving art. *Perceiving by art* means studying works of art to look for new, alternative, disturbing perceptions, meanings and ideas, being changed in your understanding, evaluation and morals. *Perceiving as art* means making your own works of art as a way of doing research, allowing new perceptions, understandings and meanings to arise (Baart, 2018b).

Conclusion

Becoming and developing yourself further as a relationally caring professional, above all, requires a formation process as a recurring detour of an ongoing practice. This process is aimed at realising formational goals that can be clustered in five core domains (see Figure 13.2). Healthcare and social work should be conceptualised as a mixed practice of relational caring with inherently moral aspects in complex organisations in late modern society. Relational caring requires that caregivers acknowledge the care receiver as someone in a predicament, to whom they should attune their practice and whom they should not abandon. Engaging in an interplay between free, open and careful phenomenological perception of the care receiver's institutional-societal situatedness, on the one hand, and knowledge from different sources and awareness of epistemic paternalism, on the other, caregivers must interpret the situation of the care receiver and their relatives with all its morally relevant aspects, and decide what they can and cannot do as political professionals. Practical wisdom, as learned from practically wise colleagues and from the professional's own experience of care done well, is essential to acting in situations in which outcomes are uncertain and there are conflicting guidelines and contradictory goals, especially in situations of complexity, ambiguity and systemic pressure. In all these five domains, caregivers and trainee caregivers need to learn and unlearn, practise and stumble, interact with other care receivers and be supervised by advanced, experienced and practically wise colleagues. It is essential that the care organisation should facilitate this, especially by offering skilled facilitators and a safe environment.

14

Epilogue: Meta-theoretical and political background theories

Motto

Why relational caring?

Instead of offering a conclusion, in this last chapter of our book we discuss the meta-theoretical and political background theories of the presence-theoretical perspective. The term 'background theory' has its origins in the philosophy of science. It is an extension of the idea that 'auxiliary hypotheses', a term coined by Henri Poincaré, are needed to make a theory 'work'. Although they are not themselves part of the theory, background theories are necessary to connect the theory in question with observations, to design experiments and to formulate testable hypotheses (Levinas and Carretero, 2010). If an observation, the testing of a hypothesis or the outcome of an experiment do not agree with the theory, coherence can be achieved by either modifying the theory or changing one or more of its background theories (cf Biesta, 2015).[1] Meta-theoretical background theories concern (cf Craig, 2013):

1. the nature, construction and justification of knowledge, different kinds of knowledge and the question of what and whose knowledge counts in care and research (*epistemology*);
2. the nature and structure of social reality and of care as part of that reality, our relation to reality and the knowability of reality (*ontology*);
3. goals and values, emergent goods and bad things, that which has proven itself to be good or bad, morality, and good care and its finality (*axiology*);
4. how we conceptualise action, of both professionals and residents, clients, pupils and patients, human agency and social structure, and how care and research must be practised (*praxeology*).

In this chapter we also discuss:

5. political background theories, partly because care itself is a political category (Tronto, 1993; 2013; Brugère, 2019), and partly because meta-theoretical theories are often co-determined by political struggles (Oksala, 2010).

The choices we make concerning meta-theoretical and political background theories stem from how we perceive good care and how care receivers are regarded, recognised and treated in good care. In this sense, practice is paramount, and not theory, and this includes background theories (Slife and Wiggins, 2009). We are continuously searching for meta-theoretical and political background theories that are helpful to understanding, practising, studying, teaching, promoting and further developing the practising of relational caring.[2] An important part of the discussions in this chapter is about how we conceive of the care receivers and their relatives. The answer to this question matters a great deal in the presence-theoretical perspective.

It makes more sense to us to discuss background theories that have to be coherent in some way with how good care is perceived, than to consider supposedly clearly defined 'paradigms', each with its own meta-theoretical assumptions, between which one would have to choose independently of how one views good care.[3] This is why we will claim, for example, that we are more teleologists than deontologists when it comes to axiology, which means that, although we are not teleologists according to the textbook definition, we are even further away from being deontologists. Nevertheless, our thinking incorporates both teleological and deontological elements.

Baart discussed the basic assumptions or postulates of the presence approach in his *A Theory of Presence*. The first is that people do not just act randomly, but that there is a logic to their motives, that they give at least some reflective direction to their actions, are subject to reason and are responsive and approachable. This assumption of reasonableness is counterfactual (2001: 767–71).

Epistemology

In our conception of care as relational caring, care is relational, situational and contextual. And it is complex, dynamic and emergent. Furthermore, care is more a conjectural approach that is aimed at something, with no prior certainty that this will be achieved. It is not an effective procedure in which a predetermined goal can be achieved with a degree of certainty by taking certain steps sequentially. Whether care is good care will have to be validated locally. We therefore need an 'epistemology of the particular' that gives space for the particular, the local and the timely. Particular cases are not 'mere manifestations of generic concepts', but can refine our understanding of more general phenomena (Tsoukas, 2009: 298).

As a consequence, relational caring depends not only on textbook knowledge but also on knowledge that is locally constructed in relationships and that is always subject to being amended. Professionals usually lean heavily on all kinds of professional, discipline-specific knowledge, including the formal knowledge of experts, the experiential and practical knowledge of practitioners and the professional's own tacit knowing. But, in addition to the professional's own knowledge, the informal knowledge and relational and embodied knowing of the resident, client, patient or pupil and their family and relatives are also important. There are thus different sources and modes of knowledge in the complex reality of relational caring in healthcare and social work. And a continuous power struggle is ongoing about which and whose knowledge should determine what should or should not be done.

The professional's professional knowledge usually takes priority over the knowledge of other parties, especially that of the care receiver and their relatives. However, the relationally caring professional should create room for

1. the informal insights of the care receiver and their relatives, for example about what will work for the care receiver;
2. their semiotic interpretations based on familiarity, for example their understanding of the meaning of the care receiver's behaviour, posture and facial expressions against the background of their shared life and history; and
3. their moral preferences and boundaries, for example about what they regard as morally appropriate concerning the continuation of the treatment.

Including these three types of knowledge curbs the professional's 'epistemic paternalism', diminishes 'epistemic injustice' and promotes a more just distribution of 'epistemic authority' (Fricker, 2007; Brister, 2012; Dotson, 2012). Being aware of cultural differences is conducive to promoting 'cognitive justice' (de Sousa Santos, 2018).

In relational caring, care receivers, as well as their relatives, are perceived as participating co-actors in care processes, with their own knowledge that is relevant to the process. They are acknowledged as unique persons, with their own inalienable identity and inner voice. It is necessary to determine not only the nature and cause of the condition that puts them in need of care, but also the meaning and significance which that condition has *for them*. Finally, care receivers are perceived as the people who provide the criteria on the spot for what good care is. Knowledge is valid and relevant when it is attuned to the care receiver's insights and uniqueness and to what is locally good and practically wise. All this stands in contrast to views that regard the knowledge of care receivers and their relatives as irrelevant, and value only general, generalised and so-called objective knowledge.

When it comes to knowledge and knowledge construction, we are more contextualists than universalists, more complexity thinkers (although we use practice theory rather than complexity theory) than reductionists, and more pluralists than paternalists.

Ontology

Relational caring presupposes a radically relational ontology (Slife, 2004; Gergen, 2009). Relationships are paramount, not entities. Persons and things are constituted by relationships. We understand reality as complex, dynamic and emergent. We do not use concepts inspired by the complexity sciences (see Chapter 6). Practice theory offers tools to 'praxeologise' reality: reality is something that is done (Schmidt, R., 2012; Nicolini, 2017). The domain of reality studied – say, the living together of mildly mentally disabled young people and their supervisors – can be conceptualised as a 'form of life', a bundle of intersecting practices that 'solves' a certain problem – for example: how to get through the day together (Kolen, 2017; cf Jaeggi, 2019). At the same time, reality also resists our interpretations. In this sense, we are more realists than constructivists.

In relational caring, care receivers are seen as relational and dependent or interdependent, as reasonable and valuable. Human beings are embodied beings who interact with each other and are constituted by this interaction, but who are at the same time vulnerable. People understand and convey meaning. It is necessary therefore for good care to be open to people's own reasonableness. Finally, people are precious and are endowed with dignity. All this stands in contrast to views that regard people as fundamentally independent, self-sufficient, autonomous persons; no rationality can be expected of some people, for instance people with advanced dementia, and they must earn their social status and a place in society.[4]

When it comes to reality, we are more critical realists than social constructivists. In fact, the term 'co-constructivists' as Morin has used it is more accurate: 'Personally, I am a co-constructivist, which means that I think we construct our perception of the world, but with the help of the world itself which, as it were, lends us a hand' (Morin, 2008: 91; cf knowledge as 'meeting the universe halfway', Barad, 1996). This corresponds with Alvesson and Kärreman's proposal to speak about 'empirical material', because it is 'co-constructed'. They assume that 'something is going on out there and there may be better or worse ways of addressing things, but also that the frameworks, preunderstandings, and vocabularies are central in producing particular versions of the world' (2007: 1265).[5]

Axiology

Relational caring is a conception of care as a moral, goal-oriented endeavour. It is not a principled approach to care, which regards care as being steered by principles such as equality, trust, reciprocity, traceability, joint ownership and role clarity. Relational caring is oriented towards an ultimate end. We therefore need an ethic that can account for a heuristic–teleological concept of action, in which action has a purpose, a tenor, an end, a *telos*. We understand 'heuristic–teleological' to mean that goals and ends are not metaphysically given a priori, defined by, for example, the essence of being human, but they have to be discovered by perceiving the action under consideration closely and critically, and perceiving what shows itself in the action as good or as a good (cf Midgley, 1988). We are therefore more non-consequentialist teleologists than deontologists. We perceive action not only in the light of its consequences but in its entirety, that is, with all the elements of bodily movement, intention, situation, consequences and goals that are inherent to it. Instead of thinking about care as action, we regard it as a practice, a practice that has an end (Nicolini and Monteiro, 2017).

Instead of principles, two conditions are essential in relational caring: relationality and finality, not as principles but more like the two focal points of an ellipse (see Chapter 10). The ultimate end of relational caring, the ultimate good that can be realised by good care, is that the care receiver finds their own, more-or-less satisfactory, relationship with the fragility of existence. Healthcare and social work can be helpful, but should not pretend, as Illich argued, that they are able to remove the necessity of coming 'to terms with pain, impairment, and death' (Illich, 1975: 90), or of living what the psychiatrist Arthur Kleinman has called, borrowing an expression from William James, 'endurance and acceptance of genuine reality' (Kleinman, 2006: 9).

Relational caring also realises immediately experienceable goods: the care receiver can show themselves and articulate their needs, desires and struggles; they are acknowledged and understood; they are counted and have a voice; they are perceived and approached within their relational network; there is someone who believes in them and who welcomes them; they are treated with courtesy. These are goods in themselves, but they also derive their goodness from their connection to the ultimate end. This connection is mediated, by so-called mediating goods. Empirical research into good practices of presence has shown that there are at least three mediating goods (Baart, 2025):

1. living and surviving as a human being, through relationally mediated access to resources, including material resources;
2. reviving as a person, through affirmation by the caregiver that the care receiver is a valued individual;
3. living together with others in public life, through recognition by society that the care receiver is a full fellow citizen.

In relational caring, care receivers are viewed as people who have to deal with the brokenness of life, which in turn is defined on the basis of the meaning and significance that this brokenness has for the persons concerned themselves. Care receivers are fellow human beings who appeal for help, human beings who are connected with each other in a web of relationships, including the responsibilities those relationships entail. Finally, care receivers are participants in inevitably ambiguous situations and practices. No caregiver is filled just with wonderful concern, no care receiver is entirely innocent, no care is only beneficial and no outcome is purely advantageous. For the relationally caring professional, the person is paramount to the problem, the appeal to the task and a sensitivity for ambiguity to the need for clarity. This stands in contrast to views which ignore, suppress or seek to smooth over tragedy, the other's appeal, and ambiguity in general.

When it comes to goals, values and goods, we are more non-consequentialist teleologists than deontologists, and more cultural moral realists than moral relativists. The latter position in particular is relevant to our conception of research, which does not aspire to value-freeness, as this does not acknowledge that the relationship that human beings have to the world is a relationship of concern (Sayer, 2011).

Praxeology

In relational caring, care is a conjectural approach that is aimed at a kind of 'goal direction' without any a priori certainty that this will be achieved. It is not regarded as an effective procedure in which a predetermined goal can be achieved with a degree of certainty by taking certain steps sequentially. This implies that, ultimately, practical wisdom – knowing how to act when rules are contradictory and outcomes are uncertain – is more important than protocols and guidelines (see Chapter 11). Taking a conjectural approach requires, and enables, the professional to mix discipline-specific knowledge and expertise with connecting-with and attuning-their-practice-to the other.

Professional care in healthcare and social work is a complex, dynamic and emergent phenomenon, in often complex organisations. We therefore need an adequate theory about care as a practice that is intersected by all kinds of other practices in complex organisations. In our view, practice theory is more helpful in this respect than theories inspired by complexity sciences (see Chapter 6).

An essential element in relational caring is the turn to particularity. It matters that the care receiver is this particular person, in this particular relational network, in this particular situation, in this particular period of their lives, in this particular context. Meeting the other in their everyday life gives more explicit knowledge and tacit knowing about them and their network, situation, period of life and context than meeting them in arranged situations. Even more importantly, everyday life, the availability of different kinds of knowledge and the formal and informal care that is given and received on a daily basis in everyday life offer more possibilities to humanise care in a more permanent way than incidental interventions. Professional care in healthcare and social work can have a huge bearing on the everyday lives of residents, clients, pupils and patients, and we therefore need a theory about everyday life (see Chapter 5).

The characteristics of relational caring also have consequences for research methodology. We need a research strategy and research methods that are able to approach the situation or practice under consideration from an engaged, 'lifeworldly' perspective. Qualitative strategies and methods as they have been developed in the behavioural and social sciences are the most obvious choices for this. Methods that are typically used in qualitative research are: open interviews, topic lists, 'tactics for generating meaning' and data matrices (Miles et al, 2019). A qualitative research strategy is generally characterised by a provisional statement of the problem that is made definitive only later, by open and unobtrusive methods of data gathering, by a methodological approach that consists of a cycle of data collection and data analysis and by a structured approach to reporting and writing of the research findings. Small-N studies are particularly interesting; they do not view particular cases as 'mere manifestations of generic concepts', but acknowledge their 'epistemic significance': they are potentially able to refine our understanding of more general phenomena (Tsoukas, 2009: 298).

Theories and theoretical concepts fulfil an indispensable role in our conception of research. 'There is nothing more practical than a good theory', as Kurt Lewin, a pioneer in social psychology, noted when he argued for close collaboration between what he called 'theoretical' and 'applied' psychology (1951). Theory can be the end product of research, but it can also be an 'instrument in the process of theory formation'. Concepts, metaphors, models, analogies and theories are not only research results but also heuristic instruments that can be used to look at other phenomena and to construct and analyse empirical material (see Chapter 6).

In relational caring, care receivers are seen as co-founders, co-actors and co-evaluators of the practice and in the practice.

When it comes to processes and practises, we are more practice theorists than action theorists. We acknowledge complexity but do not use complexity theories, and we stress practical wisdom. With regard to research, we are more qualitative researchers than quantitative or mixed-method researchers.

Politics

Care is a political category. Care practices underpin society because people are connected through them and are assigned specific positions in them. Care practices contribute to the ordering of society. Care is therefore political, in the sense of 'the political' – the actual, formal and informal organisation of society and the determination of what happens or does not happen, in cooperation, friction and struggle – not necessarily, and in fact mostly not, in the sense of 'politics' – party politics and the formal practices of representative democracy (see Chapter 8).

All kinds of concepts and ideas are circulating in healthcare and social work that are derived from outside these domains. Concepts and ideas such as the autonomous life, the free market and the supposed withdrawal of government. We are interested in how such concepts and ideas resonate in healthcare and social welfare practices. We observe, for example, that neoliberal assumptions on independence and self-reliance do not reflect the actual independence and self-reliance of vulnerable citizens. And yet, such images do inform policy, and often also practice. We have to look at how concepts and ideas derived from neoliberalism affect actual practices. This will help us to clarify issues that professionals and their managers encounter in the practices in which they work, which they manage and for which they make policies.

We have incorporated political care-ethical reflection (see Chapter 6) into our research and reflection on care practices, discourses and organisations as well as on the process of research itself. We are critical of the interpretive paradigm in which a great deal of qualitative research is currently framed, because it is based on the assumption of the singular, autonomous, self-directing individual agent who is able to give a reliable account of their authentic experiences and attributions of meaning (Garrick, 1999). Instead, researchers should become aware of 'their taken-for-granted assumptions about the lifeworld and how these assumptions have been formed through the influential discourses and power relations surrounding their practices' (Garrick, 1999: 154).

In relational caring, care receivers are recognised as interdependent citizens in a political-judicial sense; as people who have citizens' rights and obligations, in an economic-financial sense and in a social-cultural sense. Care must not be conceived of as a neoliberal market economy but as an 'economy of the gift'. We also perceive care receivers as vulnerable in several respects, but vulnerability is regarded not only as a weakness but also as a strength. Finally, we acknowledge care receivers as being resilient and recovery oriented, in the sense that they seek to find a new, personal, more or less satisfactory relationship with the fragility of existence. Their strength and energy come from being included in relational networks, having a say in relevant issues, participating in society, being allowed to exercise rights and being cared for. This stands in contrast to views that perceive care receivers as objects of care, as customers or competitors, and to views that fail to acknowledge vulnerability for what it is by asking too much of people, by accusing them or by just looking away.

The presence-theoretical perspective is a political programme, also with regard to the professional caregivers themselves. Presence addresses the desire, the enthusiasm and the initial passion of many professionals who work in care, help and support. It is a kind of empowerment for them: it articulates and legitimises their own practising of presence. Doing empirical research into their practices acknowledges them as knowers and their knowledge, tacit knowing and practical wisdom as relevant to theory development. Analysing the political aspects of their work helps them to refuse responsibilities that are not theirs.

When it comes to politics, we are more political care ethicists than neoliberal bioethicists (see Chapter 8). Bioethics was developed during the 1970s to assist medical researchers, and it stresses individual autonomy and consent. As the COVID-19 crisis has shown, it has neglected distributive justice, social contexts and the global community (Ravitsky, 2020). Care ethics has since the 1980s been developing contextual thinking about relationships and the responsibility they entail. Given that care constitutes society and care practices position people, care ethics is a political-ethical endeavour. Beyond criticising neoliberalism, a political take on care ethics should analyse how neoliberal efficiency thinking has its effect on actual practices of care in healthcare and social work.

Conclusion

In a way, practising and studying relational caring forces the practitioner and the researcher to take certain positions and reject others in epistemology, ontology, axiology, praxeology and politics. These are not fixed positions, because new situations, issues, practices and developments in society will force one to look for more adequate ideas about knowledge, the structure of social reality, good and bad, how to conceptualise acting, and the political order of society. New puzzles of good care will always arise, raise new questions and ask for new concepts, approaches and responses.

Notes

Prologue

1 Source: an article from 2017 by Anne Oude Egberink in the journal and on the website Zorg+Welzijn: https://www.zorgwelzijn.nl/magazine-artikelen/relationeel-werken-ergens-tussen-schreeuw-en-stilte/ [Accessed 16 May 2024], reproduced in Baart et al, 2018: 11–12.

2 From the analysis in Baart, 2025, cf. Beurskens et al, 2019:133–9.

Chapter 1

1 Source: a contribution from 2022 by Michelle van Tongerloo on the website De Correspondent: https://decorrespondent.nl/13106/uitgestelde-zorg-is-dure-zorg/3183522916772-9a1b48bb [Accessed 16 May 2024].

2 Source: Klaver, 2016.

3 Source: an article from 2022 by Marije van der Linde and Guus Timmerman on LinkedIn: https://www.linkedin.com/pulse/relationele-jeugdzorg-guus-timmerman-phd/, responding to: https://www.trouw.nl/binnenland/de-werkweek-van-sylvana-ik-ben-jeugdbeschermer-advocaat-mediator-en-pispaal-tegelijk~b6e98d06a/ [Both accessed 16 May 2024].

4 Source: Baart, 2001.

5 Source: Timmerman and Baart, 2016a. For more about this study, see Chapter 11.

6 Taken from Vosman and Niemeijer, 2017: 471.

7 Source: Baart and Vosman, 2015b.

Chapter 2

1 Vanessa Nurock mentioned to us that in France, when the teacher calls out the children's names, they do not say 'here' but '*présent*', meaning both I am here physically and I am a participant (personal communication, 20 March 2023).

2 Much of the literature discussed here, especially on pastoral and nursing presence, was previously considered during the process of empirical research and theory development that led to the formulation of presence theory in Baart, 2001. Although theology, and especially ecclesiology and pastoral theology, may be considered to be the 'context of discovery' of the concept of presence as we understand it, it is not its 'context of justification', which instead is constituted by empirical research of a particular caring practice; see Chapters 3 and 4.

3 A more extensive discussion of the literature about nursing presence can be found in du Plessis, 2021.

4 In Part II of this book, after having laid out the groundwork of relational caring in Chapters 9 to 11, we will shortly return to the issue of relational caring and technology.

5 In his dissertation, Andries Baart proposed a similar downwards U, from emptying to rebuilding and continuing (Baart, 1986: 223–8).

Chapter 3

1 The presence approach has been described in an almost one-thousand-page book published in Dutch (Baart, 2001). There are summary descriptions in English in Baart, 2003a and 2004d and Baart and Vosman, 2011. A favourable, detailed discussion can be found in van Heijst, 2011: 96–119. In German, the presence approach and theory is presented in Timmerman and Baart, 2016b.

2 In Baart, 2001, the two professionals in question are called 'pastor Anne' and 'pastor Bas'. Because they participated in the study as co-researchers, their real names are mentioned in the acknowledgements: Monique de Bree and Titus Schlatmann (Baart, 2001: 9).
3 Smaling has called the kind of research that Baart does 'exemplary theory-of-practice oriented research' (*exemplarisch praktijktheoretisch onderzoek*), 'provided that one does not mean a form of theoretical research and conceives "theory of practice" as Baart himself does, as containing an explicitly normative component' (Smaling, 2004: 13–14).
4 An illustration of the eight working principles in action can be found in van Heijst, 2011, 106–9.
5 Fisher and Tronto, 1990: 40, call this: 'paying attention to our world in such a way that we focus on continuity, maintenance, and repair'.

Chapter 4

1 By 'theory of practice', we do not mean a theory about the concept of 'practice'. For our purposes here, we understand 'theory' as meaning 'a sound and orderly set of insights'.
2 Compare note 6 in this chapter about poietic and stochastic techniques.
3 Chapter 3 contains a summary of what the studied professionals offer, derived from Baart, 2001: 630.
4 See Baart, 2001: 681, 713–14, 750, 798, 851–2, 857 and 860, and Baart, 2003a.
5 Within the letting mode, we distinguish between: warding, witnessing, giving in, accompanying and undergoing; see further in Chapter 9.
6 This distinction between poietic and stochastic techniques was introduced by Alexander of Aphrodisias in the second/third century CE, cf Parry, 2014; compare Aristotle's distinction between 'poièsis' and 'praxis' and Hannah Arendt's distinction between '*work*' and '*action*', cf van Heijst, 2011.

Chapter 5

1 In this book, we confine ourselves primarily to practices of care, help and support in healthcare and social work, but care also refers to management, education, care for the environment, policing, or such concepts as 'caring spaces'.
2 Similarly, Glaser and Strauss position their grounded theories 'between the "minor working hypotheses" of everyday life and the "all-inclusive" grand theories' (1967: 33).
3 Designating our studies as N=N case studies distinguishes our method from descriptive single-case studies (N=1) and multiple-case studies (N=n) – although N=N case studies as we understand them can also be about only one case. An example with one case is the study reported in Baart and Vosman, 2015a, and Baart and Timmerman, 2016: 143–4.

Chapter 6

1 See also our discussion of Gesa Lindemann's idea of theoretical concepts as heuristic devices (*Sehinstrumente*) in Chapter 5.
2 See the *Map of the Complexity Sciences* (2021) by Brian Castellani and Lasse Gerrits: https://www.art-sciencefactory.com/complexity-map_feb09.html [Accessed 16 May 2024].

Chapter 8

1 Translated excerpt from a case description by Bas Haan, in *NRC Weekend*, 15 April 2023, pp 7–10, see https://www.nrc.nl/nieuws/2023/04/14/k-29-was-een-gevaar-voor-zichzelf-en-anderen-maar-kreeg-geen-hulp-hoe-kon-het-zo-mis-gaan-in-almelo-a4161990 [Accessed 16 May 2024].
2 The expression was used in 2005 by Annelies van Heijst, who is said to have adopted it from Kees Schuyt (Baart, 2011: 17).

Chapter 9

1 cf Conradi, 2015: 117: 'Both Carol Gilligan and Joan Tronto stress how care requires that we do not "turn away from someone in need" (Gilligan, 1987: 20). Whereas Gilligan underlines the emotional pain caused by "detachment, disconnection and depersonalisation" (1987: 32; 1988: xviii), Tronto puts value on attentive assistance and support: "simply recognizing the needs of those around us, is a difficult task, and indeed, a moral achievement" (1993: 127).' In van Heijst's words, the main purpose of caring is 'the care-receivers' experience of being supported and not left on their own' (2011: 3).

2 Taken from Baart, 2025.

3 A typology of being-alone can be found in Baart, 2021b: (1) lonely, (2) socially isolated, (3) abandoned, (4) curtailed, (5) withdrawn, (6) bored, (7) rudderless, (8) unheard, (9) held hostage, (10) lost. What could help is: (1) interested attentiveness, (2) faithful availability, (3) help that really helps, (4) experiential basic care, (5) patient being-there, (6) devoted everydayness, (7) diluted seriousness, (8) an unconditional narrative space, (9) the human scale in systemic logics, (10) a fully developed position as a citizen.

4 'The fact is that many of us have been reduced to cases by the very machinery that has been instituted to care for us' (Nodding, 1984: 66).

5 Noddings writes about this in educational contexts: 'I do not need to establish a deep, lasting, time-consuming personal relationship with every student. What I must do is to be totally and nonselectively present to the student – to each student – as he addresses me. The time interval may be brief but the encounter is total' (Noddings, 1984: 180).

6 Taken from Kok, 2002: 13.

7 This is different from Noddings's use of 'completed': 'both parties contribute to the relation; my caring must be somehow completed in the other if the relation is to be described as caring' (Noddings, 1984: 4). cf Eva Feder Kittay on ethicsofcare.org: '[A genuinely normative] notion of care can perhaps best be approached from what Nel Noddings called "the completion of care". Noddings, along with Tronto, spoke of an aspect of care that few others have pursued. Tronto called it the fourth phase of care, the receiving of care, while Noddings spoke of care needing to be completed in the other. This is a profoundly important aspect of care that has been glossed over and that can, I believe, help us identify the truly normative sense of care. If care must be received as care by the one cared for, then many things that we sometimes identify with care, such as caring intentions or affect will be insufficient to be care. If care needs to be completed in the other, then actions that are overweening or paternalistic will not be taken as something desirable – as something that is really caring – by the cared for' (Kittay, 2013). However, the two notions are related. Completing care in our use of this term presupposes the completion of care in the other person.

8 cf Conradi, 2015: 123: 'As a particular way to perform supportive activities, attentiveness is a basically nonreciprocal quality that refers to an asymmetrical relationship. [...] Attentiveness is not merely the icing on the cake; it [...] is the sweetness of the cake, without which it would not be cake to begin with.' Of course, Conradi is not writing about the attentiveness of the stalker, or the control exercised by a government that systematically mistrusts citizens who rely on its help to survive.

9 Taken from Timmerman and Baart, 2016a.

10 Taken from Leest, 2016a: 22–3.

Chapter 10

1 Excerpt from Schwartz and Sharpe, 2010: 13–16.

2 There is a sense in which care is and should be self-referential, namely in the sense that the goals and quality criteria of care lie within and not outside care and can be evaluated

only from the inside, not from outside, although there are always aspects of care that can be evaluated externally, to inform the ongoing inquiry into quality of care from the inside.

3 Taken from Baart, 2001: 132. This story is told by pastor Anne. The analysis is also from Baart, 2001: 132–3.

4 This talk of an absent mother is talk from the daughter's perspective; it is not about blaming the mother for her absence. An alternative reading of this fragment, one which focuses more on Elif's own active role, can be found in van Klinken, 2012: 50–1.

5 cf the relational turn and ideas about radical relationality in psychology (Slife, 2004; Slife and Wiggins, 2009), sociology (Burkitt, 2016) and political theory (Selg, 2016; Selg and Ventsel, 2020b).

6 Taken from Andries Baart's research experience in the context of a transition and research project in a general hospital in the Netherlands in 2009–14 (Baart and Vosman, 2015b) – not previously published.

7 Taken from the research project 'Dementia from within' in 2019–21 by the Presence Foundation, commissioned by Zorgbalans, an organisation for care for older persons (Leest et al, 2021).

8 Taken from Andries Baart's research experience in the framework of a transition and research project in a general hospital in the Netherlands in 2009–14. This case fragment has also been published, in slightly different terms, in Baart et al, 2015.

9 For the concept of 'capital', derived from Bourdieu, see Chapter 8.

10 Contemporary sociology uses the term social institution to refer to 'complex social forms that reproduce themselves such as governments, the family, human languages, universities, hospitals, business corporations, and legal systems' (Miller, S., 2019).

11 See the note for Figure 10.1.

12 Taken from a North American TV series about a hospital. Title of the series and the date of broadcast of this episode are unknown. The doctor was most likely performing the so-called 'Heimlich manoeuvre' [see: https://en.wikipedia.org/wiki/Abdominal_thrusts [Accessed 16 May 2024].

13 A version of Dworkin's original formula: 'autonomy = authenticity + independence' (1976: 24).

14 Together with our colleagues Marije van der Linde and Petra Schaftenaar (van der Linde et al, 2020).

15 See note 9 in this chapter.

Chapter 11

1 Translated excerpt from a case description from 2016 by Anne Oude Egberink in the journal Zorg+Welzijn, reproduced in Baart et al, 2017: 6–7.

2 We learned from Frans Vosman to think in terms of tensions that are not eliminated but maintained; Vosman himself learned this from Paul Ricœur but gave it a twist of his own (Vosman, 2023: 37).

Chapter 12

1 Taken from Baart, 2018c: 259ff. The thematic analysis was done by Andries Baart.

2 We put CEMQUE to the test in the case of residential care for older persons in the Netherlands during the COVID-19 pandemic in Timmerman et al, 2021.

3 We have not made an exhaustive international comparison of the major quality reporting systems. We are familiar with the international literature in various disciplines such as ethics, philosophy, sociology and political science (Baart, 2018c), and we have focused on quality policies and quality systems in healthcare and social work in the Netherlands. We consider the Netherlands to be an exemplary case, due to its historically conditioned, international orientation and its receptivity to management and market thinking

(de Vries, 2007; Dwarswaard et al, 2011). Standing at the intersection of German, French and Anglo-Saxon approaches to quality, it is a country in which the deficiencies of the individual approaches are sharply exposed, the discussions are diverse and rich and the difficulties these approaches raise become sharply apparent.

4 The term 'quality awareness' originates from the fields of engineering and manufacturing (Crosby, 1979) and was adopted by ActiZ at Andries Baart's suggestion in the title of a two-year work programme (2012–14) in which he participated (Ubels, 2015).

Chapter 13

1 Taken from du Plessis and Beurskens, 2021: 25–6.

Chapter 14

1 This process can be regarded as a method of 'broad reflective equilibrium' (Daniels, 1979) between the theory of presence, background theories and 'retroductive warrants', for example the theoretical and practical fruitfulness of the theory (cf Schüssler Fiorenza, 2011). Another way of thinking about this process is to conceptualise background theories as inquiries, for instance ontology as 'an inquiry into "what happens" and "becomes ontologically revealed"' (Joronen and Häkli, 2017: 4).

2 How we conceive research (see Chapters 5 and 6) and education (see Chapter 13) consequently interacts with their respective background theories.

3 Publications about research and education usually contain at least three of the following paradigms: a positivistic or post-positivistic, interpretive or constructivist, or critical-emancipative and participatory paradigm (for example, Heron and Reason, 1997; Lincoln and Guba, 2000; Zaidi and Larsen, 2018). Literature that is inspired by the philosophy of science often contains positivism, interpretivism and critical realism (Alderson, 2020).

4 We have yet to think about the interaction with non-human and more-than-human agents (Puig de la Bellacasa, 2017; Flower and Hamington, 2022).

5 'Critical realism', as developed by Roy Bhaskar in collaboration with Andrew Sayer and others, merits a separate discussion, because it takes similar positions, not only on ontology but also on epistemology, axiology and politics (Alderson 2020). Unfortunately, we do not have the space here to do this.

References

Achterhuis, H. (1979) *De markt van welzijn en geluk: Een kritiek van de andragogie*, Baarn: Ambo. Available from: https://www.dbnl.org/tekst/acht007mark01_01/index.php.

Adams, G.S., Converse, B.A., Hales, A.H. and Klotz, L.E. (2021) 'People systematically overlook subtractive changes', *Nature*, 592(7853): 258–61. https://doi.org/10.1038/s41586-021-03380-y.

Alderson, P. (2020) *Critical Realism for Health and Illness Research: A Practical Introduction*, Bristol: Policy Press.

Alhadeff-Jones, M. (2008) 'Three generations of complexity theories: Nuances and ambiguities', *Educational Philosophy and Theory*, 40(1): 66–82. https://doi.org/10.1111/j.1469-5812.2007.00411.x.

Alvesson, M. and Kärreman, D. (2007) 'Constructing mystery: Empirical matters in theory development', *Academy of Management Review*, 32(4): 1265–81.

Alvesson, M. and Kärreman, D. (2011) *Qualitative Research and Theory Development: Mystery as Method*, London: SAGE.

Amelung, V., Stein, V., Goodwin, N., Balicer, R., Nolte, E. and Suter, E. (eds) (2017) *Handbook Integrated Care*, Cham: Springer.

Anderson, R. (2004) 'Intuitive inquiry: An epistemology of the heart for scientific inquiry', *The Humanistic Psychologist*, 32(4): 307–41.

Argyris, C. and Schön, D.A. (1974) *Theory in Practice: Increasing Professional Effectiveness*, San Francisco, CA: Jossey-Bass.

Aristotle (2013) *Aristotle on Practical Wisdom: Nicomachean Ethics VI / Translated with an Introduction, Analysis, and Commentary by C.D.C. Reeve*, Cambridge, MA: Harvard University Press.

Arvidson, P.S. (2006) *The Sphere of Attention: Context and Margin*, Dordrecht: Springer.

Aspers, P. and Kohl, S. (2013) 'Heidegger and socio-ontology', *Journal of Classical Sociology*, 13(4): 487–508.

Baart, A. (1986) 'Verhalen: De dialoog als grondmodel van het maatschappelijk activeringswerk' (PhD thesis, Erasmus University Rotterdam), Hilversum: Gooi en Sticht.

Baart, A. (1996) 'Wat heet professioneel? Naar een sterke opvatting van professionaliteit', *Journal of Social Intervention*, 5(3): 113–23.

Baart, A. (1997) 'Methodiek, de zorgbenadering en professionaliteit', in M. Verkerk (ed) *Denken over zorg: Concepten en praktijken*, Utrecht: Elsevier/De Tijdstroom, pp 205–23.

Baart, A. (2001) *Een theorie van de presentie*, Utrecht: LEMMA.

Baart, A. (2002) *Aanzetten tot een theorie van de derde partij met behulp van de presentietheorie*, Den Haag: LCO.

Baart, A. (2003a) 'The fragile power of listening', *Practical Theology in South Africa / Praktiese Teologie in Suid-Afrika*, 18(3): 136–56.

Baart, A. (2003b) 'Ongemakkelijk – zoals het hoort: In gesprek met kritische bemerkingen bij de presentietheorie', *Sociale Interventie*, 12(2): 76–94.

Baart, A. (2004a) *Aandacht: Etudes in Presentie*, Utrecht: LEMMA.

Baart, A. (2004b) 'Gebroken goed in ongebroken relaties: Theoretische notities voor de beroepspraktijk van maatschappelijke opvang', in M. Nuy and F. Brinkman (eds) *Wanorde in een mensenleven: Een bezinning op thuisloosheid*, Amsterdam: SWP, pp 137–74.

Baart, A. (2004c) 'Wat te denken geeft: Theorievorming in kwalitatief onderzoek', *Kwalon*, 9(1): 24–32.

Baart, A. (2004d) 'What makes care good care?', *Journal of Social Intervention*, 13(3): 14–26.

Baart, A. (2008) 'Over de verdringing van praktijkkennis', in F. Vosman and A. Baart (eds) *Aannemelijke zorg: Over het uitzieden en verdringen van praktische wijsheid in de gezondheidszorg* (Dual inaugural lecture, Tilburg University), Den Haag: LEMMA, pp 49–134. Available from: https://www.presentie.nl/publicaties/item/380-aannemelijke-zorg-de-uitgebreide-tekst-van-de-dubbeloratie-van-vosman-en-baart.

Baart, A. (2010) 'Case-based learning in zeven stappen', in K. Runia and R. Hortulanus (eds) *Zwerfwerken: Een evaluatieonderzoek naar de werkingskracht van presentie bij de opvang en begeleiding van zwerfjongeren*, Utrecht: Lesi, pp 151–2. https://doi.org/10.13140/RG.2.2.15282.50887.

Baart, A. (2011) *Van bewegen naar bewogenheid: Een fenomenologische verkenning van zorg geven in een politiek-ethisch perspectief* (Foundation day lecture, University of Humanistic Studies), Amsterdam: SWP.

Baart, A. (2013) 'De zorgval: Analyse, kritiek en uitzicht', in A. Baart and C. Carbo *De Zorgval*, Amsterdam: Thoeris, pp 5–128.

Baart, A. (2014a) *The Formation of the Care Ethical Practitioner*, pp 1–24. https://doi.org/10.13140/RG.2.2.16069.96487.

Baart, A. (2014b) 'Het politieke welkom aan de cultivering van kwaliteitsbewustzijn', in E. Bolt (ed) *Het cultiveren van kwaliteitsbewustzijn – leren anders te kijken, te duiden en te doen: Een onderzoek naar de werking van leermiddelen*, Utrecht: Stichting Presentie, pp 66–85.

Baart, A. (2017) *The Many Faces of Neoliberalism: Lecture at the Book Presentation 'Thomas Biebricher, Onvermoed en Onvermijdelijk'*. https://doi.org/10.13140/RG.2.2.23865.01128.

Baart, A. (2018a) 'Afterword: Discourses of care for older people in sub-Saharan Africa: Towards conceptual development', in J. Hoffman and K. Pype (eds) *Ageing in Sub-Saharan Africa: Spaces and Practices of Care*, Bristol: Policy Press, pp 183–201.

Baart, A. (2018b) *De kunst van het waarnemen en het waarnemen van de kunst* (Keynote speech, 17 April 2018). Available from: https://vimeo.com/273004704.

Baart, A. (2018c) *De ontdekking van kwaliteit: Theorie en praktijk van relationeel zorg geven*, Amsterdam: SWP.

Baart, A. (2020) 'Empirically grounded ethics of care: An argument', in F. Vosman, A. Baart and J. Hoffman (eds) *The Ethics of Care: The State of the Art*, Leuven: Peeters, pp 261–98.

Baart, A. (2021a) 'Precariousness, precarity, precariat, precarization and social redundancy: A substantiated map for the ethics of care', in M. Hamington and M. Flower (eds) *Care Ethics in the Age of Precarity*, Minneapolis, MN: University of Minnesota Press, pp 91–119. https://doi.org/10.5749/j.ctv2382dwh.8.

Baart, A. (2021b) *Wat heet eenzaam? Een essay* (2nd edn), Utrecht: Stichting Presentie. Available from: https://www.presentie.nl/images/stories/2020/AJ_Baart_2021_Wat_heet_eenzaam_2e_druk.pdf.

Baart, A. (2023) *Een precair bestaan*, Utrecht: Stichting Presentie. Available from: https://www.presentie.nl/kennisbank/essay-een-precair-bestaan-andries-baart/.

Baart, A. (2024) *Wij moeten het zeggen: Een essay over alledaagsheid, hermeneutiek en autonomie in de zorg voor wie het niet zeggen kan*, Utrecht: De Graaff.

Baart, A. (2025) *Iemand voor iemand: Handboek presentie*, Bussum: Coutinho.

Baart, A. and Carbo, C. (2013) *De Zorgval*, Amsterdam: Thoeris.

Baart, A. and Grypdonck, M. (2008) *Verpleegkunde en presentie: Een zoektocht in dialoog naar de betekenis van presentie voor verpleegkundige zorg*, Den Haag: LEMMA.

Baart, A. and Hoffman, J. (2021) 'Long-term care futures in South Africa: A different voice', in E. du Plessis (ed) *Reflecting on Presence in Nursing: A Guide for Practice and Research*, Newcastle upon Tyne: Cambridge Scholars, pp 162–98.

Baart, A. and Steketee, M. (2003) 'Wat aandachtige nabijheid vermag: Over professionaliteit en present-zijn in complexe situaties', in E. Plemper, G. van der Laan and K. van Vliet (eds) *Passie voor professionaliteit*, Utrecht: Verwey-Jonker Instituut, pp 109–24.

Baart, A. and Timmerman, G. (2016) 'Plädoyer für eine empirisch begründete Ethik der Achtsamkeit, Präsenz und Sorge', in E. Conradi and F. Vosman (eds) *Praxis der Achtsamkeit: Schlüsselbegriffe der Care-Ethik*, Frankfurt: Campus, pp 129–46.

Baart, A. and Vosman, F. (2011) 'Relationship based care and recognition: Part one: Sketching good care from the theory of presence and five entries', in C. Leget, C. Gastmans and M. Verkerk (eds) *Care, Compassion and Recognition: An Ethical Discussion*, Leuven: Peeters, pp 183–200.

Baart, A. and Vosman, F. (2015a) 'Een lastige familie die niet lastig is: Verslag van een onderzoek dat te denken geeft', in A. Baart, F. Vosman and others *De patiënt terug van weggeweest: Werken aan menslievende zorg in het ziekenhuis*, Amsterdam: SWP, pp 181–205.

Baart, A. and Willeme, F. (2010) *Van tellen naar vertellen, en terug*, Den Haag: Lemma.

Baart, A., Grypdonck, M. and Prins, C. (2015) 'Het denk- en kijkraam van opgaven en responsen: Aansluiten bij en afstemmen op de patiënt', in A. Baart, F. Vosman and others *De patiënt terug van weggeweest: Werken aan menslievende zorg in het ziekenhuis*, Amsterdam: SWP, pp 207–23.

Baart, A., Vosman, F. and others (2015b) *De patiënt terug van weggeweest: Werken aan menslievende zorg in het ziekenhuis*, Amsterdam: SWP.

Baart, A., Carbo, C., Keinemans, S. and van Dijk, B. (2007) *Kwetsbaar maar niet alleen kwetsbaar: Over het bereiken en steunen van multiproblem gezinnen, kwetsbare kinderen en tienermoeders*, Utrecht/Den Bosch: Actioma.

Baart, A., Oude Egberink, A., Ouwerkerk, M. and Peeters, H.-J. (2017) *Praktische wijsheid*, Utrecht: Stichting Presentie and Zorg+Welzijn.

Baart, A., van Dijke, J., Ouwerkerk, M. and Beurskens, E. (2011) *Buigzame zorg in een onbuigzame wereld: Presentie als transitiekracht*, Den Haag: Lemma.

Baart, A., Oude Egberink, A., Ouwerkerk, M., Peeters, H.-J. and Timmerman, G. (2018) *Relationeel werken*, Utrecht: Stichting Presentie and Zorg+Welzijn.

Balint, E. (1969) 'The possibilities of patient-centered medicine', *The Journal of the Royal College of General Practitioners*, 17(82): 269–76.

Banerjee, A. and Armstrong, P. (2015) 'Centring care: Explaining regulatory tensions in residential care for older persons', *Studies in Political Economy*, 95(1): 7–28. https://doi.org/10.1080/19187033.2015.11674944.

Banerjee, A., Armstrong, P., Daly, T., Armstrong, H. and Braedley, S. (2015) '"Careworkers don't have a voice": Epistemological violence in residential care for older people', *Journal of Aging Studies*, 33: 28–36. https://doi.org/10.1016/j.jaging.2015.02.005.

Barad, K. (1996) 'Meeting the universe halfway: Realism and social constructivism without contradiction', in L.H. Nelson and J. Nelson (eds) *Feminism, Science, and the Philosophy of Science*, Dordrecht: Springer, pp 161–94.

Barnes, M. (1997) *Care, Communities and Citizens*, Harlow: Addison Wesley Longman.

Barnes, M. (2012) *Care in Everyday Life: An Ethic of Care in Practice*, Bristol: Policy Press.

Bauman, Z. (2007) *Liquid Times: Living in an Age of Uncertainty*, Cambridge, UK: Polity Press.

Beauchamp, T.L. and Childress, J.F. (2009) *Principles of Biomedical Ethics* (6th edn), New York: Oxford University Press.

Beck, U. (1992) *Risk Society: Towards a New Modernity* [Risikogesellschaft: Auf dem Weg in eine andere Moderne, 1986] (transl M. Ritter), London: SAGE.

Benard, B. (2004) *Resiliency: What We Have Learned*, San Francisco, CA: WestEd.

Benner, P. (ed) (1994) *Interpretive Phenomenology: Embodiment, Caring, and Ethics in Health and Illness*, Thousand Oaks, CA: SAGE.

Berlyne, D.E. (1960) *Conflict, Arousal, and Curiosity*, New York: McGraw-Hill. https://psycnet.apa.org/doi/10.1037/11164-000.

Beurskens, E., van der Linde, M. and Baart, A. (2019) *Praktijkboek presentie*, Bussum: Coutinho.

Biebricher, T. (2021) *Die politische Theorie des Neoliberalismus*, Berlin: Suhrkamp.

Biesta, G. (2015) 'On the two cultures of educational research, and how we might move ahead: Reconsidering the ontology, axiology and praxeology of education', *European Educational Research Journal*, 14(1): 11–22.

Biesta, G. (2020) 'Risking ourselves in education: Qualification, socialization, and subjectification revisited', *Educational Theory*, 70(1): 89–104. https://doi.org/10.1111/edth.12411.

Biroli, F. (2020) 'Care and the new pattern of precarity', in F. Vosman, A. Baart and J. Hoffman (eds) *The Ethics of Care: The State of the Art*, Leuven: Peeters, pp 109–31.

Blokland-Potters, T. (1998) 'Wat stadsbewoners bindt: Sociale relaties in een achterstandswijk' (PhD thesis, Amsterdam University), Kampen: Kok Agora.

Bocarro, J. and Witt, P.A. (2003) 'Relationship-based programming: The key to successful youth development in recreation settings', *Journal of Park and Recreation Administration*, 21(3): 75–96.

Boeck, P.R. (2014) 'Presence: A concept analysis', *SAGE Open*, 4(1): 1–6. https://doi.org/10.1177/2158244014527990.

Bontemps-Hommen, M. (2020) 'Practical Wisdom: The Vital Core of Professionalism in Medical Practices' (PhD thesis, University of Humanistic Studies), Afferden. Available from: https://research.uvh.nl/ws/portalfiles/portal/14763241/Full+Text.pdf.

Bontemps-Hommen, C.M.M.L., Baart, A. and Vosman, F.T.H. (2019) 'Practical wisdom in complex medical practices: A critical proposal', *Medicine, Health Care and Philosophy*, 22(1): 95–105. https://doi.org/10.1007/s11019-018-9846-x.

Bontemps-Hommen, M.C.M.M.L., Baart, A.J. and Vosman, F.J.H. (2020) 'Professional workplace-learning: Can practical wisdom be learned?', *Vocations and Learning*, 13(3): 479–501. https://doi.org/10.1007/s12186-020-09249-x.

Bootsma, J. (2008) *Is het te doen? Over ethiek en methodiek van de presentiebeoefenaar in het boek 'Een theorie van de presentie' van A. Baart*, Zwolle: Christelijke Hogeschool Windesheim.

Bordin, E.S. (1979) 'The generalizability of the psychoanalytic concept of the working alliance', *Psychotherapy: Theory, Research and Practice*, 16(3): 252–60. https://psycnet.apa.org/doi/10.1037/h0085885.

Bourdieu, P. (1983) 'Ökonomisches Kapital, Kulturelles Kapital, Soziales Kapital', in R. Kreckel (ed) *Soziale Ungleichheiten*, Göttingen: Otto Schartz and Co, pp 183–98.

Bourdieu, P. (1986) 'The forms of capital', in J.G. Richardson (ed) *Handbook of Theory and Research for the Sociology of Education*, New York: Greenwood Press, pp 241–58.

Bourdieu, P. (1998) 'La precarité est aujourd'hui partout', in P. Bourdieu (ed) *Contre-feux: Propos pour servir à la résistance contre l'invasion neo-liberale*, Paris: Liber – Raison d'Agir, pp 95–101.

Brister, E. (2012) 'Distributing epistemic authority: Refining Norton's pragmatist approach to environmental decision-making', *Contemporary Pragmatism*, 9(1): 185–203. https://doi.org/10.1163/18758185-90000222.

Bröckling, U. (2007) *Das Unternehmerische Selbst: Soziologie einer Subjektivierungsform*, Frankfurt: Suhrkamp.

Bronk, K.C. (2012) 'The exemplar methodology: An approach to studying the leading edge of development', *Psychology of Well-being: Theory, Research and Practice*, 2(5): 1–10. https://doi.org/10.1186/2211-1522-2-5.

Brugère, F. (2019) *Care Ethics: The Introduction of Care as a Political Category*, Leuven: Peeters.

Burhans, L. (2008) 'What is Good Nursing Care? The Lived Meaning of Quality Nursing Care for Practicing Nurses' (PhD thesis, East Carolina University), Greenville, NC: College of Nursing, East Carolina University. Available from: http://thescholarship.ecu.edu/bitstream/handle/10342/1085/umi-ecu-1018.pdf.

Burkitt, I. (2016) 'Relational agency: Relational sociology, agency and interaction', *European Journal of Social Theory*, 19(3): 322–39. https://doi.org/10.1177/1368431015591426.

Butler, J. (2004) *Precarious Life: The Powers of Mourning and Violence*, London/New York: Verso.

Carey, T.A. (2017) *Patient-Perspective Care: A New Paradigm for Health Systems and Services*, New York: Routledge.

Cassell, E.J. (1991) *The Nature of Suffering and the Goals of Medicine*, Oxford: Oxford University Press.

Castel, R. (2003) *From Manual Workers to Wage Laborers: Transformation of the Social Question* [Les métamorphoses de la question sociale: Une chronique du salariat, 1996] (transl R. Boyd), New Brunswick, NJ: Transaction Publishers.

Charmaz, K. (2006) *Constructing Grounded Theory: A Practical Guide through Qualitative Analysis*, Thousand Oaks, CA: SAGE.

Charon, R. (2006) *Narrative Medicine: Honoring the Stories of Illness*, Oxford/New York: Oxford University Press.

Chavel, S. (2011) *Se mettre à la place d'autrui: L'imagination morale*, Rennes: Presses universitaires de Rennes.

Chouraqui, F. (2016) 'Eran Dorfman: Foundations of the everyday, shock, deferral, repetition', *Continental Philosophy Review*, 49(2): 259–65.

Christen, M., van Schaik, C., Fischer, J., Huppenbauer, M. and Tanner, C. (eds) (2014) *Empirically Informed Ethics: Morality between Facts and Norms*, Cham: Springer.

Conradi, E. (2015) 'Redoing care: Societal transformation through critical practice', *Ethics and Social Welfare*, 9(2): 113–29. https://doi.org/10.1080/17496535.2015.1005553.

Cooperrider, D.L. (2013) 'A contemporary commentary on appreciative inquiry in organizational life', in D.L. Cooperrider, D.P. Zandee, L.N. Godwin, M. Avital and B. Boland (eds) *Organizational Generativity: The Appreciative Inquiry Summit and a Scholarship of Transformation*, Bingley: Emerald Group Publishing, pp 2–67.

Craig, R.T. (2013) 'Constructing theories in communication research', in P. Cobley and P.J. Schulz (eds) *Theories and Models of Communication*, Boston, MA: De Gruyter Mouton, pp 39–57. https://doi.org/10.1515/9783110240450.39.

Crosby, P.B. (1979) *Quality is Free: The Art of Making Quality Certain*, New York: McGraw-Hill.

Daaleman, T.P., Kinghorn, W.A., Newton, W.P. and Meador, K.G. (2011) 'Rethinking professionalism in medical education through formation', *Family Medicine*, 43(5): 325–9. Available from: https://www.stfm.org/familymedicine/vol43issue5/Daaleman325.

Dancy, J. (2017) 'Moral particularism', in E.N. Zalta (ed) *The Stanford Encyclopedia of Philosophy (Winter 2017 Edition)*. Available from: https://plato.stanford.edu/archives/win2017/entries/moral-particularism/.

Daniels, N. (1979) 'Wide reflective equilibrium and theory acceptance in ethics', *The Journal of Philosophy*, 76(5): 256–82. https://doi.org/10.2307/2025881.

Davies, R., Ives, J. and Dunn, M. (2015) 'A systematic review of empirical bioethics methodologies', *BMC Medical Ethics*, 16(1): 15. https://doi.org/10.1186/s12910-015-0010-3.

de Certeau, M. (1984) *The Practice of Everyday Life* [L'invention du quotidien, I: Arts de faire, 1980] (transl S. Rendall), Berkeley, CA: University of California Press.

de Chesnay, M. and Anderson, B.A. (eds) (2019) *Caring for the Vulnerable: Perspectives in Nursing Theory, Practice, and Research* (5th edn), Burlington, MA: Jones and Bartlett Publishers.

Dean, M. (2013) *The Constitution of Poverty: Towards a Genealogy of Liberal Governance*, London: Routledge. https://doi.org/10.4324/9781315823294

Dewey, J. (1938) *Logic: The Theory of Inquiry*, New York: Holt, Rinehart and Winston.

de Jonge, E. (2015) 'Beelden van de professional: Inspiratiebron voor professionalisering' (PhD thesis, Utrecht University), Delft: Eburon.

de Jonge, E. (2018) 'Professionaliteit en neoliberalisme: Posities, paradoxen en perspectieven', *Waardenwerk*, 19(73): 71–83.

de Jonge, V., Sint Nicolaas, J., van Leerdam, M.E. and Kuipers, E.J. (2011) 'Overview of the quality assurance movement in health care', *Best Practice and Research Clinical Gastroenterology*, 25(3): 337–47. https://doi.org/10.1016/j.bpg.2011.05.001.

de Sousa Santos, B. (2018) *The End of the Cognitive Empire: The Coming of Age of Epistemologies of the South*, Durham, NC: Duke University Press.

de Veer, A.J.E., de Groot, K., Brinkman, M. and Francke, A.L. (2017) *Factsheet administratieve druk: Méér dan kwestie van tijd*, Utrecht: Nivel. Available from: https://www.nivel.nl/sites/default/files/bestanden/factsheet_administratie_druk.pdf.

de Vries, M. (2007) 'Accountability in the Netherlands: Exemplary in its complexity', *Public Administration Quarterly*, 31(3/4): 480–507. Available from: https://www.jstor.org/stable/41288300.

den Bakker, J. (ed) (2018) *Goede zorg is beweging, goede zorg vraagt beweging: Realiseren, organiseren en verantwoorden van goede zorg bij De Hagert*, Utrecht: Stichting Presentie and Trimbos instituut. Available from: https://www.presentie.nl/publicaties/item/554-goede_zorg_is_beweging.

den Uijl, H. (2022) 'Practical Wisdom in Governance: Ambiguity, Politics and Democratization in Supervising Care Institutions' (PhD thesis, Vrije Universiteit Amsterdam), Den Haag: Nederlandse School voor Openbaar Bestuur. Available from: https://research.vu.nl/en/publications/practical-wisdom-in-governance-ambiguity-politics-and-democratiza.

Dingler, C. (2016) 'Relationale Subjektivität: Zur Theoriegeschichte der Care-Ethik', in E. Conradi and F. Vosman (eds) *Praxis der Achtsamkeit: Schlüsselbegriffe der Care-Ethik*, Frankfurt: Campus, pp 93–113.

Donabedian, A. (2003) *An Introduction to Quality Assessment in Health Care*, Oxford: Oxford University Press.

Doody, O., and Noonan, M. (2016) 'Nursing research ethics, guidance and application in practice', *British Journal of Nursing*, 25(14), 803–807. https://doi.org/https://doi.org/10.12968/bjon.2016.25.14.803

Doona, M.E., Chase, S.K. and Haggerty, L.A. (1999) 'Nursing presence: As real as a Milky Way bar', *Journal of Holistic Nursing*, 17(1): 54–70.

Doona, M.E., Haggerty, L.A. and Chase, S.K. (1997) 'Nursing presence: An existential exploration of the concept', *Scholarly Inquiry for Nursing Practice*, 11(1): 3–16.

Dotson, K. (2012) 'A cautionary tale: On limiting epistemic oppression', *Frontiers: A Journal of Women Studies*, 33(1): 24–47. https://doi.org/10.5250/fronjwomestud.33.1.0024.

Drost, J.S., Reinald, A.M., Vosselman, E. and Wagensveld, K.J. (2017) 'The performativity of accounting: How performance measures mediate in a healthcare organisation', *33rd EGOS Colloquium Proceedings*, Copenhagen, pp 1–20.

du Plessis, E. (2021) 'Presence: A relational approach in nursing', in E. du Plessis (ed) *Reflecting on Presence in Nursing: A Guide for Practice and Research*, Newcastle upon Tyne: Cambridge Scholars, pp 2–19.

du Plessis, E. and Beurskens, E. (2021) 'A deeper understanding of presence through an exposure', in E. du Plessis (ed) *Reflecting on Presence in Nursing: A Guide for Practice and Research*, Newcastle upon Tyne: Cambridge Scholars, pp 20–39.

Dubet, F. (2002) *Le déclin de l'institution*, Paris: Seuil.

Dupuis, S., Gray, J., Jonas-Simpson, C., Kontos, P. and Mitchell, G. (2016) *Relational Caring* (Handout prepared for Toward Relational Care: A hands-on workshop exploring relationality through theatre presented at Walk with Me: Changing the Culture of Aging in Canada, Edmonton, Alberta. Available from: https://uwaterloo.ca/partnerships-in-dementia-care/sites/default/files/uploads/files/relational_caring-final.pdf.

Dwarswaard, J., Hilhorst, M. and Trappenburg, M. (2011) 'The doctor and the market: About the influence of market reforms on the professional medical ethics of surgeons and general practitioners in the Netherlands', *Health Care Analysis*, 19(4): 388–402. https://doi.org/10.1007/s10728-011-0166-z.

Dworkin, G. (1976) 'Autonomy and behavior control', *Hastings Center Report*, 6(1): 23–8.

Dworkin, G. (1988) *The Theory and Practice of Autonomy*, Cambridge, UK: Cambridge University Press.

Einwohner, R.L. (2011) 'Ethical considerations on the use of archived testimonies in holocaust research: Beyond the IRB exemption', *Qualitative Sociology*, 34(3): 415–30. https://doi.org/10.1007/s11133-011-9196-y.

Ellul, J. (1948) *Présence au monde moderne: Problèmes de la civilisation post-chrétienne*, Geneva: Roulet.

Engster, D. (2007) *The Heart of Justice: Care Ethics and Political Theory*, Oxford: Oxford University Press.

Engster, D. (2018) 'Moral boundaries, still', *Politics and Gender*, 14(4): 8–12. https://doi.org/10.1017/S1743923X18000417.

Engster, D. and Hamington, M. (eds) (2015) *Care Ethics and Political Theory*, Oxford: Oxford University Press.

Finfgeld-Connett, D. (2008) 'Qualitative comparison and synthesis of nursing presence and caring', *International Journal of Nursing Knowledge*, 19(3): 111–19. https://doi.org/10.1111/j.1744-618X.2008.00090.x.

Fisher, B. and Tronto, J.C. (1990) 'Toward a feminist theory of caring', in E.K. Abel and M.K. Nelson (eds) *Circles of Care: Work and Identity in Women's Lives*, Albany, NY: SUNY Press, pp 35–62.

Flower, M. and Hamington, M. (2022) 'Care ethics, Bruno Latour, and the anthropocene', *Philosophies*, 7(2): 31. https://doi.org/10.3390/philosophies7020031.

Foucault, M. (2001) *Fearless Speech* (ed J. Pearson), Los Angeles, CA: Semiotext(e).

Foucault, M. (2011) *The Courage of the Truth (The Government of Self and Others II): Lectures at the Collège de France 1983–1984* (transl G. Burchell) (ed F. Gros), New York: Palgrave Macmillan.

Frazer, E. and Lacey, N. (1994) 'MacIntyre, feminism and the concept of practice', in J. Horton and S. Mendus (eds) *After MacIntyre: Critical Perspectives on the Work of Alasdair MacIntyre*, Cambridge, UK: Polity Press, pp 265–82.

Fricker, M. (2007) *Epistemic Injustice: Power and the Ethics of Knowing*, Oxford: Oxford University Press.

Fullan, M., Quinn, J. and McEachen, J. (2017) *Deep Learning: Engage the World Change the World*, Thousand Oaks, CA: Corwin Press.

Fung, C.H., Lim, Y., Mattke, S., Damberg, C. and Shekelle, P.G. (2008) 'Systematic review: The evidence that publishing patient care performance data improves quality of care', *Annals of Internal Medicine*, 148(2): 111–23. https://doi.org/10.7326/0003-4819-148-2-200801150-00006.

Gardner, D.L. (1992) 'Presence', in G.M. Bulechek and J.C. McCloskey (eds), *Nursing Interventions: Essential Nursing Treatments*, Philadelphia, PA: W.B. Saunders, pp 191–200.

Garrick, J. (1999) 'Doubting the philosophical assumptions of interpretive research', *International Journal of Qualitative Studies in Education*, 12(2): 147–56. https://doi.org/10.1080/095183999236222.

Geller, S.M. and Greenberg, L.S. (2002) 'Therapeutic presence: Therapists' experience of presence in the psychotherapy encounter', *Person Centered and Experiential Psychotherapies*, 1(1/2): 71–86.

Geller, S.M. and Greenberg, L.S. (2012) *Therapeutic Presence: A Mindful Approach to Effective Therapy*, Washington, DC: American Psychological Association.

Georgopoulos, B.S. and Matejko, A. (1967) 'The American general hospital as a complex social system', *Health Services Research*, 2(1): 76–112.

Gergen, K.J. (2009) *Relational Being: Beyond Self and Community*, Oxford: Oxford University Press.

Gilligan, C. (1982) *In a Different Voice: Psychological Theory and Women's Development*, Cambridge, MA: Harvard University Press.

Gilligan, C. (1986) 'Reply by Carol Gilligan', *Signs*, 11(2): 324–33.

Gilligan, C. (1987) 'Moral orientation and moral development', in E.F. Kittay and D.T. Meyers (eds) *Women and Moral Theory*, Totowa, NJ: Roman and Littlefield, pp 19–33.

Gilligan, C. (1988) 'Prolog', in C. Gilligan, J.V. Ward and J.M. Taylor (eds) *Mapping the Moral Domain: A Contribution of Women's Thinking to Psychological Theory and Education*, Cambridge, MA: Harvard University Graduate School of Education, pp vii–xxxviii.

Gilligan, C. and Attanucci, J. (1988) 'Two moral orientations', in C. Gilligan, J.V. Ward and J.M. Taylor (eds) *Mapping the Moral Domain: A Contribution of Women's Thinking to Psychological Theory and Education*, Cambridge, MA: Harvard University Graduate School of Education, pp 73–86.

Glaser, B.G. and Strauss, A.L. (1967) *The Discovery of Grounded Theory: Strategies for Qualitative Research*, Chicago, IL: Aldine.

The Goals of Medicine: Setting New Priorities (Special Supplement) (1996) *The Hastings Center Report*, 26(6): S1–S27.

Goffman, E. (1970) 'On the characteristics of total institutions', in P. Worsley (ed) *Modern Sociology: Introductory Readings*, Harmondsworth: Penguin Books, pp 274–8.

González-López, G. (2011) 'Mindful ethics: Comments on informant-centered practices in sociological research', *Qualitative Sociology*, 34(3): 447–61. https://doi.org/10.1007/s11133-011-9199-8.

Goossensen, A., van Dijke, J. and Baart, A. (2014) '"Leren kennen, laten kennen": Casus en probleemformulering', in A. Goossensen (ed) *Schetsen van mismatch: Een zorgethische visie op evaluatieonderzoek*, Utrecht: Movisie, pp 18–30.

Goudsmit, A. (2005) 'De plaats van "phronese" in de huisartsgeneeskunde', *Huisarts en Wetenschap*, 48: 379–83. https://doi.org/10.1007/BF03084269.

Graham, E.L. (2002) *Transforming Practice: Pastoral Theology in an Age of Uncertainty*, Eugene, OR: Wipf and Stock.

Greve, J. and Schnabel, A. (eds) (2011) *Emergenz: Zur Analyse und Erklärung Komplexer Strukturen*, Frankfurt: Suhrkamp.

Grøthe, Å, Biong, S. and Grov, E.K. (2015) 'Acting with dedication and expertise: Relatives' experience of nurses' provision of care in a palliative unit', *Palliative and Supportive Care*, 13(6): 1547–58. https://doi.org/10.1017/S1478951513000825.

Guillemin, M. and Gillam, L. (2004) 'Ethics, reflexivity, and "ethically important moments" in research', *Qualitative Inquiry*, 10(2): 261–80. https://doi.org/10.1177/1077800403262360.

Gunawardena, C.N. (1995) 'Social presence theory and implications for interaction and collaborative learning in computer conferences', *International Journal of Educational Telecommunications*, 1(2): 147–166.

Habermas, J. (1981) *Theorie des kommunikativen Handelns, Band 1 und 2*, Frankfurt: Suhrkamp.

Habran, Y. and Battard, N. (2019) 'Caring for or caring with? Production of different caring relationships and the construction of time', *Social Science and Medicine*, 233: 78–86. https://doi.org/10.1016/j.socscimed.2019.05.043.

Harteloh, P.P.M. (2003) 'Quality systems in health care: A sociotechnical approach', *Health Policy*, 64(3): 391–8. https://doi.org/10.1016/S0168-8510(02)00183-5.

Hennink, M.M., Kaiser, B.N. and Marconi, V.C. (2017) 'Code saturation versus meaning saturation: How many interviews are enough?', *Qualitative Health Research*, 27(4): 591–608. https://doi.org/10.1177/1049732316665344.

Heron, J. and Reason, P. (1997) 'A participatory inquiry paradigm', *Qualitative Inquiry*, 3(3): 274–94.

Hewitt-Taylor, J. (2015) *Developing Person-Centred Practice: A Practical Approach to Quality Healthcare*, London: Palgrave Macmillan.

Hirschauer, S. (2008) 'Die Empiriegeladenheit von Theorien und der Erfindungsreichtum der Praxis', in H. Kalthoff, S. Hirschauer and G. Lindemann (eds) *Theoretische Empirie: Zur Relevanz Qualitativer Forschung*, Frankfurt: Suhrkamp, pp 165–87.

Honneth, A. (1995) *The Struggle for Recognition: The Moral Grammar of Social Conflicts*, Cambridge, UK: Polity Press.

Housset, E. (2003) *L'intelligence de la pitié: Phénoménology de la communauté*, Paris: CERF.

Hughes, R.G. (2008) *Patient Safety and Quality: An Evidence-Based Handbook for Nurses*, Rockville, MD: Agency for Healthcare Research and Quality. Available from: https://archive.ahrq.gov/professionals/clinicians-providers/resources/nursing/resources/nurseshdbk/nurseshdbk.pdf.

IJzerman, H. (2002) 'Een "messiaans moment" in een oude stadswijk', *Gereformeerd Theologisch Tijdschrift*, 102(2): 75–98.

Illich, I.D. (1975) *Medical Nemesis: The Expropriation of Health*, London: Calder and Boyars.

International Society for Presence Research (2000) *The Concept of Presence: Explication Statement*. Available from: https://ispr.info/about-presence-2/about-presence/.

Ives, J., Dunn, M. and Cribb, A. (2017) *Empirical Bioethics: Theoretical and Practical Perspectives*, Cambridge, UK: Cambridge University Press.

Ives, J., Dunn, M., Molewijk, B., Schildmann, J., Bærøe, K., Frith, L. et al (2018) 'Standards of practice in empirical bioethics research: Towards a consensus', *BMC Medical Ethics*, 19(1): 68.

Jacobs, G., Meij, R., Tenwolde, H. and Zomer, Y. (eds) (2008) *Goed werk: Verkenningen van normatieve professionalisering*, Amsterdam: SWP.

Jaeggi, R. (2015) 'Towards an immanent critique of forms of life', *Raisons Politiques*, 57(1): 13–29. https://doi.org/10.3917/rai.057.0013.

Jaeggi, R. (2019) *Critique of Forms of Life* [Kritik von Lebensformen, 2014] (transl C. Cronin), Cambridge, MA: Harvard University Press.

Jerak-Zuiderent, S. (2013) 'Generative Accountability: Comparing with Care' (PhD thesis, Erasmus University Rotterdam), Rotterdam.

Jerak-Zuiderent, S. (2015) 'Accountability from somewhere and for someone: Relating with care', *Science as Culture*, 24(4): 412–35. https://doi.org/10.1080/09505431.2015.1050368.

Jerak-Zuiderent, S. and Bal, R. (2011) 'Locating the worths of performance indicators: Performing transparencies and accountabilities in health care', in A. Sætnan, H.M. Lomell and S. Hammer (eds) *The Mutual Construction of Statistics and Society*, New York: Routledge, pp 224–42.

Johnson, M. (1993) *Moral Imagination: Implications of Cognitive Science to Ethics*, Chicago, IL: University of Chicago Press.

Joronen, M. and Häkli, J. (2017) 'Politicizing ontology', *Progress in Human Geography*, 41(5): 561–79.

Kal, D. (2001) 'Kwartiermaken: Werken aan ruimte voor mensen met een psychiatrische achtergrond' (PhD thesis, University of Humanistic Studies), Amsterdam: Boom.

Kaldjian, L.C. (2014) *Practicing Medicine and Ethics: Integrating Wisdom, Conscience, and Goals of Care*, Cambridge, UK: Cambridge University Press.

Kant, I. (1992) *Über den Gemeinspruch: Das mag in der Theorie richtig sein, taugt aber nicht für die Praxis. Zum ewigen Frieden: Ein philosophischer Entwurf* [original 1793], Hamburg: Felix Meiner.

Kant, I. (1998) *Groundwork of the Metaphysics of Morals* [Grundlegung zur Metaphysik der Sitten, 1785] (transl M.J. Gregor), Cambridge, UK: Cambridge University Press.

Keinemans, S. (2010) 'Eervol jong moederschap: Een studie naar de leefwereld van adolescente moeders' (PhD thesis, Tilburg University), Delft: Eburon. Available from: https://pure.uvt.nl/ws/portalfiles/portal/1298925/Proefschrift_Sabrina_Keinemans_190111.pdf.

Kekes, J. (2006) *The Enlargement of Life: Moral Imagination at Work*, Ithaca, NY: Cornell University Press.

Kemmis, S. and Grootenboer, P. (2008) 'Situating praxis in practice: Practice architectures and the cultural, social and material conditions for practice', in S. Kemmis and T.J. Smith (eds) *Enabling Praxis: Challenges for Education*, Rotterdam: Sense, pp 37–62. https://doi.org/10.1163/9789087903275_004.

Kenny, G. (2012) 'An introduction to Moustakas's heuristic method', *Nurse Researcher*, 19(3): 6–11. https://doi.org/10.7748/nr2012.04.19.3.6.c9052.

Kinsella, E.A. and Pitman, A. (eds) (2012) *Phronesis as Professional Knowledge: Practical Wisdom in the Professions*, Rotterdam: Sense.

Kittay, E.F. (2013) *Interview with Eva Feder Kittay*. Available from: https://ethicsofcare.org/eva-fedar-kittay/.

Kitwood, T.M. (1997) *Dementia Reconsidered: The Person Comes First*, Buckingham: Open University Press.

Klafki, W. (2007) *Neue Studien zur Bildungstheorie und Didaktik: Zeitgemäße Allgemeinbildung und kritisch-konstruktive Didaktik* (6th, revised edn), Weinheim: Beltz.

Klaver, K. (2016) 'Dynamics of Attentiveness: In Care Practices at a Dutch Oncology Ward' (PhD thesis, Tilburg University), Tilburg. Available from: https://pure.uvt.nl/ws/portalfiles/portal/10987382/Klaver_Dynamics_01_04_2016.pdf.

Klaver, K. and Baart, A. (2011) 'Attentive care in a hospital: Towards an empirical ethics of care', *Medische Antropologie*, 23(2): 309–24. https://doi.org/10.1177/0969733011408052.

Klaver, K. and Baart, A. (2016a) 'How can attending physicians be more attentive? On being attentive versus producing attentiveness', *Medicine, Health Care and Philosophy*, 19: 351–9. https://doi.org/10.1007/s11019-015-9669-y.

Klaver, K. and Baart, A. (2016b) 'Managing socio-institutional enclosure: A grounded theory of caregivers' attentiveness in hospital care', *European Journal of Oncology Nursing*, 22: 95–102. https://doi.org/10.1016/k.ejon.2016.04.002.

Klaver, K., van Elst, E. and Baart, A. (2014) 'Demarcation of the ethics of care as a discipline', *Nursing Ethics*, 21(7): 755–65. https://doi.org/10.1177/0969733013500162.

Kleinman, A. (2006) *What Really Matters: Living a Moral Life Amidst Uncertainty and Danger*, Oxford: Oxford University Press.

Kluxen, W. (1974) *Ethik des Ethos*, Freiburg: Alber.

Kok, E. (2002) *Dagboek van een kerk-en buurtwerkster*, Utrecht: Lemma.

Kolen, M. (2017) 'De ongekende mogelijkheid van het alledaagse: Een kwalitatief-empirische, zorgethische studie naar morele betekenissen in de alledaagse omgang tussen jongeren met een licht verstandelijke beperking en zorgprofessionals' (PhD thesis, University of Humanistic Studies), Utrecht. Available from: https://research.uvh.nl/en/publications/de-ongekende-mogelijkheid-van-het-allerdaagse-een-kwalitatief-emp.

Kozar, C.J. and Day, A. (2012) 'The therapeutic alliance in offending behavior programs: A necessary and sufficient condition for change?', *Aggression and Violent Behavior*, 17(5): 482–7. https://doi.org/10.1016/j.avb.2012.07.004.

Kuokkanen, L. and Leino-Kilpi, H. (2001) 'The qualities of an empowered nurse and the factors involved', *Journal of Nursing Management*, 9(5): 273–80. https://doi.org/10.1046/j.1365-2834.2001.00253.x.

Larmore, C. (2008) *The Autonomy of Morality*, Cambridge, UK: Cambridge University Press.

Laros, A., Fuhr, T. and Taylor, E.W. (eds) (2017) *Transformative Learning Meets Bildung: An International Exchange*, Rotterdam: Sense.

Laugier, S. (2009) 'Ethics as politics of the ordinary', *Multitudes*, 37–38(2): 80–8.

Laugier, S. (2018) 'What matters: The ethics and aesthetics of importance', in G.L. Hagberg (ed) *Stanley Cavell on Aesthetic Understanding*, Cham: Springer, pp 167–95. https://doi.org/10.1007/978-3-319-97466-8_7.

Leest, J. (2016a) *Getuige zijn: De opbrengsten van De Kracht van Ontmoeting: Een rijke ervaring*, Sittard: Huis van de Zorg.

Leest, J. (2016b) 'De troost van terpen: Over bewogenheid, inschrijfbaarheid en getuige zijn', in K. Daniëls (ed) *Trajecten van hoopverlening*, Leuven: Buurtwerk't Lampeke, pp 8–15. Available from: https://www.hoopverlening.be/#magazine.

Leest, J., Bolt, E. and van der Linde, M. (2018) *Verstandig duikelen: De complexe praktijk van sociale professionals*, Wijk bij Duurstede: Stichting Presentie.

Leest, J., Timmerman, G., van der Linde, M., van Noort, Y. and Ouwerkerk, M. (2021) *Dementie van binnenuit: Een zoektocht naar hoe het is om iemand met vergevorderde dementie te zijn*, Tielt: Lannoo Campus.

Leget, C., van Nistelrooij, I. and Visse, M. (2017) 'Beyond demarcation: Care ethics as an interdisciplinary field of inquiry', *Nursing Ethics*, 26(1): 17–25. https://doi.org/10.117/0969733017707008.

Leibfried, S. and Mau, S. (eds) (2008) *Welfare States: Construction, Deconstruction, Reconstruction*, Cheltenham: Edward Elgar.

LeVasseur, J.J. (2003) 'The problem of bracketing in phenomenology', *Qualitative Health Research*, 13(3): 408–20. https://doi.org/10.1177%2F1049732302250337.

Levinas, M.L. and Carretero, M. (2010) 'Conceptual change, crucial experiments and auxiliary hypotheses: A theoretical contribution', *Integrative Psychological and Behavioral Science*, 44(4): 288–98. https://doi.org/10.1007/s12124-010-9139-2.

Lewin, K. (1951) 'Problems of research in social psychology (1943–1944)', in D. Cartwright (ed) *Field Theory in Social Science: Selected Theoretical Papers*, New York: Harper and Brothers, pp 155–69.

Lincoln, Y.S. and Guba, E.G. (2000) 'Paradigmatic controversies, contradictions, and emerging confluences', in N.K. Denzin and Y.S. Lincoln (eds) *The SAGE Handbook of Qualitative Research* (2nd edn), Thousand Oaks, CA: SAGE, pp 163–88.

Lindblom, C.E. (1959) 'The science of muddling through', *Public Administration Review*, 19(2): 79–88.

Lindblom, C.E. (1979) 'Still muddling, not yet through', *Public Administration Review*, 39(6): 571–26.

Lindemann, G. (2008) 'Theoriekonstruktion und empirische Forschung', in H. Kalthoff, S. Hirschauer and G. Lindemann (eds) *Theoretische Empirie: Zur Relevanz qualitativer Forschung*, Frankfurt: Suhrkamp, pp 107–28.

Lindemann, G. (2009) 'Introduction: Thinking the social from the perspective of its borders [Einleitung: Das Soziale von seinen Grenzen her denken, in G. Lindemann (2009) *Das Soziale von seinen Grenzen her denken*, pp 13–35]' (transl M. Hyatt), pp 1–17. Available from: https://www.researchgate.net/publication/323401678_Lindemann_Gesa_2009_Thinking_the_social_from_the_perspective_of_its_borders_Introduction_to_the_book_Thinking_the_social_from_the_perspective_of_its_borders_English_translation_of_Das_Soziale_von_sein.

Lipman, M. (2003) *Thinking in Education* (2nd edn), Cambridge, UK: Cambridge University Press.

Loorbach, D. and Rotmans, J. (2010) 'The practice of transition management: Examples and lessons from four distinct cases', *Futures*, 42(3): 237–46. https://doi.org/10.1016/j.futures.2009.11.009.

Lorey, I. (2015) *State of Insecurity: Government of the Precarious* [Die Regierung der Prekären, 2012] (transl A. Derieg), London: Verso.

Lowenthal, P.R. (2010) 'The evolution and influence of social presence theory on online learning', in S. Dasgupta (ed) *Social Computing: Concepts, Methodologies, Tools and Applications*, Hershey, PA: IGI Global, pp 113–28.

Luria, Z. (1986) 'A methodological critique [of *In a Different Voice* (1982) by Carol Gilligan]', *Signs*, 11(2): 316–21.

MacIntyre, A. (2007) *After Virtue: A Study in Moral Theory* (3rd edn), Notre Dame, IN: University of Notre Dame Press.

Mackenzie, C. and Stoljar, N. (2000) *Relational Autonomy: Feminist Perspectives on Autonomy, Agency, and the Social Self*, Oxford: Oxford University Press.

Malloch, K., Sluyter, D. and Moore, N. (2000) 'Relationship-centered care: Achieving true value in healthcare', *Journal of Nursing Administration*, 30(7/8): 379–85.

Malterud, K., Siersma, V.D. and Guassora, A.D. (2016) 'Sample size in qualitative interview studies: Guided by information power', *Qualitative Health Research*, 26(13): 1753–60. https://doi.org/10.1177/1049732315617444.

Marchart, O. (2013) *Die Prekarisierungsgesellschaft: Prekäre Proteste, Politik und Ökonomie im Zeichen der Prekarisierung*, Bielefeld: Transcript Verlag.

Margalit, A. (1996) *The Decent Society* (transl N. Goldblum), Cambridge, MA: Harvard University Press.

McPherson, K., Headrick, L. and Moss, F. (2001) 'Working and learning together: Good quality care depends on it, but how can we achieve it?', *Quality in Health Care*, 10(Supplement 2): ii46–ii53.

Mechanic, D. (1997) 'Muddling through elegantly: Finding the proper balance in rationing', *Health Affairs*, 16(5): 83–92.

Menger, A. (2018) 'De werkalliantie in het gedwongen kader: Onderzocht bij de reclassering' (PhD thesis, Vrije Universiteit Amsterdam), Utrecht: Eburon.

Metcalfe, D., Rios Diaz, A.J., Olufajo, O.A., Massa, M.S., Ketelaar, N.A.B.M., Flottorp, S.A. and Perry, D.C. (2018) 'Impact of public release of performance data on the behaviour of healthcare consumers and providers', *Cochrane Database of Systematic Reviews*, Issue 9, Art No. CD004538. https://doi.org//10.1002/14651858.CD004538.pub3.

Midgley, M. (1988) 'Teleological theories of morality', in G.H.R. Parkinson (ed) *An Encyclopaedia of Philosophy*, London: Routledge, pp 541–67.

Miles, M.B., Huberman, A.M. and Saldaña, J. (2019) *Qualitative Data Analysis: A Methods Sourcebook: Fourth edition*, Thousand Oaks, CA: SAGE.

Mill, J.S. (2012) *On Liberty* [original 1859], New York: Cambridge University Press.

Millar, K.M. (2017) 'Toward a critical politics of precarity', *Sociology Compass*, 11(6): 1–11. https://doi.org/10.1111/soc4.12483.

Miller, K. (2014) 'Relational caring: The use of the victim impact statement by sexually assaulted women', *Violence and Victims*, 29(5): 797–813. https://doi.org/10.1891/0886-6708.VV-D-13-00056.

Miller, S. (2019) 'Social institutions', in E.N. Zalta (ed) *The Stanford Encyclopedia of Philosophy* (Summer 2019 edn). Available from: https://plato.stanford.edu/archives/sum2019/entries/social-institutions/.

Minsky, M. (1980) 'Telepresence', *Omni*, (June), 45–51.

Mitchell, G. and Agnelli, J. (2015) 'Person-centred care for people with dementia: Kitwood reconsidered', *Nursing Standard*, 30(7): 46–50. https://doi.org/10.7748/ns.30.7.46.s47.

Mol, A. (2008) *The Logic of Care: Health and the Problem of Patient Choice [De logica van het zorgen, 2006]*, London: Routledge.

Molewijk, B., Stiggelbout, A.M., Otten, W., Dupuis, H.M. and Kievit, J. (2004) 'Empirical data and moral theory: A plea for integrated empirical ethics', *Medicine, Health Care and Philosophy*, 7(1): 55–69.

Montuori, A. (2008) 'Foreword to Edgar Morin's path of complexity', in E. Morin, *On Complexity*, Cresskill, NJ: Hampton.

Moore, G. and Beadle, R. (2006) 'In search of organizational virtue in business: Agents, goods, practices, institutions and environments', *Organization Studies*, 27(3): 369–89. https://doi.org/10.1177%2F0170840606062427.

Morin, E. (2008) *On Complexity* [La complexité humain, 1994] (transl R. Postel and S.M. Kelly), Cresskill, NJ: Hampton.

Mouffe, C. (2005) *On the Political*, New York: Routledge.

Moulin, M. (2002) *Delivering Excellence in Health and Social Care: Quality, Excellence and Performance Measurement*, Buckingham: Open University Press.

Moustakas, C. (1990) *Heuristic Research: Design, Methodology, and Applications*, Newbury Park, CA: SAGE.

Nacht, S. (1963) *La présence du psychanalyste*, Paris: Presses universitaires de France.

Nicolini, D. (2012) *Practice Theory, Work, and Organization: An Introduction*, Oxford: Oxford University Press.

Nicolini, D. (2017) 'Practice theory as a package of theory, method and vocabulary: Affordances and limitations', in M. Jonas, B. Littig and A. Wroblewski (eds) *Methodological Reflections on Practice Oriented Theories*, Cham: Springer, pp 19–34.

Nicolini, D. and Monteiro, P. (2017) 'The practice approach: For a praxeology of organisational and management studies', in A. Langley, and H. Tsoukas (eds) *Handbook of Process Organization Studies*, London: Sage, pp 110–26.

Noddings, N. (1984) *Caring: A Feminine Approach to Ethics and Moral Education*, Berkeley, CA: University of California Press.

Nussbaum, M.C. (2001) *Upheavals of Thought: The Intelligence of Emotions*, Cambridge, MA: Cambridge University Press.

Nussbaum, M. (2004) 'Emotions as judgments of value and importance', in R.C. Solomon (ed) *Thinking about Feeling: Contemporary Philosophers on Emotions*, Oxford: Oxford University Press, pp 183–99.

Nussbaum, M.C. (2013) *Political Emotions: Why Love Matters for Justice*, Cambridge, MA/London: Harvard University Press/Belknap Press.

Oksala, J. (2010) 'Foucault's politicization of ontology', *Continental Philosophy Review*, 43(4): 445–66.

Olthuis, G., Kohlen, H. and Heier, J. (eds) (2014a) *Moral Boundaries Redrawn: The Significance of Joan Tronto's Argument for Political Theory, Professional Ethics, and Care as Practice*, Leuven: Peeters.

Olthuis, G., Prins, C., Smits, M., van de Pas, H., Bierens, J. and Baart, A. (2014b) 'Matters of concern: A qualitative study of emergency care from the perspective of patients, *Annals of Emergency Medicine*, 62(5): 311–19. https://doi.org/10.1016/j.annemergmed.2013.08.018.

Parry, R. (2014) 'Episteme and techne', in E.N. Zalta (ed) *The Stanford Encyclopedia of Philosophy (Fall 2014 edn)*. Available from: http://plato.stanford.edu/archives/fall2014/entries/episteme-techne/.

Pedaste, M., Mäeots, M., Siiman, L.A., de Jong, T., van Riesen, S.A.N., Kamp, E.T. et al (2015) 'Phases of inquiry-based learning: Definitions and the inquiry cycle', *Educational Research Review*, 14: 47–61. https://doi.org/10.1016/j.edurev.2015.02.003.

Perls, F.S. (1969) *Gestalt Therapy Verbatim*, Lafayette, CA: Real People Press.

Pettigrew, J. (1990) 'Intensive nursing care: The ministry of presence', *Critical Care Nursing Clinics of North America*, 2(3): 503–8.

Polanyi, M. (1958) *Personal Knowledge: Towards a Post-Critical Philosophy*, Chicago, IL: University of Chicago Press.

Polanyi, M. (1966) *The Tacit Dimension*, New York: Doubleday.

Pols, J. (2015) 'Towards an empirical ethics in care: Relations with technologies in health care', *Medicine, Health Care and Philosophy*, 18: 81–90. https://doi.org/10.1007/s11019-014-9582-9.

Porter, M.E. and Teisberg, E.O. (2006) *Redefining Health Care: Creating Value-Based Competition on Results*, Boston, MA: Harvard Business School Press.

Puig de la Bellacasa, M. (2017) *Matters of Care: Speculative Ethics in More Than Human Worlds*, Minneapolis, MN: University of Minnesota Press.

Ravitsky, V. (2020) *Post-Covid Bioethics*. Available from: https://www.thehastingscenter.org/post-covid-bioethics/.

Ray, M.A. and Turkel, M.C. (2014) 'Caring as emancipatory nursing praxis: The theory of relational caring complexity', *Advances in Nursing Science*, 37(2): 132–46.

Reckwitz, A. (2002) 'Toward a theory of social practices: A development in culturalist theorizing', *European Journal of Social Theory*, 5(2): 243–63. https://doi.org/10.1177%2F13684310222225432.

Reichenbach, R. (2014) 'Humanistic Bildung: Regulative idea or empty concept?', *Asia Pacific Education Review*, 15(1): 65–70. https://doi.org/10.1007/s12564-013-9298-1.

Ricœur, P. (1992) *Oneself as Another* [Soi-même comme un autre [1990; Gifford Lectures 1986]] (transl K. Blamey), Chicago, IL: University of Chicago Press.

Riemann, G. and Schütze, F. (1991) '"Trajectory" as a basic theoretical concept for analyzing suffering and disorderly social processes', in D.R. Maines (ed) *Social Organization and Social Process: Essays in Honor of Anselm Strauss*, New York: Aldine de Gruyter, pp 333–57.

Roeser, S. (2011) *Moral Emotions and Intuitions*, London: Palgrave Macmillan.

Rogers, C.R. (1957) 'The necessary and sufficient condition of therapeutic personality change', *Journal of Consulting Psychology*, 21(2): 95–103.

Rogers, C.R. (1980) *A Way of Being*, Boston, MA: Houghton-Mifflin.

Rosa, H. (2013) *Social Acceleration: A New Theory of Modernity* [Beschleunigung: Die Veränderung der Zeitstrukturen in der Moderne, 2005] (transl J. Trejo-Mathys), New York: Columbia University Press.

Rosenhead, J. (1998) *Complexity Theory and Management Practice*. Available from: http://faratarjome.ir/u/media/shopping_files/store-EN-1617811723-3287.pdf.

Rosenhead, J., Franco, L.A., Grint, K. and Friedland, B. (2019) 'Complexity theory and leadership practice: A review, a critique, and some recommendations', *The Leadership Quarterly*, 30(5): 101304. https://doi.org/10.1016/j.leaqua.2019.07.002.

Ruddick, S. (1989) *Maternal Thinking: Towards a Politics of Peace*, Boston, MA: Beacon Press.

Sayer, A. (2011) *Why Things Matter to People: Social Science, Values and Ethical Life*, Cambridge, UK: Cambridge University Press.

Sayer, A. (2016) 'Zugewandte Unterstützung und anteilnehmende Sorge als Weltverhältnis', in E. Conradi and F. Vosman (eds) *Praxis der Achtsamkeit: Schlüsselbegriffe der Care-Ethik*, Frankfurt: Campus, pp 351–67.

Schaftenaar, P. (2018) '*Contact gezocht: Relationeel werken en het alledaagse als werkzame principes in de klinische forensische zorg*' (PhD thesis, University of Humanistic Studies), Amsterdam: SWP.

Schaftenaar, P., van Outheusden, I., Stams, G.-J. and Baart, A. (2018) 'Relational caring and contact after treatment: An evaluation study on criminal recidivism', *International Journal of Law and Psychiatry*, 60: 45–50. https://doi.org/10.1016/j.ijlp.2018.07.011.

Scharmer, O. (2005) *Theory U: Leading From the Future as It Emerges*, San Francisco, CA: Berrett-Koehler.

Schatzki, T.R. (1996) *Social Practices: A Wittgensteinian Approach to Human Activity and the Social*, Cambridge, UK: Cambridge University Press.

Schatzki, T.R., Knorr Cetina, K. and von Savigny, E. (eds) (2001) *The Practice Turn in Contemporary Theory*, London: Routledge.

Schaufeli, W.B. (2014) 'What is engagement?', in C. Truss, R. Delbridge, K. Alfes, A. Shantz and E. Soanne (eds) *Employee Engagement in Theory and Practice*, New York: Routledge, pp 15–35.

Schilder, L. (2003) 'Presentie in maatschappelijk werk: Wenkend perspectief of terug naar af?', *Journal of Social Intervention*, 12(2): 40–9.

Schippers, K.A. and others (1990) *Kerkelijke presentie in een oude stadswijk*, Kampen: Kok.

Schmidt, J. (2022) 'Everyday ethics of dignity work: What social workers do to promote the dignity of service-users in times of austerity measures and welfare stigma', *Ethics and Social Welfare*, 16(3): 306–21. https://doi.org/10.1080/17496535.2022.2038229.

Schmidt, R. (2012) *Soziologie der Praktiken: Konzeptionelle Studien und empirische Analysen*, Berlin: Suhrkamp.

Schmidt, T. (2017) *Nie wieder Qualität: Strategien des Paradoxie-Managements*, Weilerwist: Velbrück Wissenschaft.

Schneewind, J.B. (1998) *The Invention of Autonomy: A History of Modern Moral Philosophy*, Cambridge, UK: Cambridge University Press.

Schön, D. (1983) *The Reflective Practitioner*, New York: Basic Books.

Schön, D. (1987) *Educating the Reflective Practitioner*, San Francisco, CA: Jossey-Bass.

Schüssler Fiorenza, F. (2011) 'Systematic theology: Tasks and methods', in F. Schüssler Fiorenza and J.P. Galvin (eds) *Systematic Theology: Roman Catholic Perspectives* (2nd edn), Minneapolis, MN: Fortress Press, pp 1–78.

Schutz, A. and Luckmann, T. (1973) *The Structures of the Life-World* [Strukturen der Lebenswelt] (transl R.M. Zaner and H.T. Engelhardt), Evanston, IL: Northwestern University Press.

Schwartz, B. and Sharpe, K. (2010) *Practical Wisdom: The Right Way to Do the Right Thing*, New York: Riverhead Books.

Selg, P. (2016) 'Two faces of the "relational turn"', *PS: Political Science and Politics*, 49(1): 27–31. https://doi.org/10.1017/S1049096515001195.

Selg, P. and Ventsel, A. (2020a) 'The "relational turn" in the social sciences', in P. Selg and A. Ventsel (eds) *Introducing Relational Political Analysis: Political Semiotics as a Theory and Method*, Cham: Springer, pp 15–40. https://doi.org/10.1007/978-3-030-48780-5_2.

Selg, P. and Ventsel, A. (2020b) 'Relational approach to the political: Power, governance, and democracy', in P. Selg and A. Ventsel (eds) *Introducing Relational Political Analysis: Political Semiotics as a Theory and Method*, Cham: Springer, pp 41–106. https://doi.org/10.1007/978-3-030-48780-5_3.

Sen, A. (1985) *Commodities and Capabilities*, Amsterdam: North Holland.

Sennett, R. (2008) *The Craftsman*, New Haven, CT: Yale University Press.

Sevenhuijsen, S. (1998) *Citizenship and the Ehics of Care: Feminist Considerations on Justice, Morality and Politics* [Oordelen met zorg, 1996] (transl L. Savage), London: Routledge.

Sevenhuijsen, S. (2004) 'Trace: A method for normative policy analysis from the ethic of care', in S. Sevenhuijsen and A. Švab (eds) *The Heart of the Matter: The Contributions of the Ethic of Care to Social Policy in Some New EU Member States*, Ljubljana: Peace Institute, pp 13–46.

Shojania, K.G. (2019) 'Are increases in emergency use and hospitalisation always a bad thing? Reflections on unintended consequences and apparent backfires', *BMJ Quality and Safety*, 28: 687–92. http://dx.doi.org/10.1136/bmjqs-2019-009406.

Short, J.A., Williams, E. and Christie, B. (1976). *The Social Psychology of Telecommunications*, London: John Wiley & Sons.

Sjöström, J., Frerichs, N., Zuin, V.G. and Eilks, I. (2017) 'Use of the concept of Bildung in the international science education literature, its potential, and implications for teaching and learning', *Studies in Science Education*, 53(2): 165–92. https://doi.org/10.1080/03057267.2017.1384649.

Slatman, J. (2014) 'Multiple dimensions of embodiment in medical practices', *Medicine, Health Care and Philosophy*, 17(4): 549–57. http://dx.doi.org/10.1007/s11019-014-9544-2.

Slife, B.D. (2004) 'Taking practice seriously: Toward a relational ontology', *Journal of Theoretical and Philosophical Psychology*, 24(2): 157–78. https://doi.org/10.1037/h0091239.

Slife, B.D. and Wiggins, B.J. (2009) 'Taking relationship seriously in psychotherapy: Radical relationality', *Journal of Contemporary Psychotherapy*, 39(1): 17–24. https://doi.org/10.1007/s10879-008-9100-6.

Smaling, A. (2004) 'Wat voor soort onderzoek doet Baart eigenlijk?', *Kwalon*, 9(1): 7–15.

Srinivasan, M., Wilkes, M., Stevenson, F., Nguyen, T. and Slavin, S. (2007) 'Comparing problem-based learning with case-based learning: Effects of a major curricular shift at two institutions', *Academic Medicine*, 82(1): 74–82. https://doi.org/10.1097/01.ACM.0000249963.93776.aa.

Standing, G. (2011) *The Precariat: The New Dangerous Class*, New York: Bloomsbury Academic.

Stewart, M. (2001) 'Towards a global definition of patient centred care: The patient should be the judge of patient centred care', *BMJ*, 322(7284): 444. https://doi.org/10.1136/bmj.322.7284.444.

Stolper, E., van de Wiel, M., van Royen, P., van Bokhoven, M., van der Weijden, T. and Dinant, G.J. (2011) 'Gut feelings as a third track in general practitioners' diagnostic reasoning', *Journal of General Internal Medicine*, 26(2): 197–203.

Stoopendaal, A. (2008) 'Zorg met afstand: Betrokken bestuur in grootschalige zorginstellingen' (PhD thesis, Erasmus University Rotterdam), Rotterdam.

Stoppels, S. (1996) *Gastvrijheid: Het inloopcentrum als vorm van kerkelijke presentie*, Kampen: Kok.

Straßner, V. (2005) *Die Arbeiterpriester: Geschichte und Entwicklungstendenzen einer in Vergessenheit Geratenen Bewegung*. Available from: http://nbi.sankt-georgen.de/fileadmin/redakteure/Dokumente/FAgsFs/FAgsF_43_Arbeiterpriester.PDF

Subramani, S. (2019) 'Practicing reflexivity: Ethics, methodology and theory construction', *Methodological Innovations*, 12(2). https://doi.org/10.1177%2F2059799119863276.

Surkis, J. (2012) 'When was the linguistic turn? A genealogy', *The American Historical Review*, 117(3): 700–22. https://doi.org/10.1086/ahr.117.3.700.

Sztompka, P. (2008) 'The focus on everyday life: A new turn in sociology', *European Review*, 16(1): 23–37. https://doi.org/10.1017/S1062798708000045.

Taylor, C. (1985) *Human Agency and Language: Philosophical Papers Volume 1*, Cambridge, UK: Cambridge University Press.

Taylor, C. (1989) *Sources of the Self: The Making of the Modern Identity*, Cambridge: Cambridge University Press.

Taylor, C. (1991) 'Comments and replies', *Inquiry*, 34: 237–54.

Taylor, C. (2007) *Modern Social Imaginaries*, Durham, NC: Duke University Press.

Thistlethwaite, J.E., Davies, D., Ekeocha, S., Kidd, J.M., MacDougall, C., Matthews, P. et al (2012) 'The effectiveness of case-based learning in health professional education. A BEME systematic review: BEME guide no. 23', *Medical Teacher*, 34(6): e421–e44. https://doi.org/10.3109/0142159X.2012.680939.

Thrift, N. (2004) 'Intensities of feeling: Towards a spatial politics of affect', *Geografiska Annaler: Series B, Human Geography*, 86(1): 57–8. https://doi.org/10.1111/j.0435-3684.2004.00154.x.

Tibbles, L. (1985) 'Derived consent, proxy consent', in V.L. Melnick and N.N. Dubler (eds) *Alzheimer's Dementia: Dilemmas in Clinical Research*, Totowa, NJ: Humana Press, pp 265–94. https://doi.org/10.1007/978-1-4612-5174-3_19.

Tieu, M. and Matthews, S. (2024) 'The relational care framework: Promoting continuity or maintenance of selfhood in person-centered care', *Journal of Medicine and Philosophy*, 49(1): 85–101. https://doi.org/https://doi.org/10.1093/jmp/jhad044.

Timmerman, A.B. (2011) 'Gezien de ander: Eerbied voor autonomie en authenticiteit in het pastoraat – Een kwalitatief-empirische, moraaltheologische studie' (PhD thesis, Tilburg University), Bergambacht: 2VM Uitgeverij. Available from: https://pure.uvt.nl/ws/portalfiles/portal/1337111/Timmerman_gezien_13-04-2011.pdf.

Timmerman, G. (2010) 'Respect for autonomy and authenticity: The pastor's responsiveness to the person of the pastoree', *Ethical Perspectives*, 17(2): 309–41. https://doi.org/10.2143/EP.17.2.2049268.

Timmerman, G. (2018) 'Empirically grounded ethics and Charles Taylor's relational ontology of goods', in S.C. van den Heuvel, P. Nullens and A. Roothaan (eds) *Theological Ethics and Moral Value Phenomena: The Experience of Values*, New York: Routledge, pp 49–64.

Timmerman, G. (2019) *More Self-Reliance, Less Government? Neoliberalisation in Healthcare and Social Welfare*. Available from: https://ethicsofcare.org/more-self-reliance-less-government-neoliberalisation-in-healthcare-and-social-welfare/.

Timmerman, G. and Baart, A. (2016a) *Ongeregeld goed: De huisarts aan het ziek- en sterfbed van de eigen patiënt* (Research report), Utrecht: Stichting Presentie. https://doi.org/10.13140/RG.2.2.17048.83203.

Timmerman, G. and Baart, A. (2016b) Präsentische Praxis und die Theorie der Präsenz', in E. Conradi, and F. Vosman (eds) *Praxis der Achtsamkeit: Schlüsselbegriffe der Care-Ethik*, Frankfurt: Campus, pp 190–208.

Timmerman, G. and Baart, A. (2021) 'Research methods for research on presence', in E. du Plessis (ed) *Reflecting on Presence in Nursing: A Guide for Practice and Research*, Newcastle upon Tyne: Cambridge Scholars, pp 90–109.

Timmerman, G. and Baart, A. (2022) 'The continuing formation of relational caring professionals', *Medicine, Health Care and Philosophy*, 25: 587–602. https://doi.org/10.1007/s11019-022-10104-0.

Timmerman, G. and Leest, J. (2022) 'Training actors' knowledge of the lived experience of people with advanced dementia', *Gerontology and Geriatric Medicine*, 8: 1–6. https://doi.org/10.1177/23337214221097837.

Timmerman, G. and Vosman, F. (2014) 'Steuermannskunst als empirisch begründete Metapher in der Seelsorge: Zur Methodologie und Epistemologie qualitativ-empirischer Forschung in der Moraltheologie', in W. Schaupp (ed) *Ethik und Empirie: Gegenwärtige Herausforderungen für Moraltheologie und Sozialethik*, Freiburg Schweiz/Freiburg-Wien: Academic Press Fribourg/Verlag Herder, pp 277–89.

Timmerman, G., Baart, A. and den Bakker, J. (2021) 'Cultivating quality awareness in corona times', *Medicine, Health Care and Philosophy*, 24(2): 189–204. https://doi.org/10.1007/s11019-021-10010-x.

Timmerman, G., Baart, A. and Vosman, F. (2019) 'In search of good care: The methodology of phenomenological, theory-oriented "N=N case studies" in empirically grounded ethics of care', *Medicine, Health Care and Philosophy*, 22(4): 573–82. https://doi.org/10.1007/s11019-019-09892-9.

Timmermann, M. (2010) 'Relationele afstemming: Presentieverrijkte verpleeghuiszorg voor mensen met dementie' (PhD thesis, Tilburg University), Utrecht: LEMMA. Available from: https://pure.uvt.nl/ws/portalfiles/portal/1200246/Timmermann_relationele_14-04-2011.pdf.

Tresolini, C.P. and Pew-Fetze Task Force (1994) *Health Professions Education and Relationship-Centered Care*, San Francisco, CA: Center for the Health Professions, University of California.

Tronto, J.C. (1993) *Moral Boundaries: A Political Argument for an Ethic of Care*, New York: Routledge.

Tronto, J.C. (2013) *Caring Democracy: Markets, Equality, and Justice*, New York: New York University Press.

Tronto, J. (2017) 'There is an alternative: *Homines curans* and the limits of neoliberalism', *International Journal of Care and Caring*, 1(1): 27–43. https://doi.org/10.1332/239788217X14866281687583.

Tsoukas, H. (2009) 'Craving for generality and small-N studies: A Wittgensteinian approach towards the epistemology of the particular in organization and management studies', in D.A. Buchanan and A. Bryman (eds) *The SAGE Handbook of Organizational Research Methods*, London: SAGE, pp 285–301.

Tsoukas, H. (2017) 'Don't simplify, complexify: From disjunctive to conjunctive theorizing in organization and management studies', *Journal of Management Studies*, 54(2): 132–53. https://doi.org/10.1111/joms.12219.

Tsoukas, H. and Hatch, M.J. (2001) 'Complex thinking, complex practice: The case for a narrative approach to organizational complexity', *Human Relations*, 54(8): 979–1013. https://doi.org/10.1177%2F0018726701548001.

Tzeng, H. and Yin, C. (2008) 'Patient satisfaction versus quality', *Nursing Ethics*, 15(1): 121–4. https://doi.org/10.1177/0969733007080210.

Ubels, G.M. (2015) 'Narrative accountability and quality awareness: Learning about (re)presenting narrative care', *Journal of Aging Studies*, 34: 190–8. https://doi.org/10.1016/j.jaging.2015.02.006.

Vaittinen, T. (2015) 'The power of the vulnerable body: A new political understanding of care', *International Feminist Journal of Politics*, 17(1): 100–18. https://doi.org/10.1080/14616742.2013.876301.

van de Bovenkamp, H.M., Stoopendaal, A., van Bochove, M. and Bal, R. (2020) 'Tackling the problem of regulatory pressure in Dutch elderly care: The need for recoupling to establish functional rules', *Health Policy*, 124(3): 275–81. https://doi.org/10.1016/j.healthpol.2019.12.017.

van der Geest, G. (2024) *Ze kunnen het niet zeggen: Over autonomie en afhankelijkheid in de alledaagse ondersteuning aan mensen met EVB+*, Utrecht: De Graaff.

van der Hart, O., Nijenhuis, E.R.S. and Steele, K. (2006) *The Haunted Self: Structural Dissociation and the Treatment of Chronic Traumatization*, New York: W.W. Norton.

van der Spek, J. (2010) *De kramp voorbij: Theologische noties bij zending, presentie en kerk*, Gorinchem: Narratio.

van Domselaar, I. (2021) 'Where were the law schools? On legal education as training for justice and the rule of law (against the "dark sides of legality")', *Netherlands Journal of Legal Philosophy*, 50(1): 3–12. https://doi.org/10.5553/NJLP/.000000.

van Doorn, C. (2002) 'Een tijd op straat: Een volgstudie naar (ex-)daklozen in Utrecht (1993–2000)' (PhD thesis, Utrecht University), Utrecht: NIZW.

van Elst, E. (2015) '"Poulet à la d'albufera" of hoe bereid je een bloeiende lerende gemeenschap', in A. Baart, F. Vosman and others *De patiënt terug van weggeweest: Werken aan menslievende zorg in het ziekenhuis*, Amsterdam: SWP, pp 123–38.

van Elst, E. and Baart, A. (2012) 'Hoezo implementeren? anders leren!', in C. Leget, and G. Olthuis (eds) *Menslievende zorg in de praktijk: Berichten uit het St. Elisabeth ziekenhuis*, Den Haag: Lemma, pp 79–88.

van Ewijk, H. and Kunneman, H. (eds) (2013) *Praktijken van normatieve professionalisering*, Amsterdam: SWP.

van Geffen, M. (2019) 'Kwaliteitssystemen in de Nederlandse geestelijke gezondheidszorg: Een analyse van de impact van kwaliteitssystemen op de praktijk van de zorg' (PhD thesis, Radboud University Nijmegen), Nijmegen. Available from: https://repository.ubn.ru.nl/bitstream/handle/2066/203431/203431.pdf.

van Heijst, A. (2008) *Iemand zien staan: Zorgethiek over erkenning*, Kampen: Klement.

van Heijst, A. (2011) *Professional Loving Care: An Ethical View of the Health Care Sector* [Menslievende zorg: Een ethische kijk op professionaliteit in de zorg, 2005] (transl K. Caldwell), Leuven: Peeters.

van Klinken, L. (2012) *Begrenzende presentie: Het belang van 'bottom-up' werken en het ontwikkelen van krachtige verbindingen in het sociale domein*, Master Thesis University of Humanistic Studies.

van Strien, P.J. (1993) 'The historical practice of theory construction', in H.V. Rappart, P.J. van Strien, L.P. Mos and W.J. Baker (eds) *Annals of Theoretical Psychology (Vol. 8)*, New York: Plenum Press, pp 149–227.

van Thiel, S. and Leeuw, F.L. (2002) 'The performance paradox in the public sector', *Public Performance and Management Review*, 25(3): 267–81. https://doi.org/10.2307/3381236.

van Tongeren, P. (1994) 'Narrativiteit en hermeneutiek in verband met een adequate praktische ethiek', *Ethische Perspectieven*, 4(1): 66–81.

van Tongeren, P. (1999) 'Ethiek als hermeneutiek van de morele ervaring', in J. Wils (ed) *Ethiek en hermeneutiek*, Leende: Damon, pp 217–25.

Vanlaere, L., Timmermann, M. and Grypdonck, M. (2016) 'Pflegehandeln am eigenen Körper erfahren: "Ausgesetztsein" in simulierten Situationen', in E. Conradi and F. Vosman (eds) *Praxis der Achtsamkeit: Schlüsselbegriffe der Care-Ethik*, Frankfurt: Campus, pp 231–47.

Vanlaere, L., Timmermann, M., Stevens, M. and Gastmans, C. (2012) 'An explorative study of experiences of healthcare providers posing as simulated care receivers in a "care-ethical" lab', *Nursing Ethics*, 19(1): 68–79. https://doi.org/10.1177/0969733011412103.

Verhoeven, C. (1972) *The Philosophy of Wonder: An Introduction and Incitement to Philosophy* [Inleiding tot de verwondering, 1967] (transl M. Foran), New York: Macmillan.

Veszy-Wagner, L. (1964) '*La présence du psychanalyste* by S. Nacht', *International Journal of Psycho-Analysis*, 54: 128–31.

von Bonsdorff, P. (2012) 'Aesthetics and Bildung', *Diogenes*, 59(1/2): 127–37. https://doi.org/10.1177%2F0392192112469327.

Vosman, F. (2008) 'Over het uitzieden van praktische wijsheid', in F. Vosman and A. Baart, *Aannemelijke zorg: Over het uitzieden en verdringen van praktische wijsheid in de gezondheidszorg* (Dual inaugural lecture, Tilburg University), Den Haag: LEMMA, pp 11–47. Available from: https://www.presentie.nl/publicaties/item/380-aannemelijke-zorg-de-uitgebreide-tekst-van-de-dubbeloratie-van-vosman-en-baart.

Vosman, F. (2014) 'Zorg vanuit zorgen gedacht: De veranderende ethiek in een gedecentraliseerde zorg', *Christen Democratische Verkenningen*, 2014(2): 121–7.

Vosman, F. (2016) 'Kartographie einer Ethik der Achtsamkeit: Rezeption und Entwicklung in Europa', in E. Conradi and F. Vosman (eds) *Praxis der Achtsamkeit: Schlüsselbegriffe der Care-Ethik*, Frankfurt: Campus, pp 33–51.

Vosman, F. (2018) 'The moral relevance of lived experience in complex hospital practices: A phenomenological approach', in S.C. van den Heuvel, P. Nullens and A. Roothaan (eds) *Theological Ethics and Moral Value Phenomena: The Experience of Values*, London: Routledge, pp 65–92.

Vosman, F. (2020) 'The disenchantment of care ethics: A critical cartography', in F. Vosman, A. Baart and J. Hoffman (eds) *The Ethics of Care: The State of the Art*, Leuven: Peeters, pp 17–65. Available from: https://ethicsofcare.org/the-disenchantment-of-care-ethics-a-critical-cartography/.

Vosman, F. (2023) *Surviving as a Form of Life: The Ethics of Care as a Critique of the Ideal of the Successful Life* [Overleven als levensvorm: Zorgethiek als kritiek op het ideal van het 'geslaagde leven', 2018] (transl M. Dekema, R. Brons and B. Heffernan) (Valedictory lecture, University of Humanistic Studies), Utrecht: Eburon. https://doi.org/https:/doi.org/10.60116/wujrowt9gz.

Vosman, F. and Baart, A. (2008) *Aannemelijke zorg: Over het uitzieden en verdringen van praktische wijsheid in de gezondheidszorg* (Dual inaugural lecture, Tilburg University), Den Haag: LEMMA. Available from: https://www.presentie.nl/publicaties/item/380-aannemelijke-zorg-de-uitgebreide-tekst-van-de-dubbeloratie-van-vosman-en-baart.

Vosman, F. and Baart, A. (2010) 'Frailty and care', in J. Brouwer (ed) *Successful Ageing, Spirituality and Meaning: Multidisciplinary Perspectives*, Leuven: Peeters, pp 191–206.

Vosman, F. and Baart, A. (2011) 'Relationship based care and recognition: Part two: Good care and recognition', in C. Leget, C. Gastmans and M. Verkerk (eds) *Care, Compassion and Recognition: An Ethical Discussion*, Leuven: Peeters, pp 201–27.

Vosman, F. and Baart, A. (2017) 'Ten geleide', in T. Biebricher, *Onvermoed en onvermijdelijk: De vele gezichten van het neoliberalisme*, Nijmegen: Valkhof, pp 7–16.

Vosman, F. and Niemeijer, A. (2017) 'Rethinking critical reflection on care: Late modern uncertainty and the implications for care ethics', *Medicine, Health Care and Philosophy*, 20(4): 465–76. https://doi.org/10.1007/s11019-017-9766-1.

Vosman, F., den Bakker, J. and Weenink, D. (2016) 'How to make sense of suffering in complex care practices?', in G. Spaargaren, D. Weenink and M. Lamers (eds) *Practice Theory and Research: Exploring the Dynamics of Social Life*, New York: Routledge, pp 117–30.

Vosman, F., Timmerman, G. and Baart, A. (2018) 'Digging into care practices: The confrontation of care ethics with qualitative empirical and theoretical developments in the Low Countries, 2007–17', *International Journal of Care and Caring*, 2(3): 405–23. https://doi.org/10.1332/239788218X15321005652967.

Vosselman, E. (2014) 'The "performativity thesis" and its critics: Towards a relational ontology of management accounting', *Accounting and Business Research*, 44(2): 181–203. https://doi.org/10.1080/00014788.2013.856748.

Wacquant, L. (2009) *Punishing the Poor: The Neoliberal Government of Social Insecurity [Punir les pauvres: Le nouveau gouvernement de l'insécurité sociale, 2004]*, Durham, NC: Duke University Press.

Waldenfels, B. (2004) *Phänomenologie der Aufmerksamkeit*, Frankfurt: Suhrkamp.
Waldenfels, B. (2011) *Phenomenology of the Alien: Basic Concepts* [Grundmotive einer Phänomenologie des Fremden, 2006] (transl A. Kozin and T. Stähler), Evanston, IL: Northwestern University Press.
Waldenfels, B. (2015) *Sozialität und Alterität: Modi sozialer Erfahrung*, Berlin: Suhrkamp.
Walker, M.U. (1998) *Moral Understandings: A Feminist Study in Ethics*, New York: Routledge.
Wangmo, T., Hauri, S., Gennet, E., Anane-Sarpong, E., Provoost, V. and Elger, B.S. (2018) 'An update on the "empirical turn" in bioethics: Analysis of empirical research in nine bioethics journals', *BMC Medical Ethics*, 19(1): 6. https://doi.org/10.1186/s12910-018-0246-9.
Webb, S.A. (2015) 'Social workers as "strong evaluators": Rethinking moral sources and professional identity', *International Journal of Social Science Studies*, 3(6): 143–51. https://doi.org/10.11114/ijsss.v3i6.1144.
Weerman, A. and Abma, T. (2018) 'Social work students learning to use their experiential knowledge of recovery: An existential and emancipatory perspective', *Social Work Education*, 38(4): 453–69. https://doi.org/10.1080/02615479.2018.1538335.
Wenger, E., McDermott, R. and Snyder, W.M. (2002) *Cultivating Communities of Practice: A Guide to Managing Knowledge*, Boston, MA: Harvard Business School Press.
Wilken, J.P. (2010) 'Recovering Care: A Contribution to a Theory and Practice of Good Care' (PhD thesis, Tilburg University), Amsterdam: SWP. Available from: https://pure.uvt.nl/ws/portalfiles/portal/1275835/Proefschrift_Jean_Pierre_Wilken_121110.pdf.
Woolhandler, S. and Himmelstein, D.U. (2014) 'Administrative work consumes one-sixth of US physicians' working hours and lowers their career satisfaction', *International Journal of Health Services*, 44(4): 635–42. https://doi.org/10.2190%2FHS.44.4.a.
Wyer, P.C., Alves Silva, S., Post, S.G. and Quinlan, P. (2014) 'Relationship-centred care: Antidote, guidepost or blind alley? The epistemology of 21st Century health care', *Journal of Evaluation in Clinical Practice*, 20(6): 881–9. https://doi.org/10.1111/jep.12224.
Yan, Y. (2005) 'The gift and gift economy', in J.G. Carrier (ed) *A Handbook of Economic Anthropology*, Cheltenham: Edward Elgar, pp 246–61.
Zaidi, Z. and Larsen, D. (2018) 'Commentary: Paradigms, axiology, and praxeology in medical education research', *Academic Medicine*, 93(11S), S1–S7. https://doi.org/10.1097/ACM.0000000000002384.
Zimmerman, B. (2011) 'How complexity science is transforming healthcare', in P. Allen, S. Maguire and B. McKelvey (eds) *The SAGE Handbook of Complexity and Management*, Thousand Oaks, CA: SAGE, pp 617–35.

Index

References to figures appear in *italic* type; those in **bold** type refer to tables.
References to endnotes show both the page number and the note number (28n2).

D

E

Q

Printed and bound by CPI Group (UK) Ltd, Croydon, CR0 4YY
26/05/2026
14886146-0002